P9-ELH-052

Deschutes ... ary

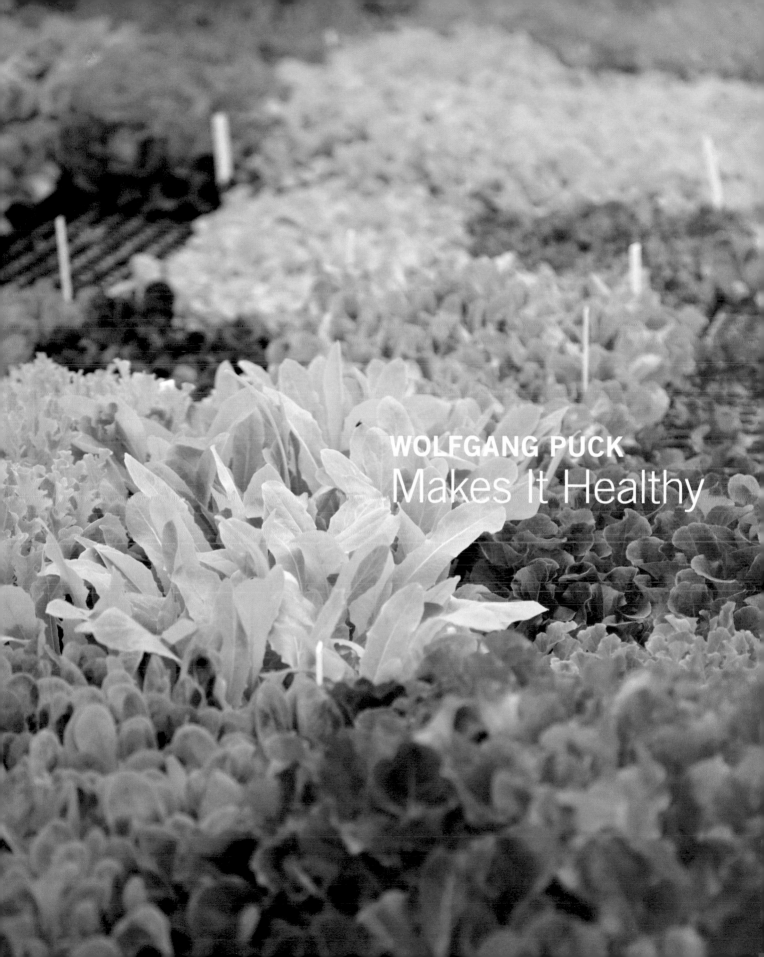

WOLFGANG PUCK
Makes It Healthy

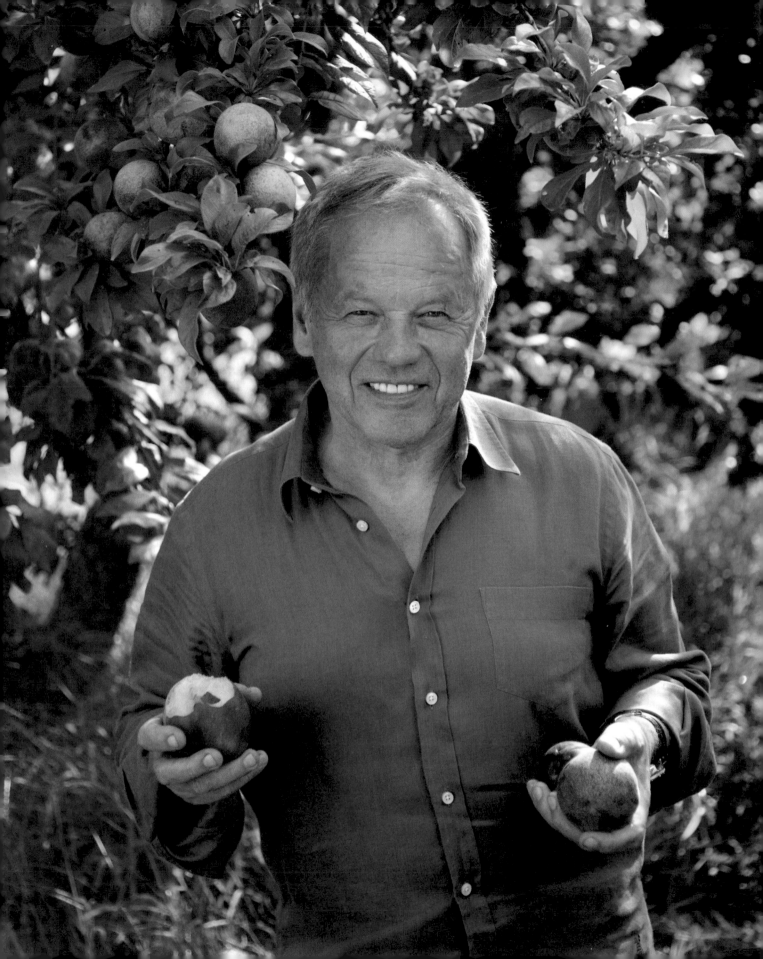

C. 1

WOLFGANG PUCK
Makes It Healthy

Light, Delicious Recipes and Easy Exercises for a Better Life

Wolfgang Puck and Chad Waterbury

with Norman Kolpas and Lou Schuler

PHOTOGRAPHS BY CARIN KRASNER

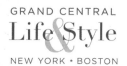

GRAND CENTRAL
Life & Style
NEW YORK • BOSTON

The information herein is not intended to replace the services of trained health professionals. You are advised to consult with your health care professional with regard to matters relating to your health, and in particular regarding matters that may require diagnosis or medical attention.

text and photographs copyright © 2014 by Wolfgang Puck Worldwide, Inc.

Illustrations copyright © 2014 by Jason Lee

All rights reserved. In accordance with the U.S. Copyright Act of 1976, the scanning, uploading, and electronic sharing of any part of this book without the permission of the publisher constitute unlawful piracy and theft of the author's intellectual property. If you would like to use material from the book (other than for review purposes), prior written permission must be obtained by contacting the publisher at permissions@hbgusa.com. Thank you for your support of the author's rights.

Photographs are by Carin Krasner.

Grand Central Life & Style
Hachette Book Group
237 Park Avenue
New York, NY 10017

www.GrandCentralLifeandStyle.com

Printed in the United States of America

Design by Gary Tooth/Empire Design Studio

Q-MA

First edition: March 2014

10 9 8 7 6 5 4 3 2 1

Grand Central Life & Style is an imprint of Grand Central Publishing.

The Grand Central Life & Style name and logo are trademarks of Hachette Book Group, Inc.

The Hachette Speakers Bureau provides a wide range of authors for speaking events. To find out more, go to www.HachetteSpeakersBureau.com or call (866) 376-6591.

The publisher is not responsible for websites (or their content) that are not owned by the publisher.

Library of Congress Cataloging-in-Publication Data
Puck, Wolfgang.
  Wolfgang Puck makes it healthy : light, delicious recipes and easy exercises for a better life / Wolfgang Puck and Chad Waterbury with Norman Kolpas and Lou Schuler.
       pages cm
  Includes index.
  ISBN 978-1-4555-0884-6 (hc) —
ISBN 978-1-4555-1761-9 (ebook) 1. Reducing diets—Recipes. 2. Exercise. 3. Cooking. I. Title.
  RM222.2.P775 2014
  641.5'635—dc23

                          2013034358

Credits

Thanks to the following stores and craftspersons for loaning some of the serving pieces that appear in the photos throughout this book.

Doug Louie: page 64.

Freehand Gallery: pages 140, 144, and 181.

Humble Ceramics: pages 132 and 233.

Mas Ojima: page 116.

Jaune de Chrome: page 138.

Medard de Noblat: pages 66 and 97.

Sierra Pecheur: page 58.

TableArt Los Angeles: pages 40, 93, 109, 111, 153, 178, 222, 240 (bowl), and 247 (underplate).

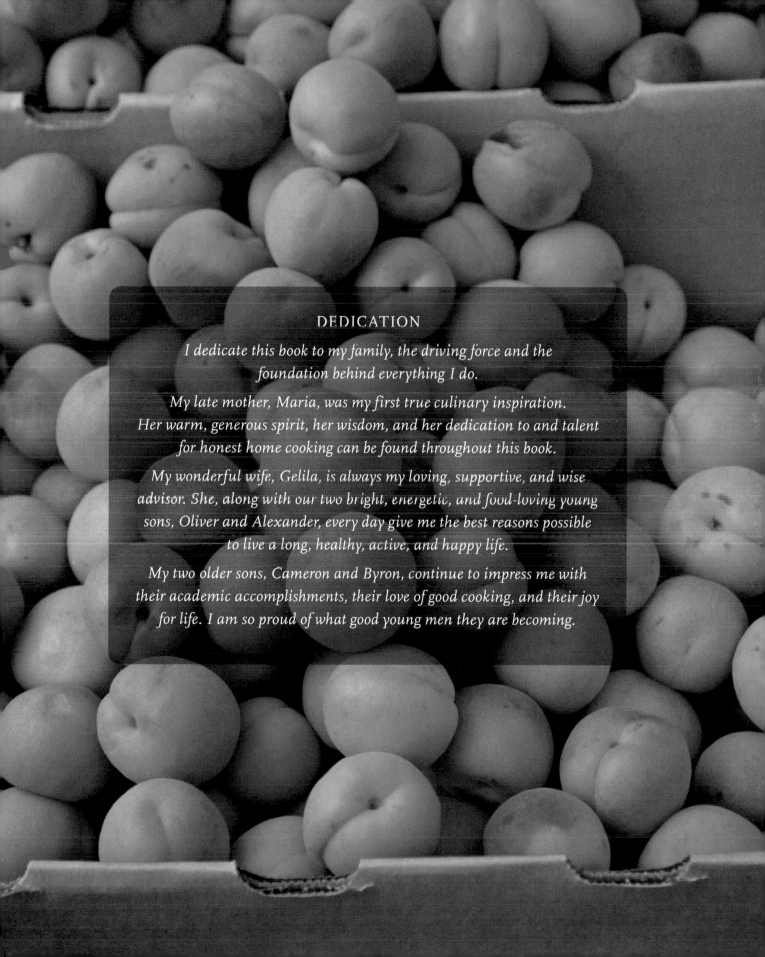

DEDICATION

I dedicate this book to my family, the driving force and the foundation behind everything I do.

My late mother, Maria, was my first true culinary inspiration. Her warm, generous spirit, her wisdom, and her dedication to and talent for honest home cooking can be found throughout this book.

My wonderful wife, Gelila, is always my loving, supportive, and wise advisor. She, along with our two bright, energetic, and food-loving young sons, Oliver and Alexander, every day give me the best reasons possible to live a long, healthy, active, and happy life.

My two older sons, Cameron and Byron, continue to impress me with their academic accomplishments, their love of good cooking, and their joy for life. I am so proud of what good young men they are becoming.

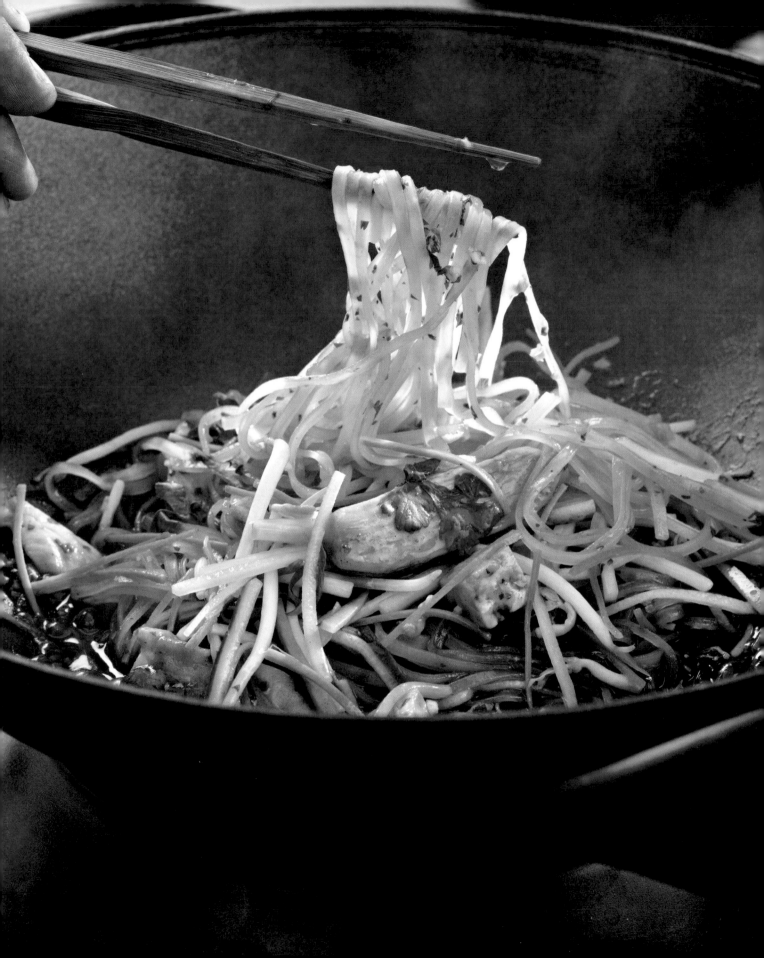

Contents

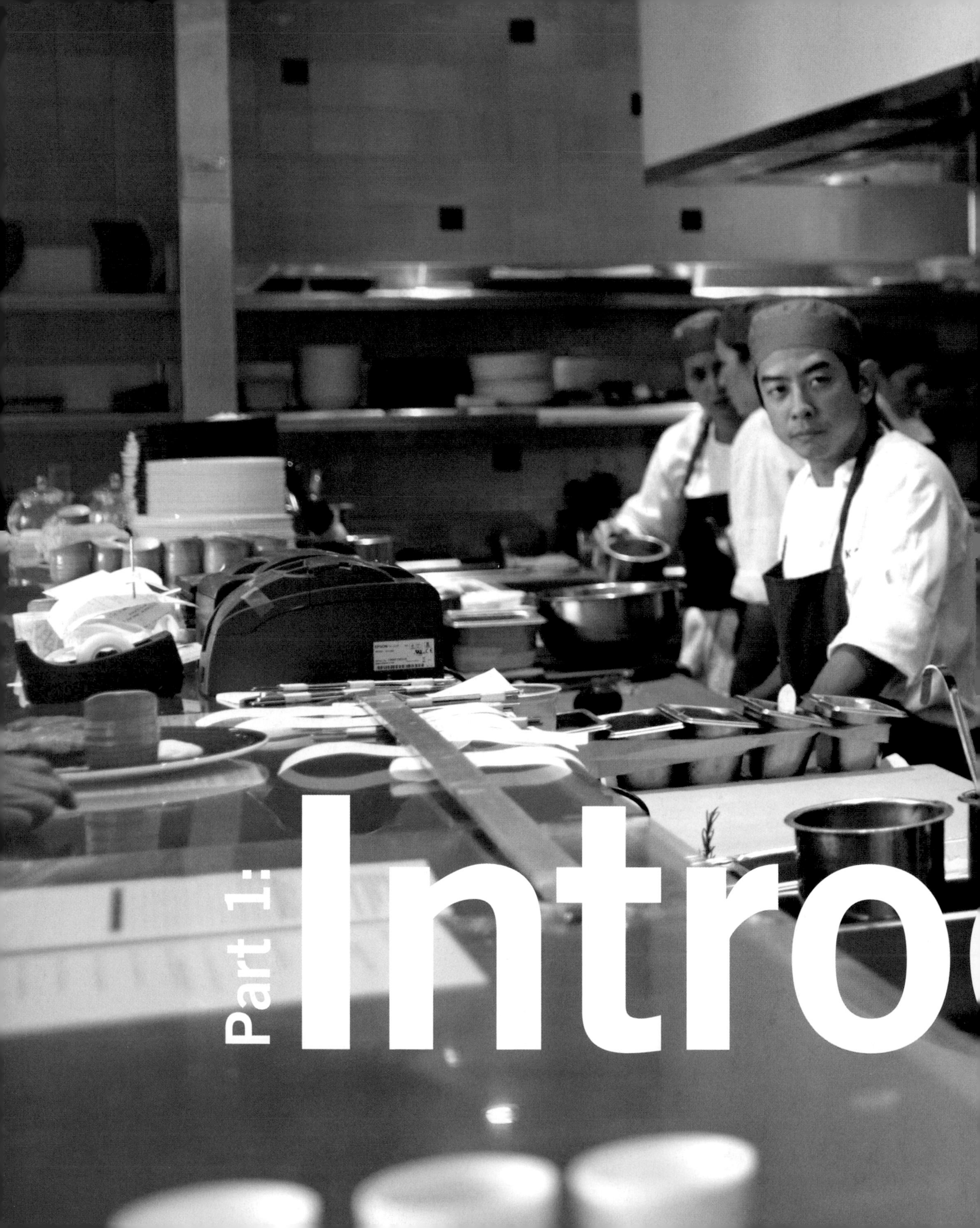

Part 1: Intro

duction

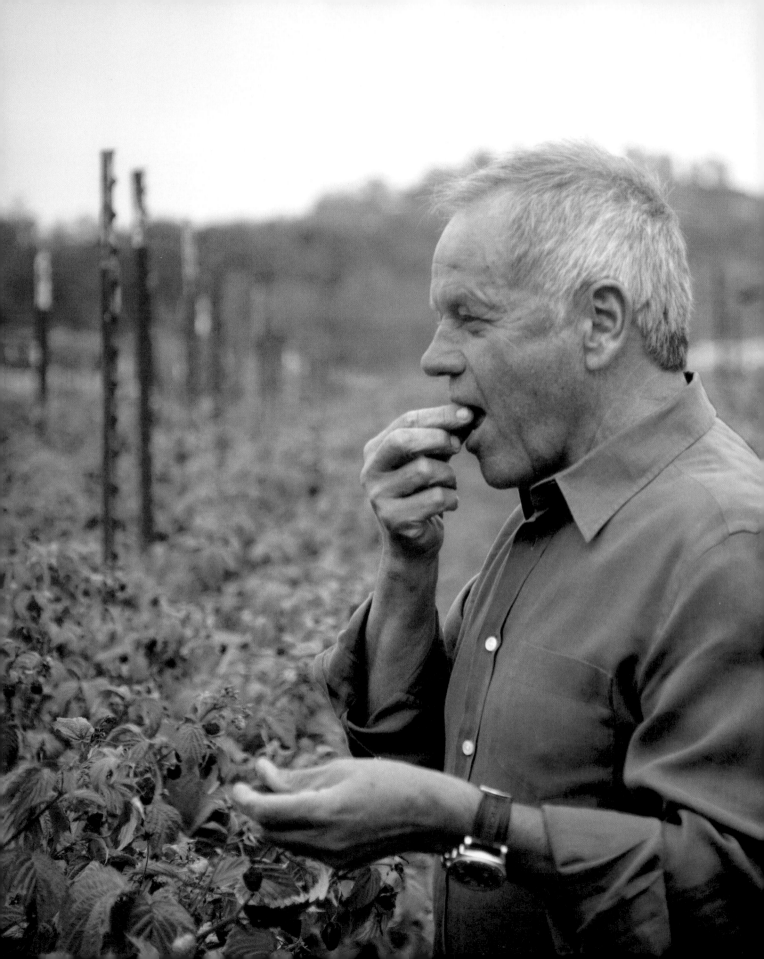

WHY I WROTE THIS BOOK

I never, ever expected to write this book. If you had suggested to me ten years ago, or even five, that my next book would focus on healthy recipes and fitness, I would've said you didn't know me very well.

I'm a chef, not a doctor or a research scientist or a registered dietitian. Of course, I read a lot about food, cooking, and eating, and I combine that with a lifetime of experience that comes from working in the kitchen, running restaurants, and seeing what people want and how they like to eat. But in recent years I've become more and more vitally concerned with ways to eat that will improve my own health and energy, as well as that of my family, my friends, and the many guests in my restaurants.

It all began to change for me in 2009. Wanting to feel healthier, I started adjusting my eating habits in simple ways—like emphasizing more fresh vegetables, fruits, and whole grains, reducing fat while maximizing flavor, and practicing moderation—that I'll explain in more detail throughout this book. And I began working with my trainer, Chad Waterbury. I was fifty-nine at the time. I had recently had a hip replacement, and I was in constant pain from an inflamed nerve in my lower back. My biggest fear was that I would have to give up skiing. That may not seem like much of a sacrifice to you, but I grew up in Austria. Skiing is what we do. Every kid skis. But lately, when I skied with my friends, I had to stop in the middle of the hill to catch my breath. Tennis is my favorite warm-weather sport, but because I'm a competitive person and I like to play with people who are better than me, it involves a lot of running, and I found I would have to sit down to rest every fifteen minutes.

It's not that I'd never tried to get in shape before. I'd tried just about everything, and most of what I did made me feel worse instead of better. The first time I exercised with a professional trainer, when I was in my thirties, I passed out. They had to carry me out of the gym. After that, I tried gym workouts, home workouts, running. I exercised with a trainer and without a trainer. The results were almost never what I hoped for. Even if I managed to lose some weight, get a little stronger, or build my endurance, the success never lasted long.

But Chad's workouts were different from any I'd tried before. During our first workout, we jumped rope, which I could only do for forty-five seconds at a stretch; did a circuit of basic calisthenics including jumping jacks, push-ups, and squats; did some boxing, with me wearing gloves and Chad holding up pads; and finished with stretching my warmed muscles. That's it. We did the entire routine in my living room, where we still work out to this day. More important, we started with a program I could realistically do, instead of a program Chad thought I should be able to do. He shared with me a simple piece of wisdom that I'd never heard before: *You can't start with an hour of training if your body is only ready for fifteen minutes.* And then we built up from where I was. A few months later, I could jump rope for ten minutes straight—and the only reason I stopped at ten was because we had to move on to another part of the workout.

EVERY DAY, PEOPLE ASK ME: "WOLFGANG, WHERE DO YOU GET ALL THIS ENERGY, AND HOW DO YOU WORK SO MANY HOURS AT YOUR AGE?" AND THEN THEY ADD: "COULD YOU BOTTLE IT, PLEASE?" THIS BOOK IS MY ANSWER TO THAT REQUEST.

About seven months after I started exercising with Chad, I went skiing in Colorado with some old friends from Austria. The difference in how I felt compared to my last ski trip was incredible. I didn't have to stop halfway down the hill for a breather. I even felt better, less lightheaded, at the high altitude. Back home in Southern California, when I played tennis, I could hit the ball for an hour straight without stopping to rest.

As you'll see, almost 90 percent of this book is what you would expect from me: recipes for great-tasting, easy-to-make food, with detailed instructions for how to prepare them in your home, and lots of general principles to help you cook and eat more healthfully, whatever you prepare or wherever you eat.

But, unlike my previous six cookbooks, I want this one also to give you the big recipe for the way I live my life today, a time when I feel I not only have more energy and more stamina than I ever had before but am also much trimmer—while also still being able to enjoy the food I love. And, as I now understand, thanks to Chad, that involves exercise.

Just as I did with exercise, I've had some less-than-satisfactory experiences with healthy eating plans. Long ago, I learned that I could lose weight on a very strict diet, and maybe it would work for three months or so. But I usually wound up feeling weaker—and as soon as I started eating normally again, even while trying to make smart food choices, I would gain the weight back, and maybe a little extra.

And let's face it: It's not reasonable for someone in my profession to stay on a strict diet. To be a good chef, I have to, and want to, sample everything in my restaurants. But that means *sample*, a small taste. If I like it, I might even have more than one taste, especially when it's a dessert. (I've always had a sweet tooth, particularly when it comes to anything with chocolate.) At any one time, I may not eat a lot; but, over the course of a day, I can sometimes consume a lot of food. It's great food—I'm always surrounded by the best ingredients, and everyone who works in my kitchens really knows how to cook well—but, since my name and reputation are so closely associated with Spago and my many other restaurants, I always have to make sure that the food meets my highest standards. I'll also have a glass or two of wine in the evening. I don't think I could be happy if I wasn't able to eat well and drink well.

The difference today is that I can eat all of my favorite foods without *overeating* anything. I feel good because of the combination of eating well and exercising. Now I want to help you achieve the same goal, to feel healthy and happy, with plenty of energy to do the things you love to do.

With that in mind, the first part of this book focuses on food. The recipes are somewhat different from what you may have seen in my previous books or ordered in my restaurants. But their style, ease, and the delicious results they deliver

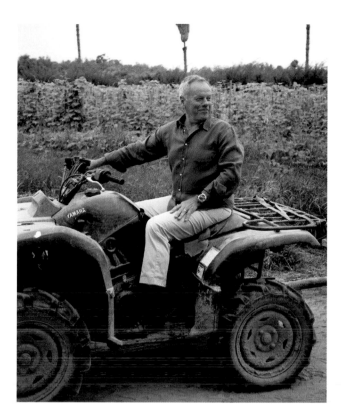

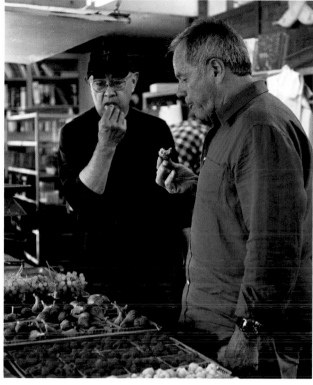

have not changed; after all, I don't believe there's any point in preparing a meal that doesn't taste great. I've worked very hard to make sure that anything you make will be a recipe I'm proud to put my name on. But, at the same time, I've made a deliberate effort to change things significantly. Fat, especially, has been reduced—usually as low as or lower than the 30 percent of total calories most experts on sound nutrition set as a benchmark. (And in some cases, where healthful ingredients are just naturally high in what are known as "good," heart-healthy fats, like the omega-3 fatty acids found in salmon and other cold-water fish, I've aimed to pair them with other ingredients or suggested side dishes that will bring down the meal's overall fat percentage.) I've reduced the salt in some of the recipes in which it makes sense to do so—or left the decision of adding salt to taste to you, since some people are more sodium-sensitive than others. (As much as possible, I also use widely available kosher salt, which is free of the additives that table salt may contain and, being coarse-grained, is lower in sodium content by volume than fine table salt.) I've also tried as much as possible to increase the amount of complex carbohydrates— for example, using whole grains and whole-grain flours instead of their refined, "white," lower-fiber counterparts.

And, maybe most important, recipe by recipe, bite by bite, I've tried to increase the amounts of healthful fresh vegetables and fruits, allowing them to play a greater role in your meals.

I want to make very clear to you, though, that I do not intend this to be what you or anyone would call a diet book. Even though these recipes represent a healthier way of eating, and will very likely help you lose weight when you eat and exercise sensibly, I am not going to tell you how much you should weigh or how much or what you should eat. Unlike the diet books you'll find everywhere, I won't make you promises of specific weight losses in a specific number of days or weeks. Those kinds of goals are best set by you and your doctor or another professional health practitioner.

Instead, what I offer you here is simply a healthier way of cooking and eating (and exercising) that will benefit you no matter what your goals might be.

In particular, the recipes and cooking instructions you'll find here will very likely bring a wider variety of healthy nutrients into your daily eating, while also helping you reduce your calorie intake by eliminating the hidden fats and empty calories found in so many foods today. And that can't help but be good for you.

Many of these recipes are simple ones that are based on the

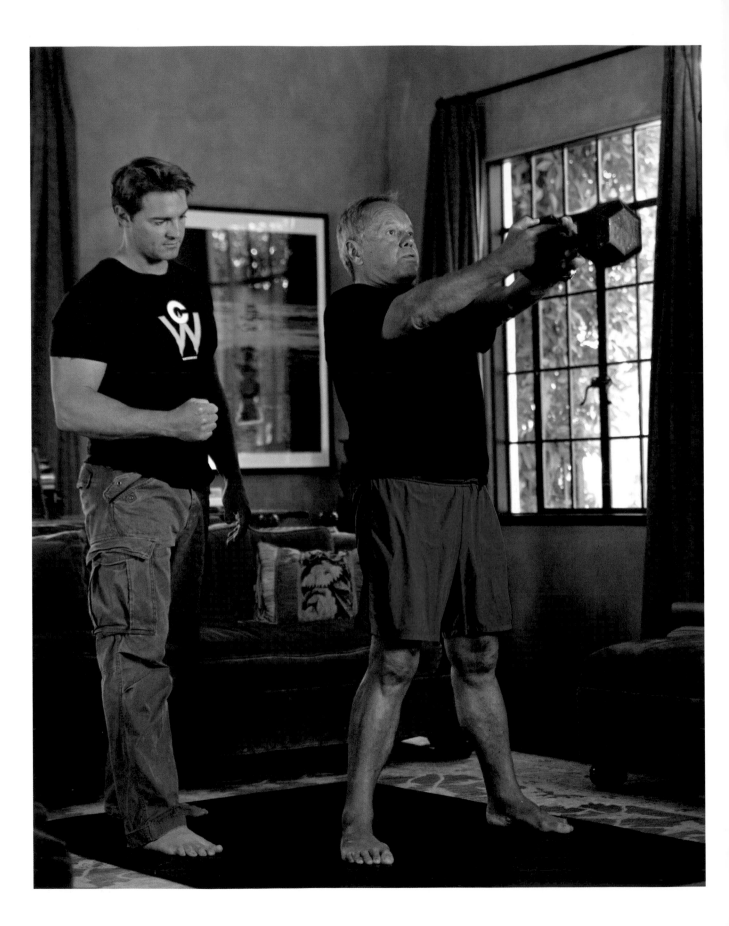

way I eat at home and cook for my own family—and sometimes they're the kinds of fresh-from-the-garden dishes my mother and grandmother cooked for me when I was a little boy. At home, I usually don't make complicated food. After all, there's an understandable difference between the dishes you find in a special-occasion restaurant and in everyday, family-style home cooking. But everything I cook at home is still great food, made with the highest-quality ingredients. If something doesn't taste good, it doesn't matter whether it's good for you. I don't want to eat anything unless it tastes great. And I don't think you should, either.

Thanks to the combination of good workouts and better eating habits, I now have more energy, more muscle, and more strength than I have in a long time. I feel less stressed and sleep better—in fact, I feel better than I have in two decades. At my age, most people would think the opposite would be true. And if I hadn't made the lifestyle changes I'm going to share with you throughout this book, that *would* be the case.

I also now weigh about twenty pounds less than I did at my heaviest. A lot of the weight I lost was in my stomach, the area of the body medical science tells us is the most dangerous place to carry excess fat. But to me that isn't even the most important benefit. What matters to me is simply that I *feel* better. I look forward to my workouts. I have more stamina than ever for my work. And best of all, I am more able to play with my children every day.

Every day, people ask me: *Wolfgang, where do you get all this energy, and how do you work so many hours at your age?* And then they add: *Could you bottle it, please?* This book is my answer to that request.

That's why exercise is such an important part of this book, along with the food. It reflects the fact that I have now made exercise an important part of my lifestyle. And I don't do it for the exercise itself. Yes, I like being stronger, but I've never cared about being able to lift a lot of weight, or flexing my muscles in the mirror. For me, that's not real life.

The reason I exercise is that I want to be good at what I like to do. And what I like to do, more than anything else, is cook.

I grew up watching my mother and grandmother cook. I started my first apprenticeship in a restaurant kitchen when I was fourteen. Since then, I've been on my feet for ten to twelve hours a day, six days a week, month after month, year after year.

The workouts in this book not only helped me lose fat but they also improved my core strength and my stamina, making it easier for me to stand for long hours. Today, I need less sleep than I did just a few years ago. I travel more than ever. My businesses have all grown larger, and I open more new restaurants every year all over the world, which only adds to my hectic travel schedule. And yet, I feel less fatigued. I spend more time with my wife and children, eating breakfast with my boys every morning that I'm in town, before I take them to school; and having dinner with my family almost every evening. One of my sons even sometimes joins me for my morning workouts with Chad. None of that would be possible without the energy I get from my workouts and from the benefits of a healthier, more reasonable way of eating.

My goal with this book is to help you achieve what I've achieved: a better, more sustainable, and more enjoyable lifestyle. I want to help you enjoy your food, your fitness, and your time with your loved ones. I want to share with you the kinds of meals and exercises that can enhance your own life. If that describes your goals, too, then let's get started.

MY GUIDE TO DELICIOUS, HEALTHY COOKING

To me, food should nourish the body, mind, and soul alike. It's a complete experience that activates and engages every one of your senses.

You could definitely use the word *healthy* to describe the way I love to eat today, and the way I prefer to cook for myself and my family. I prepare and eat food that is mostly low in fat, low in sodium, and higher in complex carbohydrates, recipes featuring generous amounts of the freshest in-season vegetables and fruits that I can find. And that kind of delicious, healthy food, in combination with regular exercise under the training of Chad Waterbury, makes me feel better and more energetic than I have ever felt in my life.

But, to tell you the truth, I don't really think about food and cooking as "healthy" or "unhealthy." Instead, I usually think in terms of "good food" or "bad food."

What do I mean by *good* food? It's the result of good

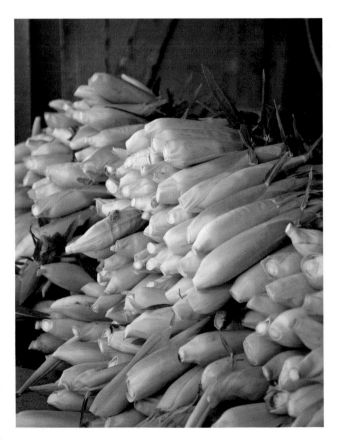

cooking. And good cooking starts with the finest-quality ingredients you can find: fresh produce; the best seafood, poultry, and meat; whole grains and beans; flavorful, heart-healthy cooking oils; and vibrant seasonings. Back in the kitchen, good cooking continues with recipes and methods that highlight and intensify the natural flavors and textures of those ingredients without masking them, resulting in food that tastes absolutely delicious.

Compare that ideal to so many of the foods today that are considered "bad" for us, particularly processed rather than fresh ingredients and products, whether people cook them at home or buy them in convenience stores or at fast-food restaurants. The aim of such foods seems to be to mask sometimes poor-quality ingredients with far too much of the things we human beings crave—fat, sugar, and salt—in spite of the fact that too much of those substances can damage our health. Those kinds of foods often remind me of creations from a mad scientist's lab, especially when you read the list of hard-to-pronounce chemical ingredients on their labels. Today, so many foods like that have turned eaters into addicts.

By contrast, I believe that food that is good for you can also be the kind of food that you will love and crave. Start with high-quality ingredients and cook them with simplicity, intelligence, and creativity, and they can taste even more delicious and be every bit as crave-able as the bad foods so many people find hard to avoid.

Good, healthy food can be convenient, too. It's easy to make, once you understand a few simple guidelines. On the following pages (as well as in the "Wolfgang's Healthy Tips" that appear with each recipe in this book), I'll share with you my approach to good, healthy, delicious cooking. I'll explain how easy it can be to cook smartly for better health. And I'll share my personal inspirations for getting creative in the kitchen to produce meals that will excite you, your family, and your friends so much that you'll want to cook and eat like this all the time.

THE GOALS OF GOOD, HEALTHY COOKING AND EATING

Over the years, I've devised my own secrets to preparing healthy food. Before I get into more detail about ingredients and cookware and cooking methods and so on, I would like to share a few broader observations about how to make the most delicious healthy meals—and the wisest choices—possible.

MAKE FRESH PRODUCE AND WHOLE GRAINS THE STARS. Not so long ago, if you asked someone what they planned to have for dinner on a particular night, their answer would probably be something like, "I'm having steak tonight," or "I think I'll have fish tonight." Today, I like to make seasonal produce the star of the plate: vegetables from the farmers' market or a good greengrocer, leafy salad greens, ripe fruits in desserts or even in some main dishes. It's hard to overeat or gain weight from vegetables. I also add more whole grains to my meals; high in fiber and generally low in fat and calories, whole grains fill you up more quickly and deliver more nutrients than processed grains. And if you aim to eat a rainbow of different colorful vegetables and fruits, you'll get a wide variety of healthy nutrients. Whole grains and legumes, along with fruits and vegetables, are also rich sources of fiber.

EAT REGULAR BUT SMALLER PORTIONS OF SEAFOOD, POULTRY, AND MEAT. Yes, animal proteins may seem like the featured players, since most people still define main courses by the proteins they contain. But, while we need regular protein to provide our bodies with the building blocks they need to function, we don't need too much. I now try to limit my protein portions to 4 to 6 ounces per serving, a healthier balance to the other items on my plates, and I aim for lower-fat choices like fresh fish, skinless chicken, leaner cuts of red meat. You can also get good protein from non-animal sources by regularly eating beans and lentils, nuts, dairy products (unless you're a vegan, of course), and whole grains.

CUT DOWN ON FATS—AND CHOOSE GOOD FATS. The broad consensus today seems to be that a healthy diet limits calorie intake to just under a third from fat. I've made that a goal for all of my recipes—that their calories are 30 percent or less from fat. A few are a bit higher in fat—some simply because cutting the fat too much would compromise good flavor, but mostly because they feature fish that are rich in heart-healthy omega-3 fatty acids, such as salmon, or because they include heart-healthy olive oil or other heart-healthy fats, including other vegetable oils, avocado, or nuts. Regardless, that limitation on fat calories need not apply to every bite of food you put in your mouth—it should be your average intake over a meal or a day. So, if you're going to choose to make and eat something that's slightly higher in fat, average out your intake by serving it with something much lower in fat or eating lower-fat dishes the rest of the day.

LIMIT SODIUM. Yes, there is too much salt (the diet's main source of sodium) in much of the food people eat today, especially in processed foods. Although some people are more sensitive to sodium than others, it's generally a good idea to cut down on how much salt you eat for the sake of cardio-vascular health. But it's also a simple fact that salt helps enhance the taste of many foods. Throughout this book, I've aimed to cut down on salt. As explained in individual recipes, I've found many other ways to enhance and intensify the natural flavors of ingredients. When I feel salt is needed, I usually (but not always) say to add it "to taste," leaving its addition and quantity to your own discretion and personal dietary needs. (Ingredients added to taste, without specific quantities, are not included in the nutritional analyses that follow each recipe.) Bear in mind, though, that many foods naturally include sodium. If you're on a sodium-restricted diet, do your own calculations and make your choices based on your doctor's guidelines.

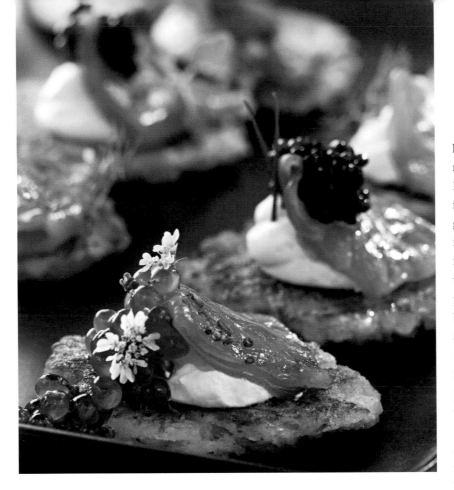

CHOOSE VARIETY. Nutrition experts tell us that the best way to eat for optimum health, regardless of whether you're a carnivore, a vegetarian, a vegan, or someone following other dietary guidelines, is to eat a wide variety of foods. Whether you do it over the course of a meal, a day's eating, or a week, aim to eat as many different kinds of vegetables, fruits, grains, lean proteins, and low-fat dairy products as possible. Doing this will help ensure that your body gets as much as possible of the many different nutrients it needs.

HIGHLIGHT AND INTENSIFY NATURAL FLAVORS AND TEXTURES. The more flavor and texture there is in a dish, the more pleasure and excitement it delivers with every bite or spoonful, and the more likely you are to slow down and savor it. How can you not eat more slowly to experience the bright crunch and freshness of a salad vegetable, the chewiness and earthiness of a sautéed mushroom, the way lively seasonings complement a moist and delicate morsel of fish, the pure and intense fruit essence that bursts from a cloud-like spoonful of surprisingly low-fat soufflé? And, as scientists and lay-persons alike have known for decades, when you eat more slowly, you generally eat less, since it takes at least twenty minutes of eating for your brain to recognize that your hunger is satisfied.

PRESENT FOOD BEAUTIFULLY. We eat with our eyes before food ever enters our mouths, so I always try to make the food I eat look as beautiful as possible on the plate. That doesn't mean you have to carve vegetables into flowers, or make intricate mosaics of ingredients. In fact, I don't like my food to look too fussy. But, as you'll see in the photographs throughout this book, and read in the final paragraphs of the recipe instructions, I do like to give some thought to making each plate of food a pleasure to look at, arranging it casually, but artfully, on attractive serving dishes and garnishing it simply but beautifully. (For example, when I'm at the farmers' market, I can't resist buying all sorts of pesticide-free organic flowers, many of them herb blossoms, to use as garnishes. I add these spontaneously to all sorts of dishes, and you'll see such flowers in many of the photos.) Stop to admire a beautiful plate of food and you can't help but eat it more slowly and enjoy it more. I'm also aware that, according to psychologists, food served on a smaller plate will look like a more generous portion, tricking your brain into thinking you're eating more. So I try to avoid using tableware that is so large it dwarfs the food.

PREPARE MEALS THAT SATISFY. In the end, if the food you eat doesn't satisfy you, you're going to want to eat more. The healthy food I prepare has big flavors, interesting textures, and lots of variety, and it looks beautiful. From your first sight of it on the plate to your very last bite, it's a satisfying experience that you will want to slow down and savor. As I said before, it should nourish the body, the mind, and the soul.

A NOTE ON NUTRITIONAL ANALYSES

Accompanying each recipe in this book, you'll find a listing of key "Nutrition Facts" per serving. (Note that these nutritional analyses are, by their nature, approximate, since no two specimens of a particular ingredient will be precisely identical. Also, ingredients added "to taste" or listed as "optional" are not included in a recipe's analysis.) You can use this information to help you plan and keep track of your own dietary goals, whatever they might be, that you've set with your doctor or other health advisor. Here, I'd like to review briefly the items I include in those listings.

CALORIES: The calorie, defined in the laboratory as how much energy it takes to raise the temperature of 1 gram of water by 1°C, is the basic measurement of the amount of energy supplied by any food. Note that fats, by weight, are more than twice as calorie-dense (9 calories per gram) as proteins or carbohydrates (4 calories per gram)—another good reason to limit fat intake.

CALORIES FROM FAT: This caloric number will help you determine at a glance how many of the calories in a particular dish come from fat.

TOTAL FAT: The total number of fat grams in a given dish. Some fat is needed in the diet, though, as fats play several key roles in keeping our bodies functioning healthily. Note that some fats are more or less beneficial to your health than others (see column to the right). The recipes in this book do not make use of so-called "trans fats," found in hydrogenated vegetable oil products such as vegetable shortening or stick margarine as well as manufactured foods containing such fats. These have been found to elevate blood cholesterol levels.

SATURATED FAT: These fats come from animal sources, including animal proteins, whole-fat dairy products, egg yolks, cocoa butter, and tropical oils such as coconut. Although they sometimes provide rich, distinctive flavor, they should be used in limited quantities, as they contribute to raised blood cholesterol levels.

MONOUNSATURATED FAT AND POLYUNSATURATED FAT: These types of fats—both monounsaturated (from olive, canola, and peanut oils, avocados, and nuts) and polyunsaturated (other plant-derived oils)—have been found to be heart-healthy and help to lower cholesterol when consumed in moderation.

CHOLESTEROL: Present in animal fats, this substance plays a key role in the body's cellular functioning. But too much cholesterol can increase the risk of cardiovascular disease.

SODIUM: There is too much salt (the diet's main source of sodium) in much of the food people eat today, especially in processed foods. Although some people are more sensitive to sodium than others, it's generally a good idea to try to cut down on how much salt you eat for the sake of cardiovascular health.

TOTAL CARBOHYDRATE: There are two types of carbohydrates. "Simple" carbohydrates provide quick energy and come from refined sugar, honey, fruits, and dairy products. "Complex" carbohydrates, also commonly known as "starches," come from grains, flours and pastas, potatoes, starchy or sweet vegetables, and beans; requiring digestion, they release energy more slowly to the body, and also provide beneficial vitamins, minerals, and fiber.

DIETARY FIBER: This indigestible plant substance contributes to good health in several important ways. "Soluble" fiber from fruits, dried beans and peas, oatmeal, and barley helps regulate blood sugar levels, reduces blood cholesterol, and helps elimination. "Insoluble" fiber from vegetables and whole grains like wheat also contributes to gastrointestinal health.

SUGARS: The carbohydrate sugar on its own—whether refined sugar, honey, syrups, or sugary preserves—provides no nutrients, just energy. That's why it's often referred to as a source of "empty calories." As much as possible, I try to add sweetness to recipes through the sugars naturally present in nutritious fruits.

PROTEIN: Made up of the building blocks known as amino acids, protein is essential for the growth and repair of our bodies, for carrying nutrients to cells, and for helping to regulate body functions. Simply put, it's essential to eat enough protein for good health. Animal proteins, preferably from lower-fat, heart-healthy choices, provide the full range of amino acids the human body needs. Vegetarians and vegans can still get sufficient protein from beans, legumes, and whole grains, preferably eaten together to provide all the necessary amino acids.

SHOPPING FOR INGREDIENTS

Buying good, healthy ingredients is so much easier today than it was even a decade ago. More and more supermarkets emphasize quality ingredients. They've enlarged their produce departments and expanded their offerings of fresh seafood, poultry, and meat choices. And new farmers' markets seem to be popping up in neighborhoods across the nation, making it more and more possible for everyone to buy good-quality, in-season produce—and sometimes eggs, dairy products, and other ingredients—grown a relatively short distance away.

As much as possible, I try to buy produce that is organically and sustainably farmed, as well as proteins that come from farms practicing sustainable and cruelty-free methods. I'm not going to go into the politics or ethics of those issues here, especially at a time when some people simply cannot afford to pay the higher prices such products often carry. But I will say that organic, sustainably and responsibly produced ingredients can sometimes be higher in quality and nutritional value, as well as often, in my opinion, tasting better than their mass-produced counterparts. And the more people who demand and buy such ingredients, the more farmers will want to grow them and the more likely the prices are to become accessible to everyone.

When it comes to shopping for my family at home, I like to follow the traditional European style. That is, as much as possible our meals combine pantry staples that keep for a long time without refrigeration, such as dried pastas, whole grains, dried beans, canned tomatoes, dried herbs and spices, healthy oils, and so on; refriger-ated staples that keep for several days, such as dairy products and eggs; and fresh ingredients you buy within a day or two of a meal, including vegetables and fruits, seafood, poultry, and meat. Such an approach helps make sure that you're eating foods at their peak of flavor and texture and that you get a good variety of ingredients and nutrients. It also helps you avoid one of the saddest aspects of cooking in the Western world today: waste, the amount of food that is thrown out instead of being eaten.

It would take a book in itself to give you tips on how to buy the best of every single ingredient you might like to cook. But most such decisions usually boil down to a matter of common sense: If it looks good and smells good—and tastes good if you're offered a taste— it probably is good. Beyond that bit of wisdom, let me share a few more tips on how to get the best out of your shopping excursions.

VEGETABLES AND FRUITS

Whenever possible, I like to shop at local farmers' markets, which are widespread in sunny Southern California and appearing more and more fre-quently everywhere. In fact, doing that is a favorite and regular Sunday morning excursion for my two young sons and me. At the farmers' market, you're more likely to get a wider variety of good-quality, fresh, in-season produce that was grown within a relatively short drive of the market, and probably find more organic choices. And the growers, who often tend their own stalls, generally offer tastes of what they're selling. That doesn't happen as often in supermarkets, where some ingredients have traveled greater distances, even across international borders and oceans. More and more, however, I'm happy to see that the success of farmers' markets is influencing big chain markets, where you'll see more products labeled "organic" or "local," and also be offered more tastes while shopping. I must confess, I enjoy snacking my way through a farmers' market—and what healthy snacks they usually are!

BEANS AND LEGUMES

These pantry staples, which keep well for months when stored in an airtight container away from light and heat, are invaluable sources of healthy protein, carbohydrates, and fiber—especially for those who are following vegetarian or vegan diets. I always like to keep a variety at hand to use not just in main courses but also in soups, salads, and side dishes. Also in this category, but found in the refrigerated section of your market, is protein-rich tofu, the custard-like bean curd made from soybeans.

SEAFOOD, POULTRY, AND MEAT

As much as possible, I like to buy these animal proteins within a day or so of cooking them. I decide on the dish I plan to cook, and then go shopping specifically for the featured ingredient. (If you like to, or have to, shop less frequently, animal proteins also keep well in the freezer for several months when wrapped in airtight freezer bags.) Whether you buy your seafood, poultry, or meat in a supermarket or from a specialty store, always choose products that look and smell clean and fresh, without any suspicious discolorations or "off" odors. Just about any seafood choice will be a good one for healthy eating; even those fish that are higher in fat, such as salmon and tuna, are rich in omega-3 fatty acids, which medical studies have found to benefit the heart. As for poultry, healthy, lower-fat cooking becomes easier thanks to the skinless pieces widely sold today, whether of lower-fat breast meat or slightly richer dark meat. And many cuts of red meat can be healthier

choices, too, when eaten in moderation; look for leaner cuts with the least amount of visible "marbling" of fat, and trim away as much fat as you can before cooking, or ask a butcher to do the trimming for you at the time of purchase.

GRAINS, PASTAS, AND FLOURS

If I served brown rice in one of my restaurants even ten years or so ago, it was very possible that several guests a day would say to the server, "What is this? A health food place?" Today, brown rice—with its fiber- and nutrient-rich hull and germ still attached—is much more widely enjoyed, not just for its dietary benefits but also for its nutty flavor and chewy texture. I always have brown rice at home, stored in my pantry in an airtight container, along with a selection of other healthy whole grains that can bring such delicious variety to soups,

salads, side dishes, and main dishes, including the ancient Incan grain quinoa; farro, an ancient ancestor of wheat long used in Italy; and, of course, all-American wild rice. More and more pastas are available in whole-grain varieties, too; and not just whole wheat pastas but those made from other grains—such as brown rice, oats, or corn—for pasta lovers who are avoiding foods containing gluten. I also include whole grains in the flours and meals I keep on hand for baked goods, including whole wheat flour, oat flour, oatmeal, cornmeal, rice flour, and spelt flour. Look in the baking, grains, or specialty foods aisles of many mainstream markets today, and you'll be surprised by the variety available. Do a quick Internet search and you'll see how easily you can order all kinds of whole grains, too, which will arrive at your door in a matter of days.

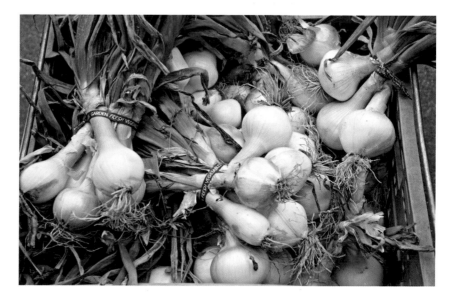

OILS AND FATS

As you'll see from just a quick glance through the recipes in this book, good extra-virgin olive oil is one of my favorite fats for cooking. Not only does it impart a delicious flavor, even when used in small amounts, but it also has been found to be a heart-healthy form of fat. That's not to say that I completely avoid butter and other animal fats; I just use them very occasionally and sparingly for the touch of rich flavor they can impart without making a dish overly indulgent. And, when I need the stick-resistant properties of oil or fat for browning or for baking, but don't need its flavor or richness or its calories, I'll often use nonstick cooking spray, which is virtually fat free and stores well in the pantry.

DAIRY AND EGGS

I love dairy products, whether it's a touch of steamed milk in my morning *espresso macchiato*, a light dusting of freshly grated Parmesan on some pasta, or a nibble of good cheese at the end of a meal. But I also realize that many of my favorite dairy products are also rich sources of the kinds of fats that aren't really good for you. So I try to choose reduced-fat or nonfat options whenever possible, and to make smart substitutions for the cream or whole eggs that enrich so many of the kinds of recipes that people love. In egg dishes, for example, I've learned to substitute egg whites for at least some of the yolks, leaving a yolk or two in a recipe to contribute its familiar and welcome rich flavor and color. I've also found that low-fat buttermilk and nonfat plain yogurt—especially the very thick and rich-tasting Greek style—can provide a lot of the richness and body our palates normally associate with cream. So I keep smart ingredients like these on hand in my refrigerator, or put them on my shopping list when I'm planning to make a recipe that will benefit from them.

SUGARS

I learned an interesting lesson years ago the first time I visited Asia, where I have several restaurants and plan to open more. Chocolate lover that I am, I eagerly tried the best products I could find there—and was immediately surprised to discover that they were noticeably less sweet than those we eat in North America and in Europe. I realized that different cultures learn from an early age to like different levels of sweetness in their foods, just as they learn to like or dislike different levels of other flavors. And, even as grown-ups, we can relearn to like our sweets less sweet. So I don't shun sugar completely in my delicious, healthy cooking—I just use sugar and other sweeteners more sparingly than I used to. Do that yourself, and over time you'll get used to foods tasting less sweet, and like them that way. (Of course, if you're dealing with diabetes, you'll make your own smart decisions with your doctor's guidance.) I also prefer to use brown sugar and honey, primarily because they have more complex, rich, and satisfying flavors that also go better with whole grains and other wholesome ingredients. As you'll see in many of the dessert recipes in this book, I rely a lot on fresh seasonal fruit to provide much, if not all, of the dessert's sweetness.

SALTS

Especially if your doctor has warned you to cut your sodium intake, salt is something to add to your food judiciously—and certainly something we could all stand to consume less of. Even though salt can help highlight the flavors of certain foods and bring them into sharper focus, you can adjust to using less salt in your food just as you can adjust to less sugar. That's why many of the recipes in this book give no specific quantities when they call for salt (or other salty or high-sodium seasonings such as soy sauce), and instead tell you to add it to taste. (Note, too, that ingredients added to taste are not included in the nutritional analyses that accompany the recipes.) Try to add as little as possible to reach the point at which the food tastes good to you. Still, unless you are specifically trying to avoid salt, it's good to have it in your pantry. I like to use good-quality sea salt or flakes of French *fleur de sel*, which have a more complex flavor from the additional minerals present and can satisfy a craving for a hint of salt with just a small pinch. I also like kosher

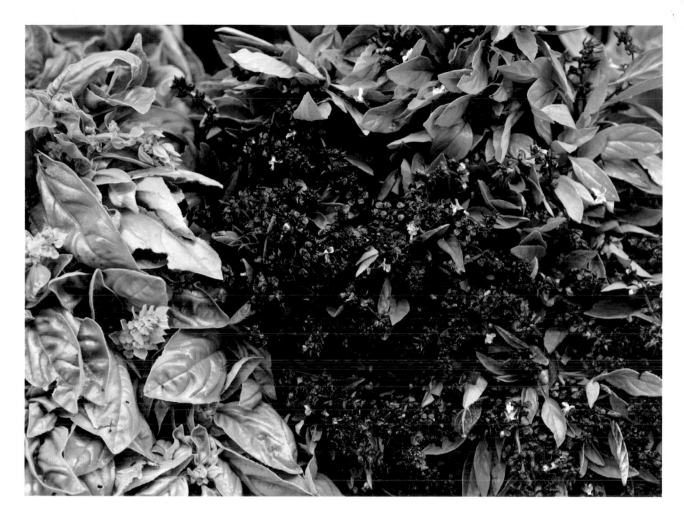

salt; generally, you can use less kosher salt to get the desired seasoning than you would table salt.

HERBS AND SPICES

These are some of the most potent ingredients for delicious, healthy cooking. Herbs (the flavorful, aromatic fresh or dried leaves of certain plants) and spices (the usually dried aromatic seeds, barks, roots, or rhizomes—underground stems—of certain plants) do so much to make the food you cook taste delicious. I like to keep a good selection of dried herbs and spices in my pantry, to cover a wide range of the kinds of recipes I most like to cook; and, with time, you can build up your own collection. That said, I never buy my seasonings in larger quantities than I'm likely to use in a few months, as dried herbs and spices gradually lose their flavor over time, even when properly stored in airtight containers in a cupboard at room temperature. As for fresh herbs, which brighten so many savory and sometimes sweet dishes, I make them a regular purchase on my trips to farmers' markets or the supermarket produce aisle, and keep them in the refrigerator produce bin with their stems wrapped in a damp paper towel to extend their freshness.

EQUIPPING YOUR KITCHEN

I'm not going to bombard you with long lists of all the cookware you need, since this isn't a book about how to set up your first kitchen. In the instructions for every recipe in this book, I tell you what cooking equipment you need to prepare it, giving specific measurements if the precise size or volume of the cookware has a significant effect on the recipe's outcome (such as the size of dishes for baking the soufflés on pages 252–255), or providing a more general idea of the size ("large," "medium," or "small") if slight variations will not affect the dish. Chances are, you already have most of the equipment you need.

There are certain items, however, that will definitely help you in your efforts to cook healthier food. And I'd like to review some key choices with you here.

POTS AND PANS

In my own cooking at home, and in my restaurant kitchens, I mainly use stainless-steel pots and pans. The best stainless-steel pots and pans have thick, three-layer bonded bottoms that sandwich a disc of heavy aluminum between the stainless steel. Such pans conduct heat extremely well and evenly, browning food perfectly, and are virtually nonstick if you preheat them and coat them with just a little oil, fat, or nonstick cooking spray. (It's important, too, to clean stainless steel with warm, soapy water right after use, to remove any residue easily from its still-warm cooking surface.) You can also use cookware with nonstick coatings, but these require special care to help keep their nonstick surfaces intact. To preserve the nonstick qualities of these pans, avoid using utensils that might scratch the coating, such as metal spatulas, and do not cook over too-high temperatures. In some cases, especially when a recipe calls for cooking eggs in an omelet pan or cooking foods on a griddle, I may specifically prefer to use a pan with a nonstick surface.

SMALL APPLIANCES

So many different kinds of small electric countertop appliances make meal preparation easier, efficiently performing specialized cooking functions without the need for heating up your stove. I don't think you need to own every kind of small appliance there is, especially since many people have kitchens with limited space. But it's worth looking into a few little machines.

My favorite among these is the **electric pressure cooker,** a virtually foolproof device that dramatically speeds up cooking and intensifies flavor by cooking low-fat, healthy foods under the greater atmospheric pressure and intensified heat that builds up in a tightly and safely sealed cooking chamber. It can cook soups and stews and grain dishes in a matter of minutes, and makes the purest, most intensely flavored, clearest broths you can imagine. Modern electric pressure cookers eliminate all the guesswork: Just assemble the ingredients as a recipe instructs, securely seal the safety-locked lid, and set the timer. The pressure cooker heats up, starts the timer as soon as full pressure is reached, and cooks for the desired time. You can then allow the pressure to release naturally through the safety valve or open the valve for quicker release as the specific recipe requires.

I also like **electric steamers.** Yes, you can buy all kinds of stovetop steamers in which a perforated basket holds food above a pan of simmering water; but such setups often require you to pay attention so that the water doesn't boil away or the food overcook. Injection steamers allow greater control, containing water chambers, heating elements, and timers for more carefree cooking. Some models even include multilayered cooking trays for preparing several

HEALTHY COOKING METHODS

dishes at the same time; and others build up a little extra pressure on their own (much less than a pressure cooker, though), speeding up cooking a bit and enhancing flavor by driving seasonings into the food.

Several other small electric appliances can make healthy food preparation more efficient. These include **hinged contact grills** and **panini makers** with ridged nonstick plates that cook foods on both sides at once, producing results in half the time and also draining away excess fat in the process. **Electric nonstick woks** are ideal for cooks who like the convenience and creativity of stir-frying. And an **electric reversible nonstick griddle-grill** makes it easy and quick to prepare healthy foods in quantity, from turkey burgers to fish fillets to pancakes and French toast.

You can use so many different methods for cooking foods healthily. Of course, you won't find any deep-frying or shallow-frying in this book; they just involve too much fat. But each of the methods reviewed here can play a special role in creating meals that taste as delicious as they are good for you.

STEAMING

Cooking food by surrounding it with steam in a covered container is one of the lowest-fat cooking methods there is. And steamed food can be anything but bland. By marinating ingredients, coating them with seasonings, or adding aromatic seasonings to the boiling liquid that flavor and scent the steam itself, you can create surprisingly complex-tasting, delicious results without any added fat. You can steam in a perforated and covered steamer basket over a pan or pot of simmering water on the stovetop, or use a counter-top injection steamer (see opposite).

POACHING

Gently simmering foods to doneness and tenderness is a time-honored way to cook without fat. As with steaming, you can also easily flavor the cooking liquid—whether water, broth, juice, or some other fluid—with seasonings of your choice. I generally like to poach in a wide, shallow pan with just enough liquid to cover the ingredients, so they're easier to see, to test for doneness, and to remove when they're ready. Always keep poaching liquid at a gentle simmer; the higher temperature

of an active boil can toughen proteins.

BOILING

Cooking food in a large pan or pot filled with boiling water is one of the best ways to prepare vegetables, pasta, and other ingredients. Always make sure you have a large enough pot to hold the food comfortably and circulating freely in a generous quantity of water. Too little water in a not-large-enough pan will make the water stop boiling and the cooking temperature drop.

BRAISING AND STEWING

These two related moist-heat cooking methods differ mostly in the size of the ingredients and the proportion of solids to liquids. In braising, larger pieces of food are gently simmered in a relatively small amount of liquid, which then reduces to become a flavorful sauce. Stewing involves smaller, often bite-size pieces of food gently simmered in a larger quantity of liquid; the solids and liquid are served together in bowls. (In fact, stews often differ from soups mostly in that the solids for soups are cut up even smaller.) Whether you prepare a braise

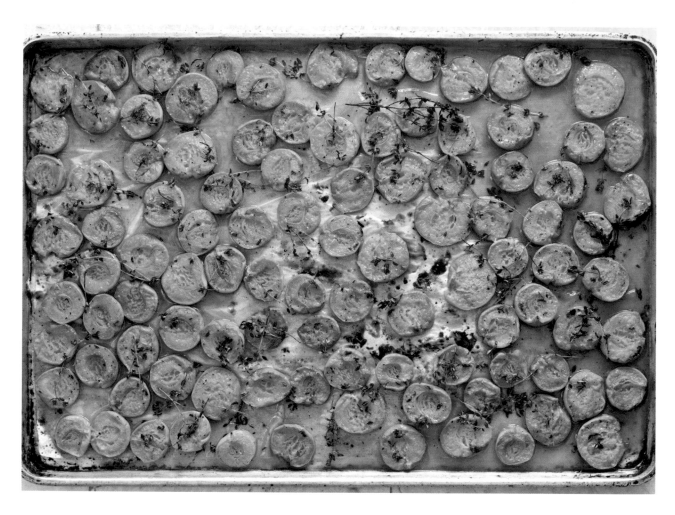

or a stew, there are many ways to make them good and healthy: starting with lower-fat proteins and lots of vegetables; browning the solids first in a small amount of oil or fat to develop more flavor; choosing low-fat, flavorful cooking liquids; and, if necessary, skimming liquefied fat from the surface during cooking.

SAUTÉING AND STIR-FRYING

Quickly searing food in a hot pan helps to caramelize its surface, developing a more intense flavor. Sautéing quickly cooks relatively small or thin pieces of food and is basically the same principle as stir-frying in the curved surface of a wok. You don't really need much fat to

sauté or stir-fry—just the lightest coating of healthy olive oil, for example, or a spritz of nonstick cooking spray will usually do, especially if you're using a pan with a nonstick coating.

GRILLING AND BROILING

Both these methods involve exposing relatively thin pieces of food—such as fish fillets, boneless and skinless chicken breasts, steaks or cutlets, or sliced vegetables—to an intense direct-heat source below or above the cooking grid on which the food is placed. You don't really need any extra fat for this method beyond what little you might add to a marinade or to help keep food from sticking. And the speed of

grilling or broiling helps create a flavorful brown surface on food and cook it through quickly without drying it out.

ROASTING

In roasting, the dry heat of an oven completely surrounds food, slowly penetrating it while also browning its surface to a crisp and flavorful finish. Seasonings rubbed onto the surface help flavor the food, mingling with the juices that bubble to its surface as the food heats up. The lightest coating of oil can help the seasonings adhere and also promote browning, while adding not too many calories relative to the number of servings a large roast can yield.

A NOTE ON MEAL PLANNING AND NUTRITION

As I have noted, I don't think of this book as a diet or weight-loss book. Instead, I consider it a lifelong way to cook, eat, and exercise for better health. If, however, you use this book in combination with the guidance you receive from your personal health professional, you will increase the likelihood that you will reach and maintain your ideal weight.

Although some of my recipes, especially those for main dishes, include suggestions for good side dishes to go with them, I am deliberately not including suggested menu plans. In many ways, the days of formal three-course menus—first course, main dish (plus sides), and dessert—seem long gone. People in restaurants and at home alike enjoy a greater variety of dishes and styles of cooking at every meal. Sometimes, they'll compose a menu just of small plates. Or they'll have a big stew or pilaf full of vegetables, grains, and proteins, with a salad on the side. Or they'll begin a meal with tastes inspired by Asian cuisine, only to go on to something Italian- or French-inspired.

That is the spirit in which I would like you to use this book. Let your meal and menu planning be dictated by the season and what vegetables and fruits look freshest at your market; the weather, with lighter and cooler dishes for warmer weather, and warmer, more robust meals for colder times of year; the occasion, whether casual and convenient or a special occasion worthy of more elaborate cooking; and, simply, your mood and what you feel like. Start by picking the main dish, if you like, and then build a complementary menu around it. Or select your starter first, and see where it might lead. Or make up a menu entirely of appetizers. Or choose the dessert you're craving, and then work your way backward!

In the end, aim for balance and variety, and I'm sure you'll be pleased.

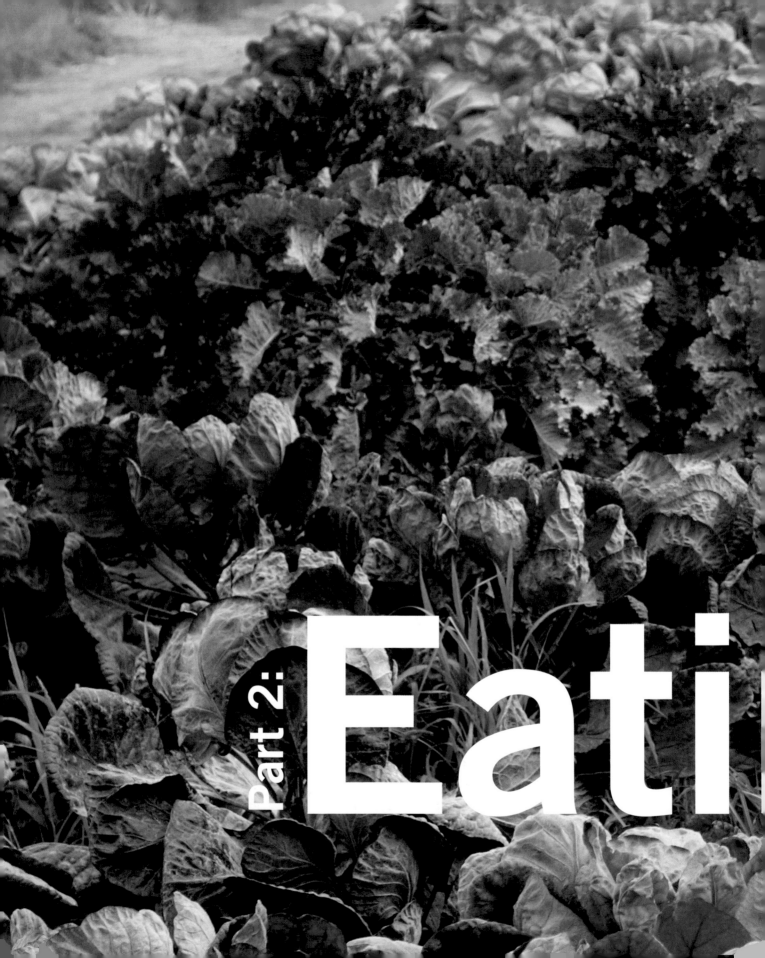

Part 2: Eati

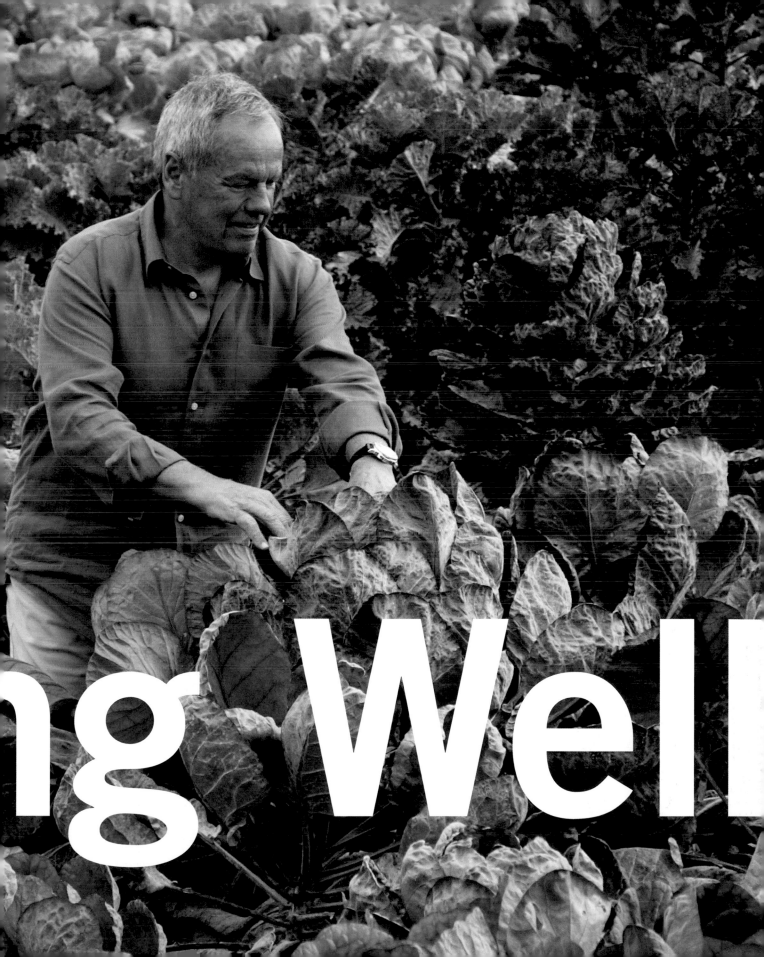

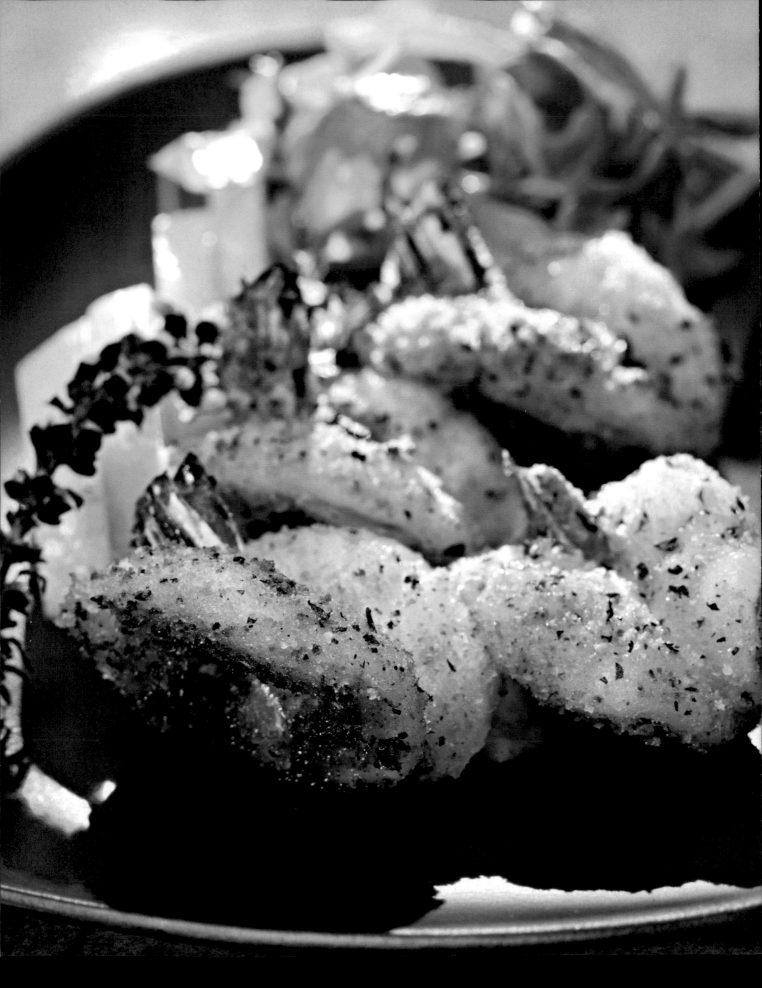

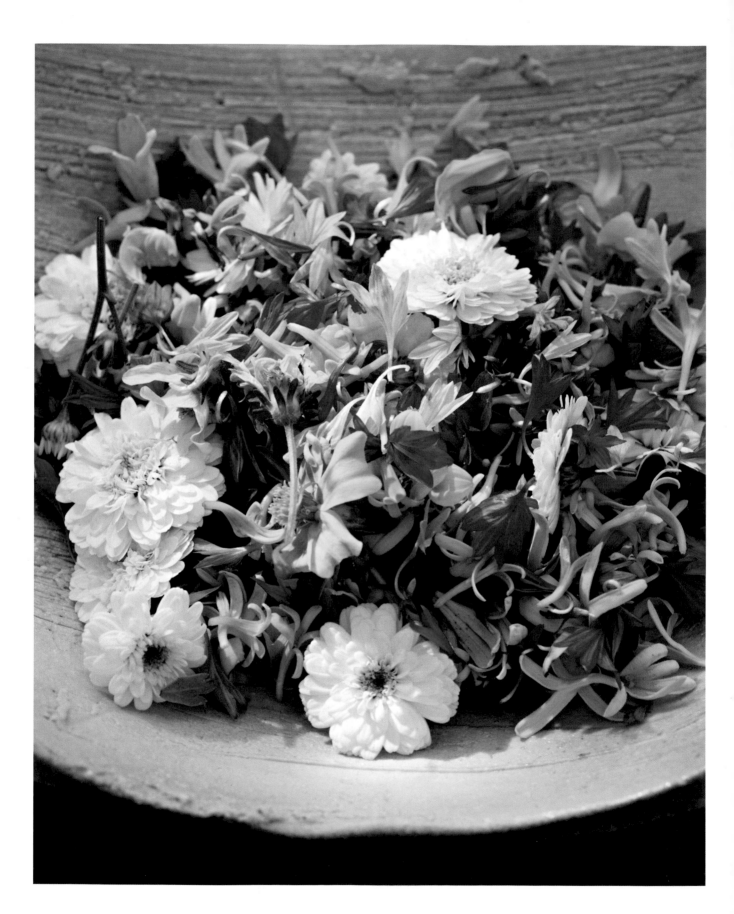

APPETIZERS

It's not surprising that one of the most popular ways to dine out these days is to order a wide assortment of small plates for everyone to share. And who doesn't love being invited to cocktail or buffet parties where you get to sample all kinds of different dishes?

Appetizers offer you wonderful ways to introduce variety to your menu. Choose a recipe that features ingredients different from your main dish, yet complementary to its seasonings or cooking method, and you'll go a long way toward creating the sense that you have dined well—and even more so when the foods you serve have been selected and prepared in ways that promote wellness, as the recipes in this chapter do. Remember: The more variety there is in a meal, the more we slow down to appreciate it all, and the less food it takes to chase hunger away.

You'll find a diverse range of appetizers in this chapter. (And, of course, many of the soups on pages 49–69, salads on pages 73–97, and side dishes on pages 177–213 could also be served as appetizers.) If you like, you might even want to try composing complete meals from several of these dishes alone.

→ Asparagus with Citrus-Mustard-Yogurt Sauce

→ Bruschetta with Heirloom Tomatoes, Red Chile, and Fresh Basil

→ Steamed Whole Artichokes with Green Goddess Dressing

→ Red Snapper Crudo with Fresh Salsa

→ Butterflied Baked Shrimp with Herbed Bread Crumbs and Roasted Garlic Lemon Yogurt Aioli

→ Buckwheat Blini with Smoked Whitefish

→ Griddled Potato Pancakes with Smoked Fish

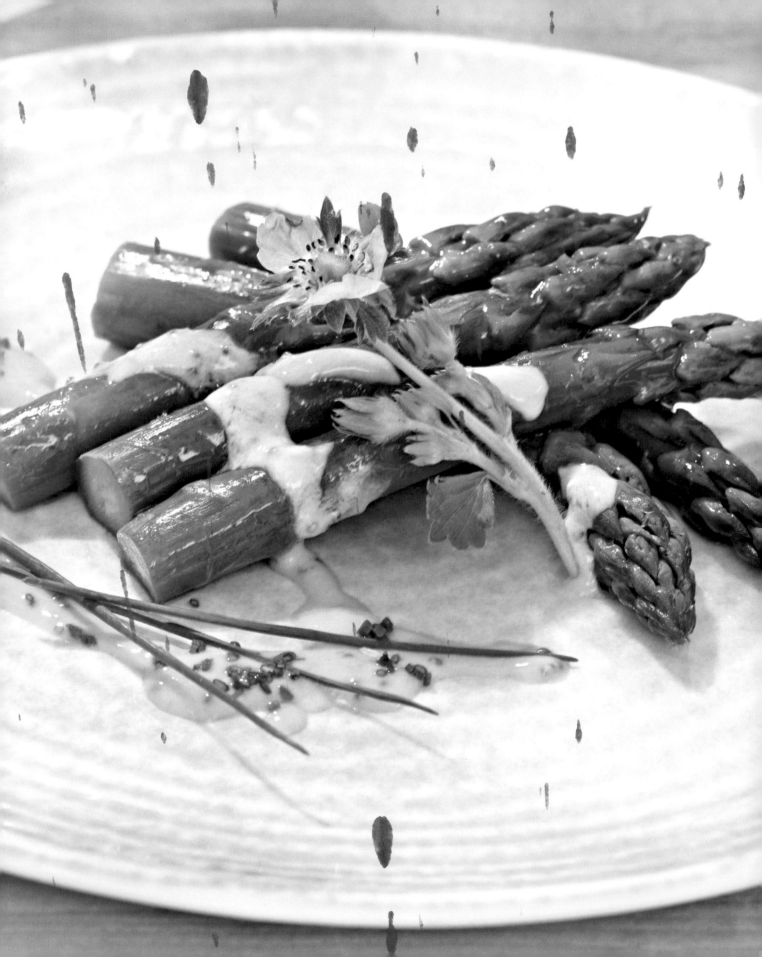

Asparagus with Citrus-Mustard-Yogurt Sauce

SERVES 4

Chilled cooked asparagus spears are traditionally served in French cuisine as an elegant appetizer accompanied by an oil-rich vinaigrette or a sauce based on mayonnaise and cream. This recipe offers all the classic pleasure with almost none of the fat.

2 pounds jumbo asparagus, tough stalk ends snapped off

2 cups fresh orange juice, strained of pulp

½ cup fresh lemon juice

2 tablespoons grainy mustard

½ teaspoon kosher salt

¼ teaspoon freshly ground white pepper

1 cup nonfat plain Greek yogurt

Fresh chives, some finely chopped, some left whole, for garnish

In a pot large and wide enough to submerge all the asparagus horizontally, bring salted water to a boil. Add the asparagus and cook until al dente (tender but still slightly crisp), about 5 minutes for jumbo spears (3 minutes for pencil thin spears) from the time the water returns to a boil.

Meanwhile, fill a large bowl with ice cubes and water. As soon as the asparagus is done, drain it and submerge the spears in the ice water to stop the cooking process. Drain well, transfer to a platter, cover with plastic wrap, and refrigerate until ready to serve.

In a medium saucepan, combine the orange and lemon juices and bring to a brisk simmer over medium heat. Cook until the juice has reduced to ½ cup, about 20 minutes. Transfer the juice reduction to a heatproof bowl set inside a larger bowl filled with ice and stir occasionally until thoroughly cooled.

Stir the mustard, salt, and pepper into the chilled juice reduction. Add the yogurt and stir with a whisk until well blended. Cover the bowl with plastic wrap and refrigerate until ready to serve.

At serving time, arrange the asparagus spears on four chilled serving plates, dividing the asparagus equally. Spoon a little of the sauce over each serving and garnish with chives. Pass the extra sauce at the table.

WOLFGANG'S HEALTHY TIPS

→ Feel free to use regular plain nonfat yogurt instead of Greek yogurt, though you'll get a slightly less creamy consistency.

→ Try the sauce as a dip for fresh or blanched and chilled vegetable crudités.

Nutrition Facts Per Serving: Calories: 148; Calories from Fat: 5; Total Fat: 0.65g; Saturated Fat: 0.16g; Monounsaturated Fat: 0.24g; Polyunsaturated Fat: 0.25g; Cholesterol: 0mg; Sodium: 147mg; Total Carbohydrate: 27.41g; Dietary Fiber: 5.67g; Sugars: 18.09g; Protein: 12.60g

Bruschetta with Heirloom Tomatoes, Red Chile, and Fresh Basil

SERVES 4

One of the most popular of appetizers can also be one of the healthiest—sun-ripened tomatoes, well seasoned and heaped on top of toasted bread. This version is even healthier, reducing the oil and adding whole-grain bread.

Tomato Topping:

5 medium sun-ripened heirloom tomatoes

⅓ cup thinly shredded fresh basil leaves

½ tablespoon balsamic vinegar

½ tablespoon extra-virgin olive oil

½ teaspoon kosher salt, plus more as needed

¼ teaspoon freshly ground black pepper, plus more as needed

¼ teaspoon red pepper flakes, plus more as needed

Bread Base:

8 slices baguette-style whole-grain or multigrain rustic bread, each about ½ inch thick

1 or 2 large garlic cloves, halved

1½ tablespoons extra-virgin olive oil

To Assemble:

1 tablespoon balsamic vinegar

3 tablespoons thinly shredded fresh basil leaves

Preheat the broiler or grill.

Prepare the Tomato Topping: With a sharp knife, halve each tomato vertically, cutting down through the core at its stem end. Cut a v-shaped notch on either side of the core in each half to remove the core. Coarsely cut the tomato halves into ½-inch dice.

In a medium bowl, combine the diced tomatoes, basil, vinegar, oil, salt, black pepper, and red pepper flakes. With a fork or spoon, gently stir the ingredients together until thoroughly combined. Taste and, if necessary, adjust the seasonings. Set this mixture aside at room temperature.

Prepare the Bread Base: Broil or grill the bread slices until golden brown on both sides. With the cut side of a garlic clove half, generously rub one side of each toasted bread slice. With a basting brush, very lightly brush the garlic-rubbed side of each slice with the oil. Place the slices on a serving platter or individual plates with their garlicky sides up.

Assemble the dish: Using a slotted spoon to drain off excess liquid, divide the tomato mixture evenly among the bread slices, mounding it neatly but casually on top of each slice. Drizzle with the balsamic vinegar, garnish with the shredded basil, and serve immediately.

WOLFGANG'S HEALTHY TIPS

→ Look for a longer, narrower whole-grain loaf to get the right size of slices. Or cut slices from a wider loaf, then cut each slice crosswise in half.

→ Just a touch of olive oil, together with some balsamic vinegar, helps to dress the tomato mixture; for an even leaner topping, leave out the oil.

→ As an hors d'oeuvre before a bigger meal, this recipe yields twice as many servings.

Nutrition Facts Per Serving: Calories: 278; Calories from Fat: 90; Total Fat: 10.05g; Saturated Fat: 1.51g; Monounsaturated Fat: 5.74g; Polyunsaturated Fat: 2.80g; Cholesterol: 0mg; Sodium: 272mg; Total Carbohydrate: 41.65g; Dietary Fiber: 5.95g; Sugars: 7.52g; Protein: 7.17g

Steamed Whole Artichokes with Green Goddess Dressing

SERVES 4

A pressure cooker makes it extra fast and easy to steam whole artichokes. If you want to cook them on the stovetop instead, simply put them with the other ingredients in a large nonreactive pot, bring to a boil, and simmer until tender enough for a leaf from the center to pull out easily, 30 to 45 minutes depending on size.

4 large artichokes

1 lemon, cut into 4 center slices each ¼ inch thick, remaining cut ends reserved

1 cup dry white wine

1 cup homemade Vegetable Stock (page 274), good-quality canned low-sodium vegetable broth, or water

½ tablespoon whole coriander seeds

½ tablespoon whole black peppercorns

1 bay leaf

1 cup Low-Fat Green Goddess Dressing (page 279), for serving

First, trim the artichokes: With a sharp serrated knife, cut off the stem ends and a little bit of the base to form flat bottoms. Steadying each artichoke on its side on a cutting board, slice off the top third of the narrower petal end. With kitchen shears, snip off any remaining sharp petal tips. With the reserved lemon ends, gently rub all the cut edges of the artichokes to keep them from oxidizing.

In a pressure cooker, combine the white wine, stock or water, coriander, peppercorns, and bay leaf. Stand the artichokes upright, side by side, inside the cooker. Place a lemon slice on top of each artichoke.

Close the pressure cooker, bring to full pressure, and cook the artichokes for 10 minutes, until tender.

Release the pressure. Remove the artichokes and let them cool slightly. Serve hot, warm, or chilled, accompanied by Low-Fat Green Goddess Dressing in individual ramekins for dipping. Be sure to provide side plates or bowls, or a larger communal one, for discarding petals as eaten (see sidebar).

WOLFGANG'S HEALTHY TIPS

→ Artichokes, along with being low calorie and low fat, satisfy hunger because they take so long to eat. If you've never eaten one before, start by pulling a petal from near the bottom. Dip its fleshy base into the dressing and then scrape off the flesh between your teeth before discarding the petal. Continue, working round and round and up the artichoke. When you get to the fuzzy "choke" at the center, scrape out and discard it with a spoon. Then, with a fork and knife, cut up and eat the artichoke's heart, dipping each bite into the dressing.

→ Low-Fat Green Goddess Dressing in this recipe replaces the traditional melted butter, oil-rich vinaigrette, or mayonnaise usually served with artichokes. If you like, substitute one of the other light dressings found on pages 275–280.

Nutrition Facts Per Serving (including dressing): Calories: 120; Calories from Fat: 10; Total Fat: 1.23g; Saturated Fat: 0.24g; Monounsaturated Fat: 0.76g; Polyunsaturated Fat: 0.22g; Cholesterol: 0mg; Sodium: 220mg; Total Carbohydrate: 17.27g; Dietary Fiber: 6.82g; Sugars: 4.21g; Protein: 6.31g

Red Snapper Crudo with Fresh Salsa

SERVES 4

It's surprising that eating fresh raw seafood seemed a novelty not so long ago, considering how much people everywhere love it today. And that's good news when you look at how healthy this appetizer, inspired by both Mediterranean (*crudo* means "raw" in Italian) and Mexican cooking, can be. Look in Latino markets and well-stocked greengrocers for a fresh banana leaf to line the serving platter, if you like. Keep the snapper fillet well chilled in the refrigerator until serving time.

¼ cup fresh lime juice, from 2 to 3 limes

1 tablespoon fresh lemon juice

1 tablespoon bottled Mexican chile sauce, such as Tapatío or Cholula brands

¼ cup chopped fresh cilantro leaves

½ small red onion, cut into ¼-inch dice

½ to 1 jalapeño, halved, stemmed, seeded, deveined, and cut into ¼-inch dice

1 medium ripe tomato, halved, cored, seeded, and cut into ¼-inch dice

½ medium Japanese cucumber, cut into ¼-inch dice (to yield 1 cup)

Kosher salt

Freshly ground black pepper

1 head butter lettuce, leaves separated, thoroughly rinsed, and patted dry

Banana leaf (optional)

¾ pound fresh sushi-grade red snapper fillet

In a mixing bowl, stir together the lime juice, lemon juice, chile sauce, cilantro, onion, jalapeño, tomato, and cucumber. Season to taste with salt and pepper.

Line a serving platter with the lettuce leaves (or set them aside in a separate bowl if you have a banana leaf to line the platter). Cut the fish fillet crosswise into thin slices and arrange them overlapping on the platter. Spoon the fresh salsa over the fish down the center of the platter. Serve immediately, encouraging guests to transfer portions to individual plates to eat with a fork and knife, or to fold slices of the fish and some salsa inside lettuce leaves to eat out of hand.

WOLFGANG'S HEALTHY TIPS

→ This recipe makes the already light preparation even lighter still by eliminating the oil sometimes used in the salsa.

→ Including some fresh cucumber in the salsa mixture makes the crudo extra refreshing and healthful. Try adding small dice of other fresh salad vegetables, such as celery, bell pepper, or jicama, the crispy, snowy-white root so popular in Mexico.

→ You'll find fish labeled "sushi-grade" in the seafood department of good-quality supermarkets. If yours doesn't offer red snapper, look for yellowtail or ask the fishmonger for another recommendation, such as ahi tuna.

Nutrition Facts Per Serving: Calories: 72; Calories from Fat: 3; Total Fat: 0.43g; Saturated Fat: 0.13g; Monounsaturated Fat: 0.10g; Polyunsaturated Fat: 0.20g; Cholesterol: 10mg; Sodium: 64mg; Total Carbohydrate: 9.55g; Dietary Fiber: 2.21g; Sugars: 4.01g; Protein: 7.98g

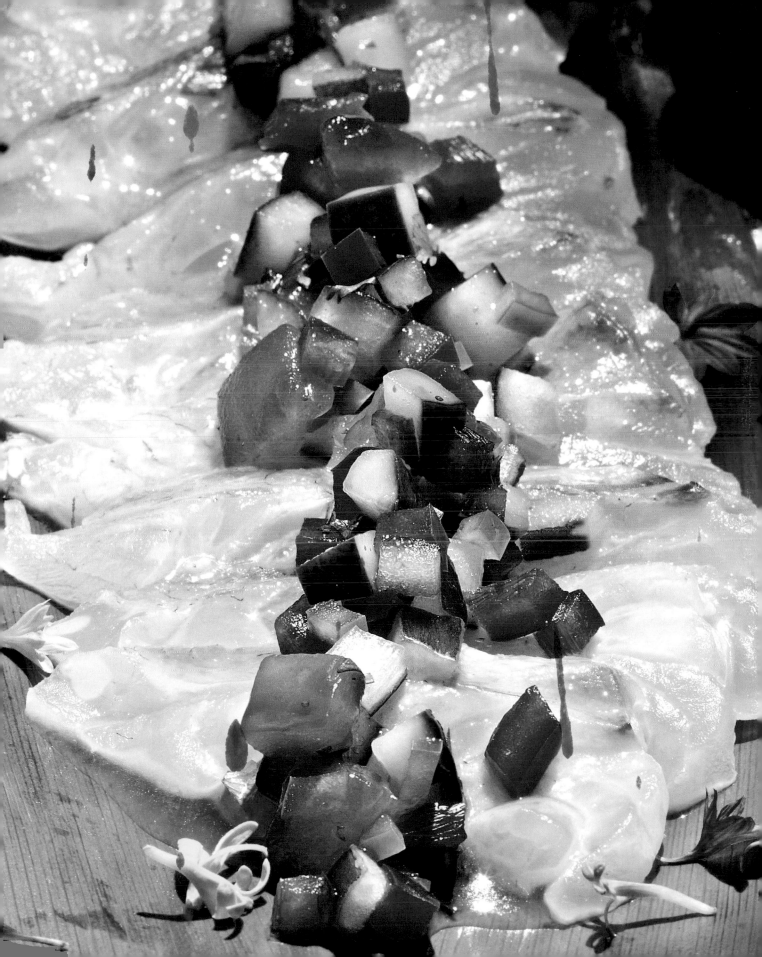

Butterflied Baked Shrimp with Herbed Bread Crumbs and Roasted Garlic Lemon Yogurt Aioli

SERVES 4

I first served a version of this appetizer years ago at Ma Maison in Hollywood. Today, I make it much lighter and even more flavorful by replacing the butter with olive oil and adding a refreshing arugula salad. The quick, easy, and delicious sauce is reminiscent of aioli but replaces the mayonnaise with nonfat yogurt.

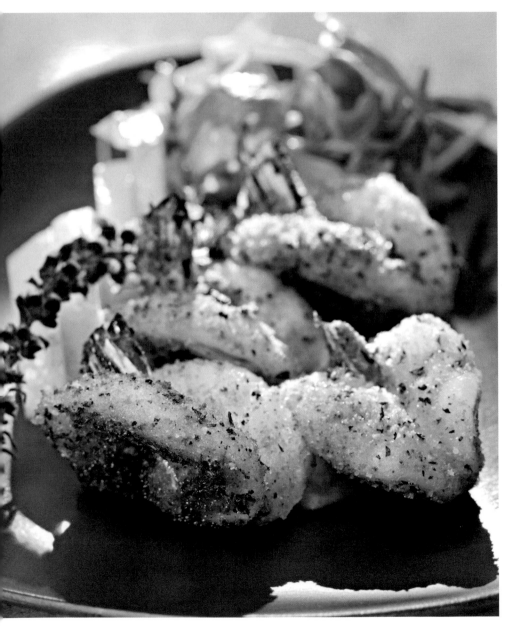

Butterflied Baked Shrimp:

¾ cup fresh bread crumbs

16 fresh extra-large shrimp (about ¾ pound), peeled and deveined, tails left on

Kosher salt

Freshly ground black pepper

1½ tablespoons chopped fresh basil leaves

1½ tablespoons chopped fresh oregano leaves

1½ tablespoons chopped fresh flat-leaf parsley leaves

2 teaspoons chopped fresh thyme leaves

2 teaspoons minced garlic

¼ teaspoon ground Espelette pepper or hot paprika

2 tablespoons extra-virgin olive oil

4 cups packed baby arugula leaves, rinsed well and patted dry

Juice of ½ lemon

Roasted Garlic Lemon Yogurt Aioli:

¾ cup nonfat plain Greek yogurt

4½ tablespoons mashed Roasted Garlic, homemade (page 284) or store-bought

1½ tablespoons fresh lemon juice

½ teaspoon honey

Pinch of cayenne pepper

Pinch of freshly ground black pepper

Kosher salt

To Assemble:

Lemon wedges, for garnish

Preheat the oven to 400°F.

Prepare the Butterflied Baked Shrimp: Evenly spread the bread crumbs on a rimmed baking sheet and toast them in the oven until golden brown, about 10 minutes, watching very carefully to make sure they don't burn. Remove them from the oven, transfer to a mixing bowl, and set aside to cool. Raise the oven temperature to 500°F.

With a small, sharp knife, butterfly each shrimp by slicing along the length of its outer curve where the vein was removed, cutting about half to two-thirds of the way down through it, from just in front of the tail to the head end; be careful not to cut all the way through. Turn the shrimp over and gently make three very shallow slits across the other side, perpendicular to the length of the shrimp, to prevent it from curling during cooking. Lightly season each shrimp on both sides with salt and black pepper. Set aside.

Add the basil, oregano, parsley, thyme, garlic, and Espelette pepper to the bowl with the cooled bread crumbs. Season to taste with salt and black pepper and toss well to combine.

Brush a large ovenproof skillet with 1 tablespoon of the oil to coat the bottom. Press the open side of each shrimp down in the oil in the skillet, and then dredge it in the bread crumb mixture, pressing down firmly so the crumbs stick to and coat the shrimp well. Place all the shrimp, bread crumb side up, in the skillet in a single layer. Bake until the shrimp are just cooked through, turning pink and white, and the bread crumbs are a deep golden brown, about 5 minutes.

While the shrimp are baking, put the arugula leaves in a large bowl, add the remaining 1 tablespoon oil and the lemon juice, season with salt and black pepper, and toss well. Divide the arugula evenly among four serving plates, mounding it on one side.

Prepare the Roasted Garlic Lemon Yogurt Aioli: In a medium bowl, combine the yogurt, Roasted Garlic, lemon juice, honey, cayenne, black pepper, and salt to taste. Stir well.

Assemble the dish: Arrange 4 shrimp, bread crumb side up, on each plate alongside the arugula. Serve immediately with lemon wedges, passing the aioli at the table for guests to help themselves.

WOLFGANG'S HEALTHY TIPS

→ For a special presentation, after butterflying the shrimp and before coating them with the bread crumb mixture, I like to cut a small slit along the center of each shrimp and then curl the fins of the tail end back and push them through the slit to give the shrimp an attractive, compact shape.

→ Although I usually serve this as an appetizer for a dinner party, you can also double the portion size and offer it as a light but very satisfying main course.

→ Make this with crumbs from whole-grain bread, if you like, to add more fiber per serving.

→ The Espelette pepper I call for in the crumb coating is a traditional Basque seasoning, often labeled *piment d'Espelette*. Noticeably spicy but not too hot, it adds extra-satisfying excitement to every bite. Look for it in specialty food stores, well-stocked supermarkets, or online; or substitute hot paprika.

Nutrition Facts Per Serving: Calories: 217; Calories from Fat: 70; Total Fat: 7.83g; Saturated Fat: 1.32g; Monounsaturated Fat: 5.21g; Polyunsaturated Fat: 1.30g; Cholesterol: 36mg; Sodium: 351mg; Total Carbohydrate: 26.14g; Dietary Fiber: 2.20g; Sugars: 6.71g; Protein: 10.71g

Buckwheat Blini with Smoked Whitefish

SERVES 4

This classic appetizer or party hors d'oeuvre—bite-sized pancakes topped with luxurious-tasting smoked fish—can be surprisingly healthy. Try it with whatever kind of smoked fish you prefer.

Blini:

¼ cup all-purpose flour

3 tablespoons buckwheat flour

1 tablespoon minced fresh dill

½ teaspoon kosher salt

½ teaspoon freshly ground black pepper

½ cup good-quality beer, at room temperature

1 tablespoon unsalted butter, melted

2 large egg whites

Nonstick cooking spray

To Assemble:

¼ cup low-fat sour cream

½ cup minced red onion

4 ounces smoked whitefish, skin and all bones removed, flesh flaked by hand

Freshly ground black pepper

Small fresh dill sprigs or 1 tablespoon minced fresh dill, for garnish

Preheat the oven to its lowest setting.

Prepare the Blini: In a medium bowl, combine the all-purpose and buckwheat flours, minced dill, salt, and pepper. Add the beer and melted butter and stir to combine.

In a separate, clean bowl, whisk the egg whites (or beat them with a hand mixer) until they form stiff peaks. With a rubber spatula, gently fold the egg whites into the batter just until incorporated.

Heat a heavy nonstick skillet or a stovetop griddle over medium-high heat (or preheat an electric countertop griddle to medium high). Spray lightly with nonstick cooking spray. With a 2-ounce ladle, pour the batter onto the skillet or griddle to form 2- to 3-inch pancakes, taking care not to overcrowd the cooking surface. Cook the blini until their undersides are browned, 2 to 3 minutes. With a spatula, flip the blini and cook until browned on the other side, 1 to 2 minutes more. Transfer the blini to a baking sheet large enough to hold them in a single layer and keep them warm in the oven while you cook any remaining batter. (You should have 12 to 16 blini in all.)

Assemble the dish: Arrange the blini on a heated serving platter or individual serving plates—or on the still-warm countertop griddle, with its temperature turned to the lowest setting. Spread a thin layer of the sour cream over each blini. Sprinkle with the minced onion and arrange flakes of smoked whitefish on top. Grind a little black pepper over the blini and garnish with dill.

> **WOLFGANG'S HEALTHY TIPS**
>
> → Just a couple of simple changes— egg whites in place of whole eggs in the batter, nonstick cooking spray instead of butter on the griddle, reduced-fat sour cream—bring the calories from fat in this dish within standard healthy-eating guidelines.
>
> → The blini would also be delicious with thin shavings of lean smoked ham or smoked turkey breast on top.

Nutrition Facts Per Serving: Calories: 158; Calories from Fat: 45; Total Fat: 5.02g; Saturated Fat: 3.19g; Monounsaturated Fat: 1.48g; Polyunsaturated Fat: 0.35g; Cholesterol: 21mg; Sodium: 363mg; Total Carbohydrate: 14.18g; Dietary Fiber: 1.19g; Sugars: 1.18g; Protein: 11.37g

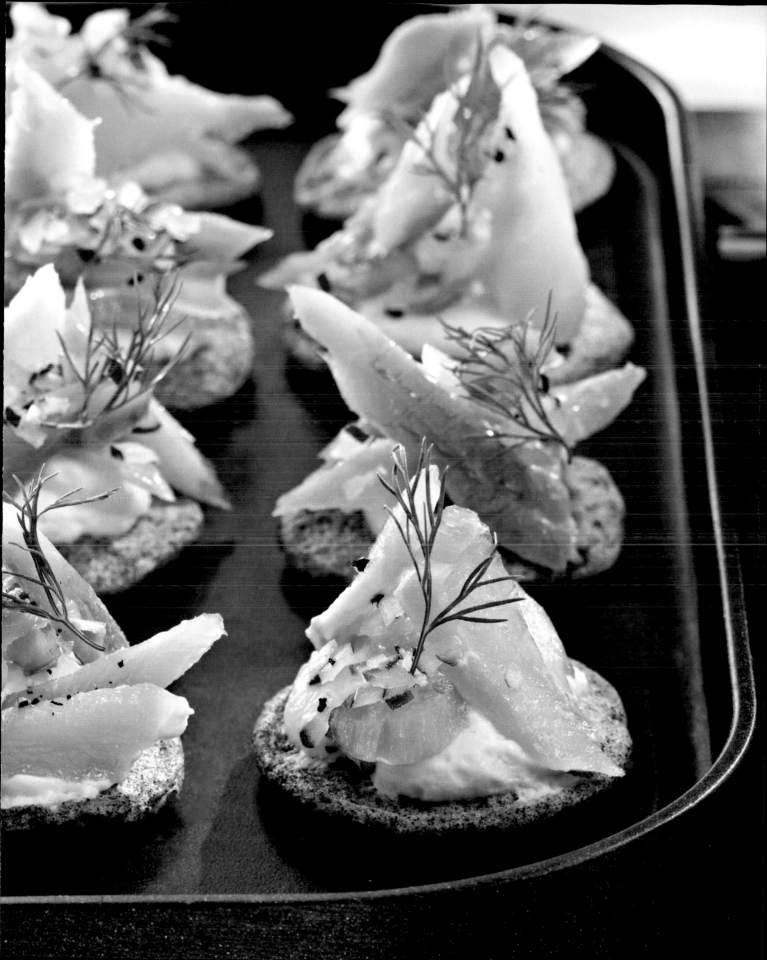

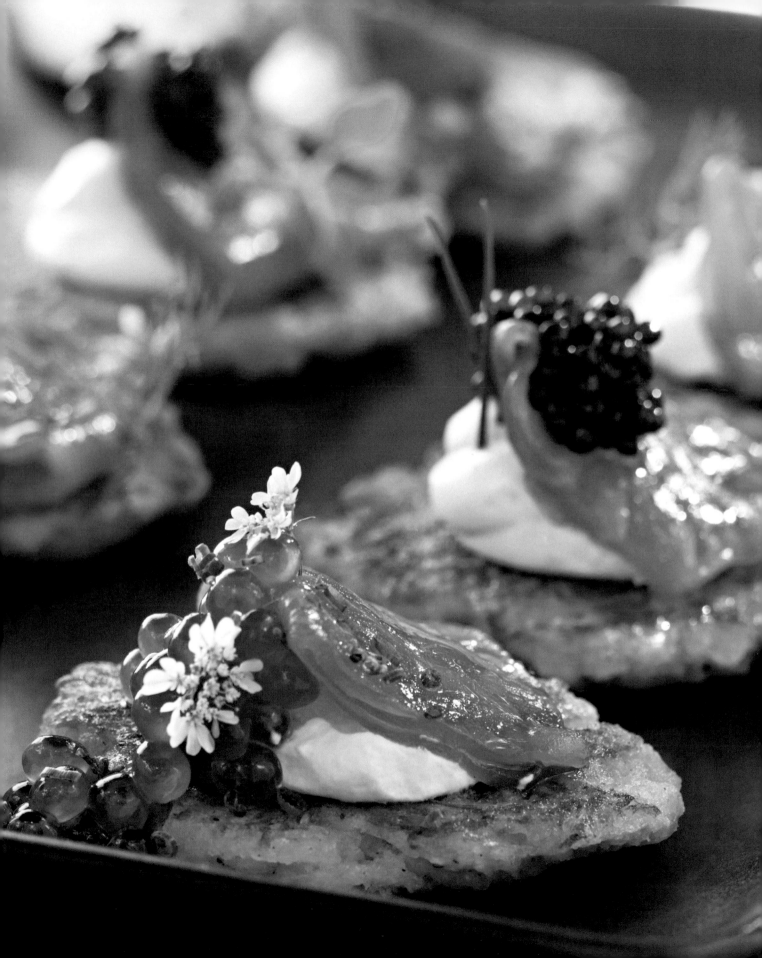

Griddled Potato Pancakes with Smoked Fish

SERVES 4

As most people know them, potato pancakes are thick discs that have been shallow-fried or deep-fried in oil. But you can still get delicious, crispy, and much lighter results by cooking thin potato pancakes on a nonstick griddle. I like to top mine with smoked fish and a little seasoned low-fat sour cream.

1 pound russet baking potatoes

1 small yellow onion

1 large egg, beaten

½ teaspoon baking powder

¾ teaspoon kosher salt, plus more as needed

¼ teaspoon freshly ground black pepper, plus more as needed

Nonstick cooking spray

¼ cup low-fat sour cream

1 tablespoon chopped fresh dill

1 teaspoon fresh lemon juice

½ pound smoked sturgeon, trout, whitefish, or salmon, any skin or bones removed, flesh separated into large flakes or cut into bite-size pieces

¼ cup salmon roe or caviar, for garnish (optional)

1 tablespoon finely chopped fresh chives, for garnish

1 lemon, cut into wedges

Preheat the oven to its lowest setting. Set a baking dish in the oven.

Line a large bowl with a clean kitchen towel.

Using the fine holes of a box grater/shredder (or a food processor fitted with the grating disc), grate the potatoes. Transfer the grated potato to the prepared bowl. Grate in the onion.

Twist the towel around the potato-onion mixture and squeeze out as much liquid as you can. (Alternatively, you can pick up the mixture by handfuls and squeeze out the liquid.)

Transfer the mixture to a clean bowl. Add the egg, baking powder, salt, and pepper and stir with a fork until well blended.

Heat a large nonstick griddle or skillet over medium-high heat. Spray with non-stick cooking spray. With a metal table-spoon, carefully place spoonfuls of the potato mixture on the griddle, spacing them about 1 inch apart and pressing down on the mixture to flatten them to a thickness of no more than ¼ inch.

Cook the pancakes until deep golden-brown and crispy, 3 to 5 minutes per side. If you have more potato mixture left to cook, or don't plan to serve the pancakes right away, transfer the pancakes to the baking dish in the oven to keep warm while you cook the remaining pancakes.

In a small bowl, stir together the sour cream, chopped dill, and lemon juice. Season to taste with salt and pepper.

To serve, transfer the potato pancakes to a warmed platter or individual serving plates. Spoon a little of the sour cream mixture onto each pancake and top with pieces of smoked fish. If you like, add a little salmon roe or caviar. Garnish with chives. Serve immediately, with lemon wedges for squeezing.

WOLFGANG'S HEALTHY TIPS

→ For even lower-fat results, replace the whole egg with an equivalent amount of nonfat real egg product, found in cartons in the refrigerated case at your supermarket.

→ As well as being offered as a sit-down appetizer, they're excellent served as a tray passed or buffet hors d'oeuvre, accompanied by Champagne or other sparkling wine. For such an occasion, I recommend including the optional salmon roe or caviar garnish.

→ I also like to serve these as a brunch dish.

Nutrition Facts Per Serving: Calories: 327; Calories from Fat: 48; Total Fat: 5.34g; Saturated Fat: 2.29g; Monounsaturated Fat: 2.39g; Polyunsaturated Fat: 0.66g; Cholesterol: 96mg; Sodium: 570mg; Total Carbohydrate: 44.04g; Dietary Fiber: 3.38g; Sugars: 2.95g; Protein: 25.29g

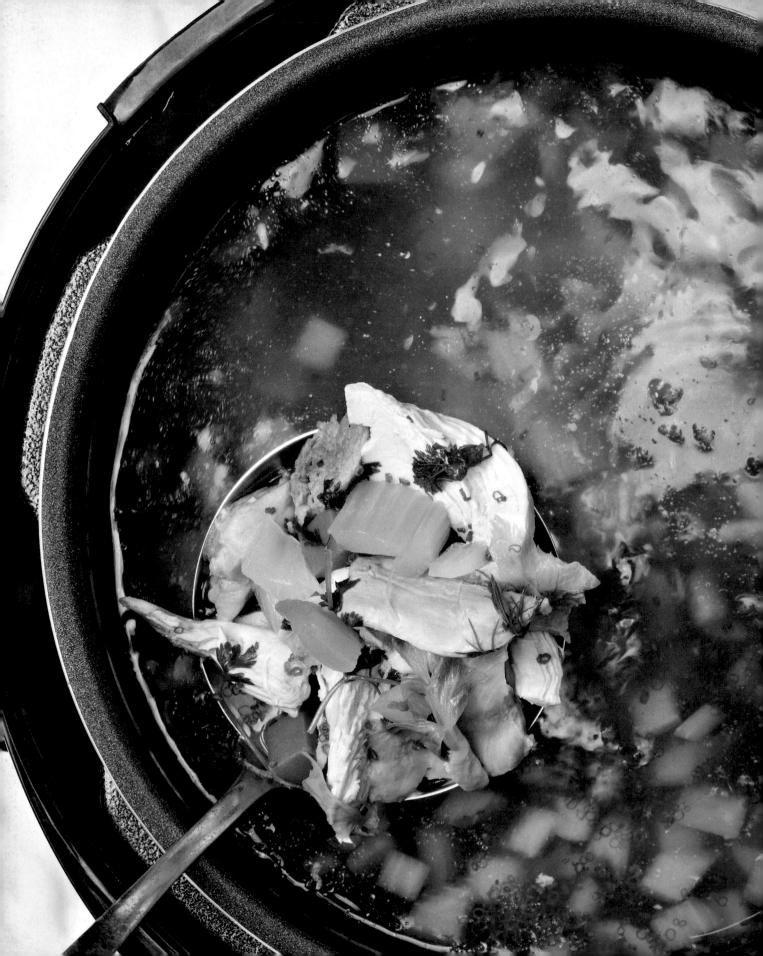

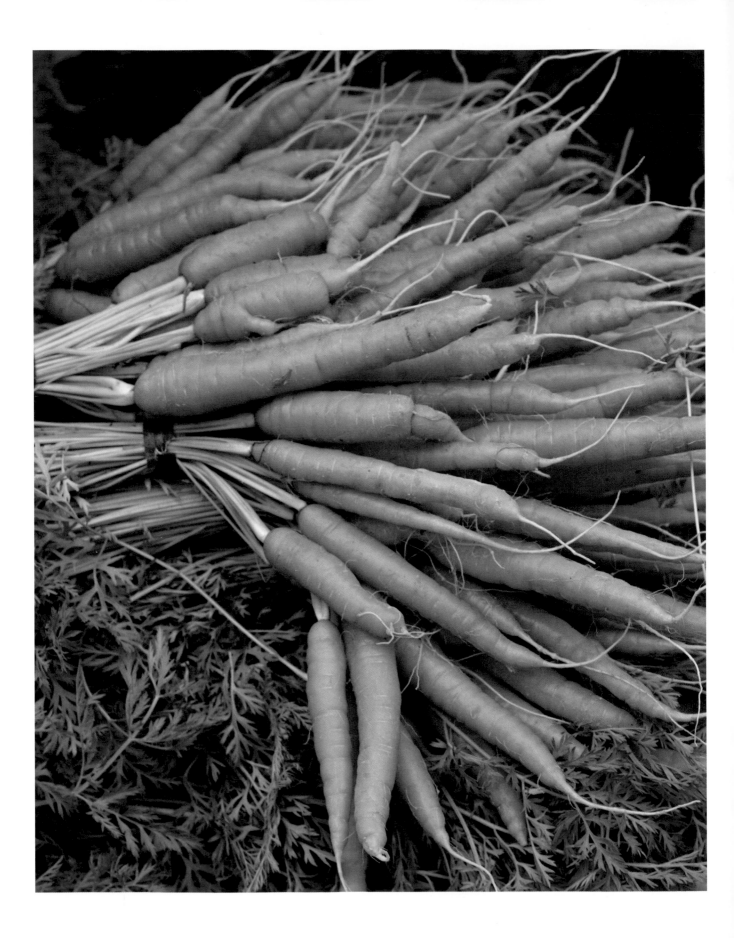

SOUPS

Some studies have shown that people who regularly start meals with soup have an easier time controlling their weight. Why? Not only because a delicious bowl of healthy soup helps to fill you up at the start of a meal but also because it makes you slow down and enjoy it spoonful by spoonful, so your appetite is well on its way to being satisfied before you even reach the next course. In fact, a hearty bowl of soup accompanied by a salad and some crusty bread could become a meal in its own right.

Of course, that benefit means nothing if a soup is packed with butter, cream, and other high-fat ingredients. That's just one reason why I like to make my soups more simply. Fortunately, the techniques used to make good, healthy soups concentrate the flavors of the soups' key ingredients, so there's no real need to fortify their flavors in other ways.

Try the soups in this chapter and you'll see what I mean. Some of them are incredibly simple and quick to make—in fact, a few require virtually no cooking. Others take a little longer, especially those that need gentle simmering to turn dried beans or whole grains tender.

And all of them will help send you away from the table feeling satisfied and happy.

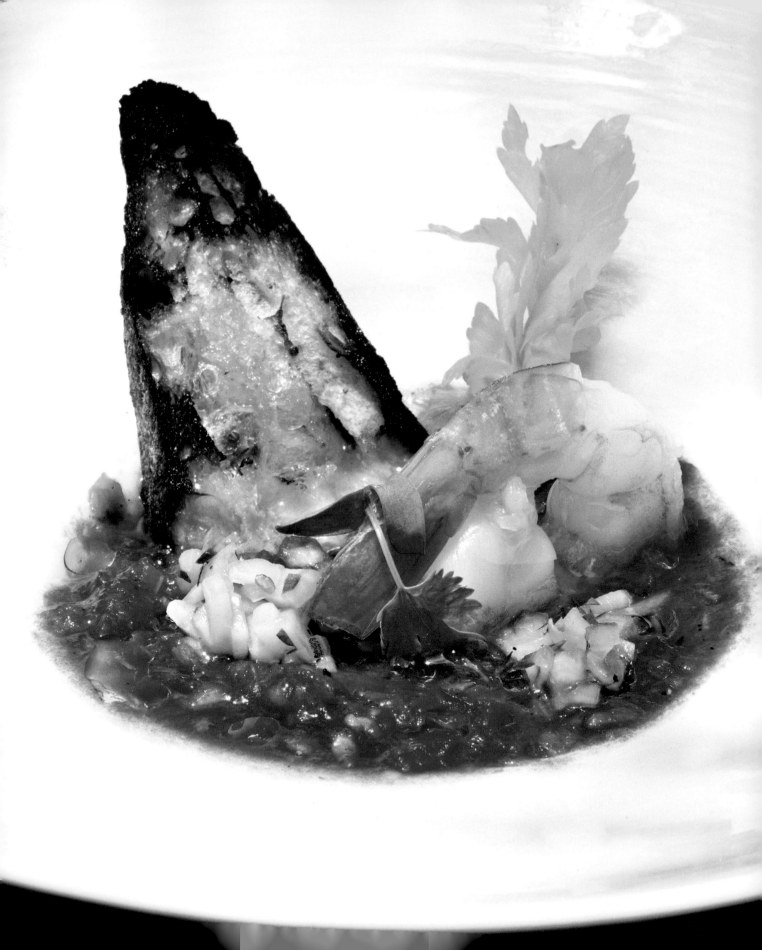

Gazpacho with Cucumber Relish and Shrimp

SERVES 4

The Spanish cold vegetable soup, best in summer when sun-ripened tomatoes are at their sweetest, most flavorful peak, traditionally starts with a base of bread and olive oil. This healthier version is just vegetables, vegetables, and more vegetables—plus chilled cooked shrimp that could help the soup double as a light lunch dish.

Gazpacho:

4 medium sun-ripened tomatoes (about 1¼ pounds), cored and quartered

1 medium English (hothouse) cucumber, peeled, seeded, and cut into 1-inch pieces

1 small red, yellow, or green bell pepper, stemmed, seeded, and quartered

1 stalk celery, cut into 1-inch pieces, leaves reserved for garnish

½ jalapeño, roasted, peeled, stemmed, seeded, deveined (see page 289), and quartered

1 tablespoon sherry vinegar

1 tablespoon sugar

1 cup tomato-based mixed vegetable juice or tomato juice

1 to 2 tablespoons tomato paste

1 teaspoon kosher salt

¼ teaspoon freshly ground black pepper

Cucumber Relish:

½ medium English (hothouse) cucumber, peeled and seeded

2 tablespoons finely chopped red onion

½ tablespoon fresh lime juice

Kosher salt

Freshly ground black pepper

To Assemble:

½ pound cooked, peeled, and deveined medium shrimp

Fresh cilantro leaves, for garnish

4 teaspoons extra-virgin olive oil

Prepare the Gazpacho: Put all the vegetables and the roasted jalapeño in a stainless-steel, glass, or ceramic bowl. Stir in the vinegar and sugar, cover with plastic wrap, and refrigerate for 6 to 8 hours or overnight, stirring once or twice.

In a food processor fitted with the stainless-steel blade, process the cut-up vegetables with the vegetable juice, working in batches if necessary to avoid overcrowding, until the vegetables are pureed but still have some texture. Return the mixture to the bowl.

Stir in 1 tablespoon of the tomato paste along with the salt and pepper. Taste and adjust the seasonings. If the tomato flavor isn't strong enough, stir in more tomato paste. Cover and chill in the refrigerator until ready to serve.

Prepare the Cucumber Relish: Quarter the cucumber lengthwise and thinly slice the quarters crosswise. In a medium bowl, combine the cucumber slices, onion, and lime juice. Season with salt and pepper to taste, and toss to combine.

Assemble the Dish: Ladle the soup into chilled bowls. Top each bowl evenly with the shrimp, cucumber relish, cilantro leaves, and reserved celery leaves. Lightly drizzle each serving with 1 teaspoon of the olive oil.

WOLFGANG'S HEALTHY TIPS

→ The light drizzle of olive oil gives each serving a beautiful fragrance. But feel free to leave it out if you want the soup to be almost fat free.

→ If you're watching your cholesterol intake, leave out the shrimp for a wonderful vegan soup.

→ I like to serve a slice of well-grilled or toasted crusty bread, lightly drizzled with good olive oil, to dunk in each bowl. With few added calories, it helps a simple bowl of soup feel like a complete (but light) meal.

Nutrition Facts Per Serving: Calories: 160; Calories from Fat: 44; Total Fat: 4.96g; Saturated Fat: 0.81g; Monounsaturated Fat: 3.39g; Polyunsaturated Fat: 0.76g, Cholesterol: 71mg; Sodium: 423mg; Total Carbohydrate: 19.63g; Dietary Fiber: 3.71g; Sugars: 12.87g; Protein: 10.85g

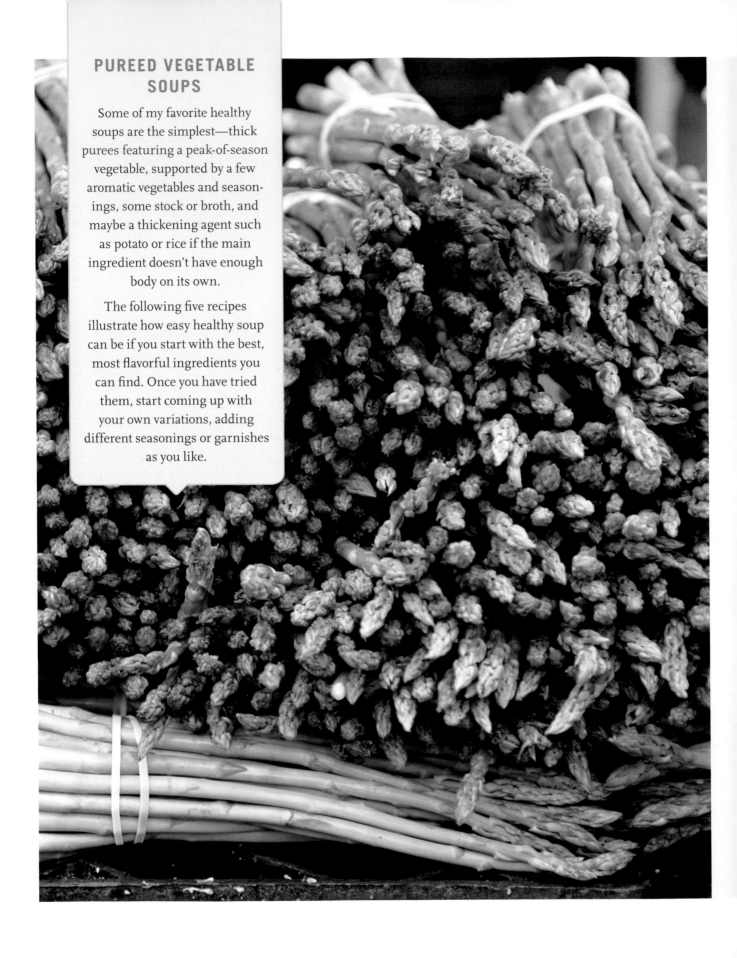

PUREED VEGETABLE SOUPS

Some of my favorite healthy soups are the simplest—thick purees featuring a peak-of-season vegetable, supported by a few aromatic vegetables and seasonings, some stock or broth, and maybe a thickening agent such as potato or rice if the main ingredient doesn't have enough body on its own.

The following five recipes illustrate how easy healthy soup can be if you start with the best, most flavorful ingredients you can find. Once you have tried them, start coming up with your own variations, adding different seasonings or garnishes as you like.

Asparagus Soup

SERVES 8

Beautiful green asparagus stars in this springtime soup. Quickly cooling the pureed soup over ice helps to preserve its bright color, whether you serve the soup chilled or reheat it.

2½ pounds pencil-thin asparagus, trimmed

1 tablespoon extra-virgin olive oil

1 tablespoon unsalted butter

1 medium leek, white and light green parts only, slit lengthwise, thoroughly rinsed, and finely chopped

2 garlic cloves, finely chopped

6 cups homemade Chicken Stock (page 271), Vegetable Stock (page 274), or good-quality canned low-sodium broth

2 tablespoons honey

1 teaspoon kosher salt, plus more as needed

¼ teaspoon freshly ground white pepper, plus more as needed

1 tablespoon fresh lemon juice

1 tablespoon chopped fresh flat-leaf parsley or chives

Cut off and reserve 1½-inch-long tips from 8 of the asparagus spears. Chop the remaining stalks and tips into ¼-inch pieces.

In a large nonreactive saucepan, heat the oil over medium heat. Add the butter. When it foams, add the leek and garlic, reduce the heat to low, and sauté, stirring frequently and taking care not to let them brown, until the leek is translucent and very tender, 7 to 10 minutes.

Stir in the stock, honey, salt, and white pepper. Raise the heat to medium high, bring to a simmer, and continue simmering for 5 minutes.

Stir in the asparagus, reserving the 8 tips, and cook until tender, 3 to 5 minutes.

Remove the pot from the stove. In a food processor or blender, working in batches to avoid overfilling, and following the manufacturer's instructions for working carefully with hot liquids to avoid spattering, puree the soup; or puree the soup in the pot using an immersion blender. In batches, strain the soup through a fine-mesh strainer over a large bowl, pressing it through with a rubber spatula and then discarding any solids left in the strainer.

Transfer the soup to a heatproof bowl set inside a larger bowl partially filled with ice and water. Stir until completely cool. Cover and refrigerate for several hours.

Before serving, bring a small saucepan of salted water to a boil. Meanwhile, fill a small bowl with ice cubes and water. Add the reserved asparagus tips to the boiling water and cook until tender-crisp, 2 to 3 minutes. Drain and immediately immerse the tips in the ice water to stop the cooking process. Drain well.

Stir the lemon juice into the soup. Serve the soup chilled, or reheat it gently in a saucepan over low heat. Taste and adjust the seasonings with more salt and white pepper, as needed, before ladling into chilled or heated bowls. Garnish each bowl with an asparagus tip and a sprinkling of fresh parsley or chives.

WOLFGANG'S HEALTHY TIPS

➜ Once chilled, the soup can also be frozen in individual containers to enjoy hot or cold later.

➜ For a light luncheon main-course soup, garnish each serving with some cold cooked flaked crabmeat or baby shrimp and serve lemon wedges alongside to squeeze over the seafood.

➜ Use vegetable stock and replace the butter with more olive oil for a vegan version.

Nutrition Facts Per Serving: Calories: 102; Calories from Fat: 28; Total Fat: 3.18g; Saturated Fat: 1.23g; Monounsaturated Fat: 1.61g; Polyunsaturated Fat: 0.35g; Cholesterol: 3mg; Sodium: 712mg; Total Carbohydrate: 14.38g; Dietary Fiber: 4.24g; Sugars: 8.76g; Protein: 6.88g

Broccoli Soup

SERVES 8

Fresh broccoli makes a beautiful, delicious, healthy pureed soup. The secret to keeping its color bright green is to avoid overcooking and to chill the soup right away after pureeing. A little fresh lemon juice also helps keep the color a vivid green and sparks up the flavor.

2½ pounds broccoli, trimmed

1 tablespoon extra-virgin olive oil

1 tablespoon unsalted butter

1 medium leek, white and light green parts only, slit lengthwise, thoroughly rinsed, and finely chopped

2 garlic cloves, finely chopped

7 cups homemade Chicken Stock (page 271), Vegetable Stock (page 274), or good-quality canned low-sodium broth

3 tablespoons honey

1 teaspoon kosher salt, plus more as needed

¼ teaspoon freshly ground white pepper, plus more as needed

2 tablespoons fresh lemon juice

1 tablespoon chopped fresh chives

Cut off and reserve 8 small, attractive florets from the broccoli. Chop the remaining broccoli into ¼-inch pieces.

In a nonreactive saucepan, heat the oil over medium heat. Add the butter. When it foams, add the leek and garlic. Reduce the heat to low and sauté, stirring frequently and taking care not to let them brown, until the leek is translucent and very tender, 7 to 10 minutes.

Stir in the stock, honey, salt, and white pepper. Raise the heat to medium high, bring to a simmer, and continue simmering for 5 minutes.

Stir in the broccoli and cook until tender, about 5 minutes.

Remove the pot from the stove. In a food processor or blender, working in batches to avoid overfilling, and following the manufacturer's instructions for working carefully with hot liquids to avoid spattering, puree the soup; or puree the soup in the pot using an immersion blender. In batches, strain the soup through a fine-mesh strainer over a large bowl, pressing it through with a rubber spatula and then discarding any solids left in the strainer.

Transfer the soup to a heatproof bowl set inside a larger bowl partially filled with ice and water. Stir until completely cool. Cover and refrigerate for several hours.

Before serving, bring a small saucepan of salted water to a boil. Meanwhile, fill a small bowl with ice cubes and water.

Add the reserved broccoli florets to the boiling water and cook until tender-crisp, 2 to 3 minutes. Drain and immediately immerse the florets in the ice water.

Stir the lemon juice into the soup. Serve the soup chilled, or reheat gently in a saucepan over low heat. Taste and adjust the seasoning with more salt and white pepper, as needed, before ladling into chilled or heated bowls. Garnish each bowl with a broccoli floret and a sprinkling of the fresh chives.

WOLFGANG'S HEALTHY TIPS

→ It's worth making a soup like this in quantity, ladling whatever you don't eat within a day or two into 1- or 1½-cup freezer containers, ready to reheat in the microwave or on the stovetop.

→ Serve larger portions as the main dish in a light lunch, accompanied by a salad and some whole-grain bread.

→ If you're trying to keep dairy out of your diet, use another tablespoon of olive oil in place of the butter; and use vegetable stock instead of chicken stock for a vegetarian or vegan version.

→ If you eat dairy and want to add more calcium and protein, garnish the soup with a dollop of nonfat plain regular or Greek yogurt.

Nutrition Facts Per Serving: Calories: 122; Calories from Fat: 28; Total Fat: 3.14g; Saturated Fat: 1.21g; Monounsaturated Fat: 1.62g; Polyunsaturated Fat: 0.31g; Cholesterol: 3mg; Sodium: 569mg; Total Carbohydrate: 18.85g; Dietary Fiber: 3.96g; Sugars: 9.88g; Protein: 7.14g

Butternut Squash Soup

SERVES 8

You won't believe how rich and indulgent this low-fat soup looks and tastes, from its deep golden-orange color to its velvety texture and creamy (but cream-free) flavor to the crunchy, tangy-sweet garnish.

1 tablespoon vegetable oil

1 small white onion (about 4 ounces), peeled, trimmed, and finely diced

½ teaspoon ground cinnamon

¼ teaspoon ground ginger

¼ teaspoon freshly grated nutmeg

1 large butternut squash (about 3¾ pounds), halved, peeled, seeded, and cut into 1-inch cubes

1 large acorn squash (about 1¼ pounds), halved, peeled, seeded, and cut into 1-inch cubes

2 tablespoons honey

6 cups homemade Chicken Stock (page 271), Vegetable Stock (page 274), or good-quality canned low-sodium broth

1 sprig fresh rosemary

½ teaspoon kosher salt, plus more as needed

⅛ teaspoon freshly ground white pepper, plus more as needed

1 tablespoon unsalted butter

1 tart-sweet, crisp apple (such as Granny Smith), peeled, cored, and cut into ¼-inch dice

¼ cup dried cranberries

2 teaspoons lemon juice

½ tablespoon dark brown sugar

2 tablespoons coarsely chopped walnuts or pecans, toasted (see page 289)

Heat a pressure cooker with the lid off. Add the oil and the onion and sauté, stirring frequently, just until the onion begins to turn golden, 3 to 5 minutes. Add the cinnamon, ginger, and nutmeg and sauté, stirring, until fragrant, about 1 minute more. Add the cubed squash and the honey and cook, stirring, until the squash begins to soften, about 5 minutes.

Add the stock, rosemary, salt, and white pepper. Secure the lid on the pressure cooker and bring to pressure, following the manufacturer's instructions. Cook under pressure for 8 minutes.

Release the pressure. When fully released, remove the lid. Remove and discard the rosemary. In a food processor or blender, working in batches to avoid overfilling, and following the manufacturer's instructions for working carefully with hot liquids to avoid spattering, puree the soup; or puree the soup in the pressure cooker using an immersion blender. Taste and adjust the seasoning, as needed, with more salt and pepper. Keep warm.

In a medium nonstick skillet, melt the butter over medium heat. Add the apple, cranberries, lemon juice, and sugar and cook, stirring occasionally, until the apple is tender, 5 to 7 minutes. Stir in the walnuts or pecans.

To serve, ladle the soup into individual heated bowls. Spoon some of the apple-cranberry mixture onto the center of each serving.

WOLFGANG'S HEALTHY TIPS

→ Store any extra servings in the refrigerator for up to 3 days, or freeze in individual-portion containers.

→ If you don't plan to serve all the soup at once, make only as much of the garnish as you'll need, since the apples and walnuts will have the best texture freshly prepared. Make more of the garnish when you reheat the refrigerated or frozen soup, or simply garnish with some minced fresh herbs.

→ For a vegan version, use vegetable stock and sauté the apple mixture in a little vegetable oil in place of the butter.

Nutrition Facts Per Serving: Calories: 219; Calories from Fat: 56; Total Fat: 6.25g; Saturated Fat: 1.87g; Monounsaturated Fat: 2.22g; Polyunsaturated Fat: 2.16g; Cholesterol: 9mg; Sodium: 281mg; Total Carbohydrate: 36.85g; Dietary Fiber: 4.29g; Sugars: 16.61g; Protein: 6.67g

Springtime Pea Soup

SERVES 8

To those who have only had wintertime split-pea soup made from the dried legumes, a bright green bowl of soup made from fresh (or frozen) peas is a revelation. It has the sweet, subtle taste of springtime, wonderfully light and flavorful.

2 tablespoons extra-virgin olive oil

1⅓ cups finely chopped white onion

8 cups homemade Chicken Stock (page 271), Vegetable Stock (page 274), or good-quality canned low-sodium broth

2 teaspoons kosher salt, plus more as needed

½ teaspoon freshly ground white pepper, plus more as needed

2½ tablespoons honey

3⅓ pounds shelled fresh English peas or defrosted frozen peas (about 9 cups)

1 tablespoon lemon juice

In a nonreactive pot, heat the olive oil over medium heat. Add the onion, reduce the heat to low, and cook, stirring occasionally, until the onion is translucent and very tender but not yet turning brown, 5 to 7 minutes.

Add the stock, salt, white pepper, and honey and bring to a boil. Boil for 5 minutes. Raise the heat to high, add the peas and boil rapidly until the peas are tender, about 2 minutes. With a slotted spoon, remove a couple of tablespoons of peas to reserve as a garnish

Remove the pot from the heat. In a food processor or blender, working in batches to avoid overfilling, and following the manufacturer's instructions for working carefully with hot liquids to avoid spattering, puree the soup; or puree the soup in the pot using an immersion blender. In batches, strain the soup through a fine-mesh strainer over a large bowl, pressing it through with a rubber spatula and then discarding any solids left in the strainer. Stir in the lemon juice. Taste and season with additional salt and white pepper, if necessary. Return the soup to the pan and gently reheat. Serve immediately, garnished with the reserved peas.

> WOLFGANG'S HEALTHY TIPS
>
> → Do not let the pureed soup sit on the stovetop for too long, or it will slowly discolor. If you do not plan on serving it right away, place the pot in an ice bath to cool down the soup as quickly as possible to retain the color. Just before serving, reheat the soup and add the lemon juice, or serve cold.
>
> → Feel free to freeze leftover soup in individual-serving containers to reheat and serve warm or thaw and serve cold.
>
> → Frozen peas are a rarity among vegetables in that the frozen variety can taste almost as good as freshly cooked in certain recipes.
>
> → For a light main-course lunchtime soup, garnish big bowlfuls with some cooked fresh crabmeat. Garnish each bowl with a spoonful of nonfat plain yogurt seasoned to taste with lemon juice and zest, chopped fresh basil and mint, and a little salt and freshly ground white pepper.
>
> → Make the soup with vegetable stock for a vegan version.

Nutrition Facts Per Serving: Calories: 236; Calories from Fat: 46; Total Fat: 5.12g; Saturated Fat: 0.98g; Monounsaturated Fat: 3.22g; Polyunsaturated Fat: 0.92g; Cholesterol: 3mg; Sodium: 250mg; Total Carbohydrate: 35.93g; Dietary Fiber: 8.83g; Sugars: 17.71g; Protein: 12.20g

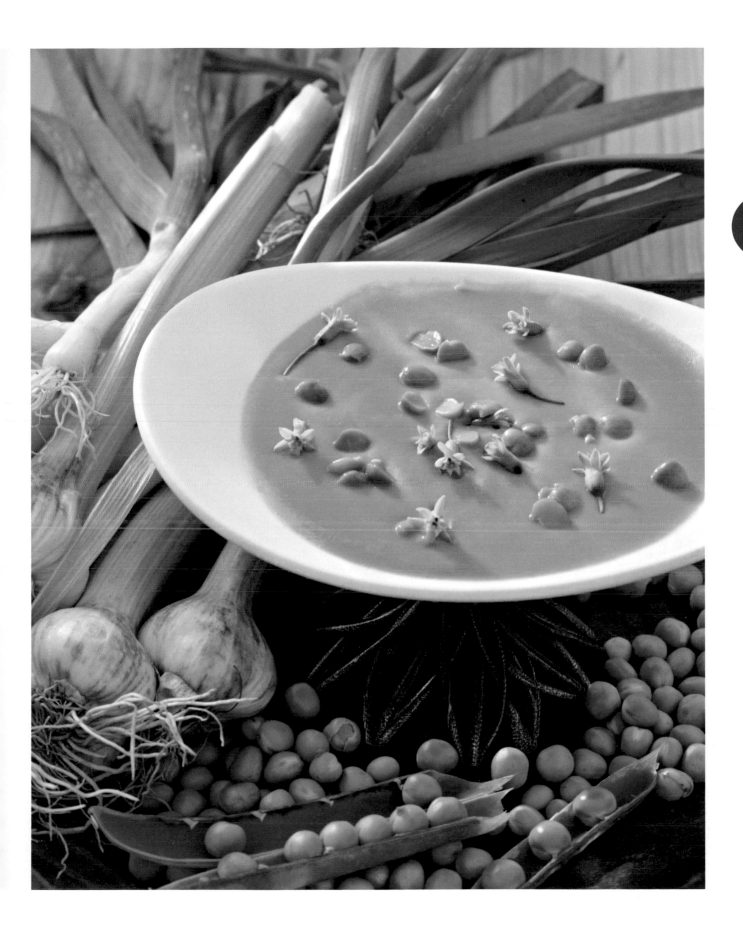

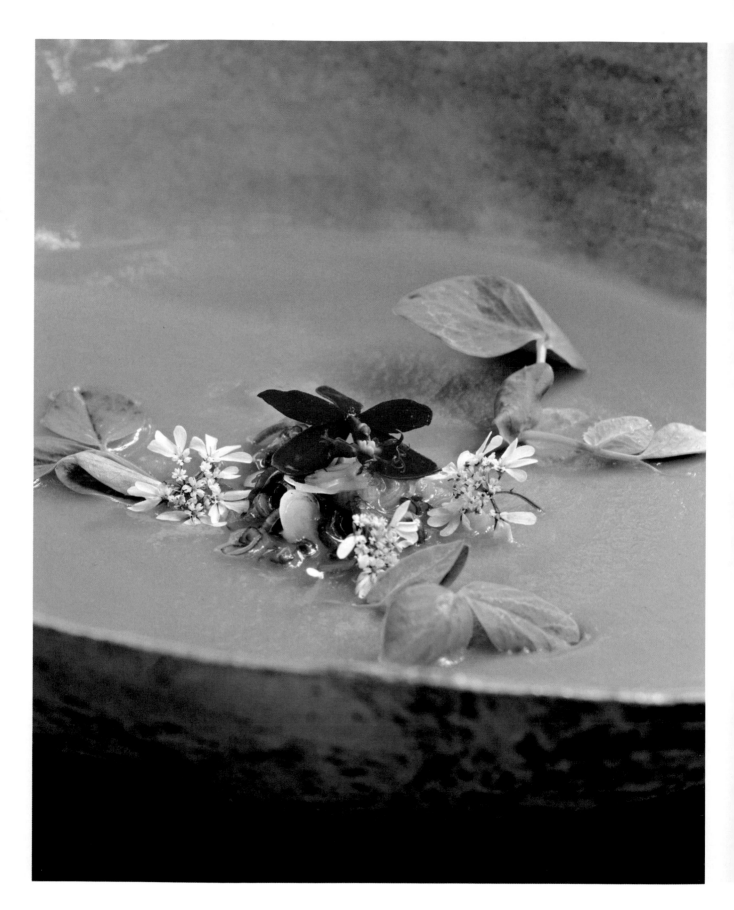

Carrot and Ginger Soup

SERVES 8

This low-fat soup tastes especially rich thanks to the body that results from slowly cooking and then pureeing the fresh carrots. I love the spicy-sweet flavor fresh ginger adds, but you could cut the amount in half if you prefer.

¼ cup peanut oil or vegetable oil

1 pound orange carrots, cut crosswise into ¼-inch-thick slices

1 pound yellow carrots (or additional orange carrots), cut crosswise into ¼-inch-thick slices

1 pound white carrots (or additional orange carrots), cut crosswise into ¼-inch-thick slices

1 tablespoon minced garlic

1 tablespoon minced fresh ginger

2 tablespoons minced scallion, white part only, green parts reserved for garnish

1 tablespoon kosher salt, plus more as needed

½ teaspoon freshly ground white pepper, plus more as needed

½ teaspoon turmeric

7 tablespoons honey, plus more as needed

12 cups homemade Vegetable Stock (page 274) or good-quality canned low-sodium vegetable broth, plus more as needed

Juice of ½ lemon

3 tablespoons thinly sliced scallion greens (reserve from above) or micro pea tendrils and edible flowers

In a stockpot, heat the oil over medium-high heat. Add the sliced carrots and sauté, stirring frequently, until they start to caramelize around the edges, 7 to 10 minutes. Stir in the garlic, ginger, and scallion whites and sauté, stirring frequently, just until glossy and fragrant but not yet browned, 1 to 2 minutes.

Add the salt, white pepper, turmeric, and honey and sauté, stirring constantly, for 2 minutes. Add the stock and bring to a boil. Reduce the heat to maintain a steady simmer and cook until the carrots are very tender, about 40 minutes.

Remove the pot from the heat. In a food processor or blender, working in batches to avoid overfilling, and following the manufacturer's instructions for working carefully with hot liquids to avoid spattering, puree the soup; or puree the soup in the pot using an immersion blender. In batches, strain the soup through a fine-mesh strainer over a large bowl, pressing it through with a rubber spatula and then discarding any solids left in the strainer.

Rinse out and dry the stockpot, return the soup to it, and stir in the lemon juice. If the soup seems too thick, stir in additional stock to achieve a thick and creamy, but still fluid, consistency. Taste and adjust the seasoning, if necessary, with more salt, white pepper, and honey.

To serve, ladle the soup into heated bowls. Garnish with scallion greens or pea tendrils.

WOLFGANG'S HEALTHY TIPS

→ For the finest, fullest flavor, buy the best carrots, preferably organic, that you can find at your local farmers' market.

→ I find that the salt in this recipe helps balance the sweetness of the carrots and honey. But if you're watching your sodium intake, use less salt than what is called for in the ingredient list, and then season (or not) to taste.

→ Serve the soup in little espresso or sake cups as an hors d'oeuvre for a winter party. Or offer it as a cold soup when the weather is hot.

→ Store individual portions in freezer containers to have ready to microwave for a quick, healthy first course at dinner, or to enjoy with crusty whole-grain bread and a salad for a complete lunch.

Nutrition Facts Per Serving: Calories: 187; Calories from Fat: 31; Total Fat: 3.53g; Saturated Fat: 0.65g; Monounsaturated Fat: 1.59g; Polyunsaturated Fat: 1.30g; Cholesterol: 0mg; Sodium: 1,825mg; Total Carbohydrate: 34.52g; Dietary Fiber: 5.16g; Sugars: 24.41g; Protein: 6.77g

My Mother's Garden Vegetable Soup

SERVES 4

From the end of June to October, my mother would walk out the kitchen door of my childhood home in the Austrian town of Sankt Veit, at 10 in the morning, into the garden. By 12:30 we would have fresh vegetable soup for lunch. Her recipe is still one of my favorites—and it's so healthy!

1 small leek, white parts only, split lengthwise, thoroughly washed with cold running water, and patted dry

½ medium onion

1 stalk celery

1 medium carrot

1 medium potato

1 medium zucchini

12 green beans, trimmed

3 tablespoons extra-virgin olive oil

4 cups homemade Chicken Stock (page 271), Beef Stock (page 272), Vegetable Stock (page 274), or good-quality canned low-sodium broth

Kosher salt

2 ripe tomatoes, peeled, seeded (see page 288), and coarsely chopped

10 pieces sun-dried tomato, thoroughly drained

10 fresh basil leaves

2 medium garlic cloves

Freshly ground black pepper

Cut the leeks, onion, celery, carrot, potato, zucchini, and green beans into ¼-inch dice, keeping them all separate from one another.

In a large saucepan, combine 1½ tablespoons of the olive oil with 1½ tablespoons water. Add the leek and onion and sauté over medium-low heat until all the water has evaporated and the vegetables are tender but not yet beginning to brown, about 5 minutes.

Add the celery, carrot, potato, stock, and salt to taste. Raise the heat to high and bring to a boil. Reduce the heat to maintain a gentle boil and cook, uncovered, for 30 minutes.

In a food processor fitted with the metal blade, combine the chopped tomatoes, sun-dried tomatoes, basil, garlic, and remaining 1½ tablespoons olive oil. Pulse the machine until the mixture is pureed. Transfer to a sauceboat or bowl and set aside.

About 5 minutes before the soup is done, stir the diced zucchini and green beans into the pan and continue cooking until all the vegetables are tender.

Season the soup with salt and pepper to taste. Stir the pureed tomato mixture into the soup or pass it separately for each person to add to taste. Ladle the soup into a tureen or individual bowls and serve.

WOLFGANG'S HEALTHY TIPS

→ Unlike the other recipes in this chapter, this one yields just four servings, because it's so quick to make and its flavors are at their very best enjoyed fresh.

→ With its big, fresh flavors, sometimes a generous bowl of this healthy soup, accompanied by some crusty bread, is all the lunch I need. I also like it to start a casual dinner.

→ This recipe was just a starting point for my mother, the basis for soup that could change every day depending on what she harvested from the garden. You can treat your farmers' market, supermarket, or home garden the same way. I especially liked it when my mother added chopped wild mushrooms that we found in the nearby forest; you could use any of the many varieties of mushroom now sold in markets.

Nutrition Facts Per Serving: Calories: 171; Calories from Fat: 56; Total Fat: 6.26g; Saturated Fat: 0.96g; Monounsaturated Fat: 4.39g; Polyunsaturated Fat: 0.92g; Cholesterol: 0mg; Sodium: 608mg; Total Carbohydrate: 23.72g; Dietary Fiber: 4.36g; Sugars: 7.53g; Protein: 7.11g

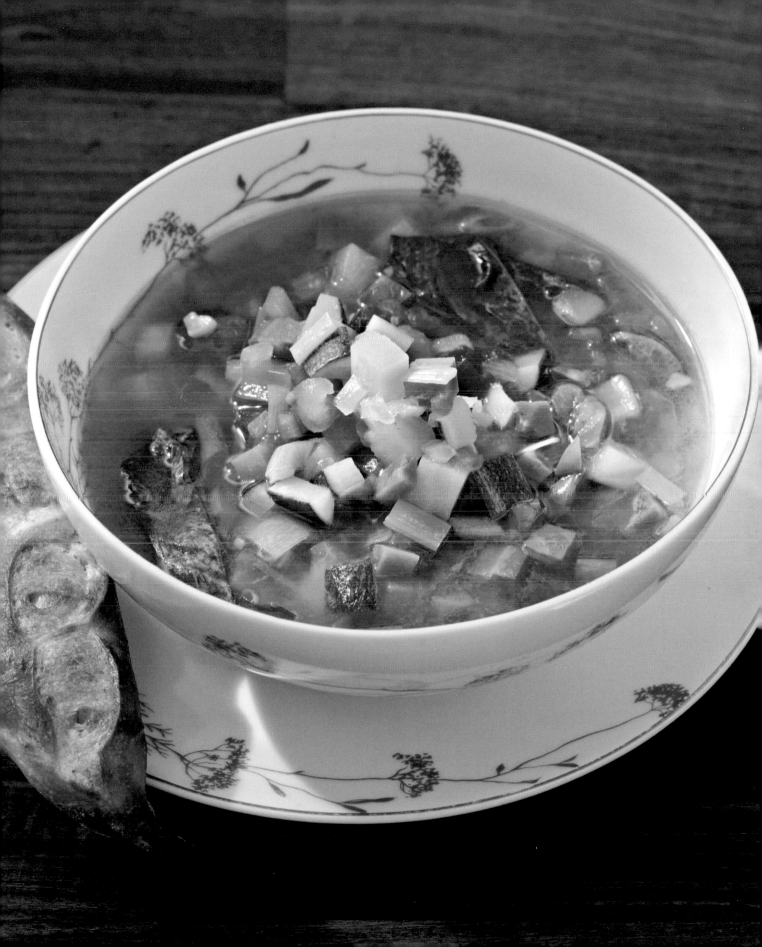

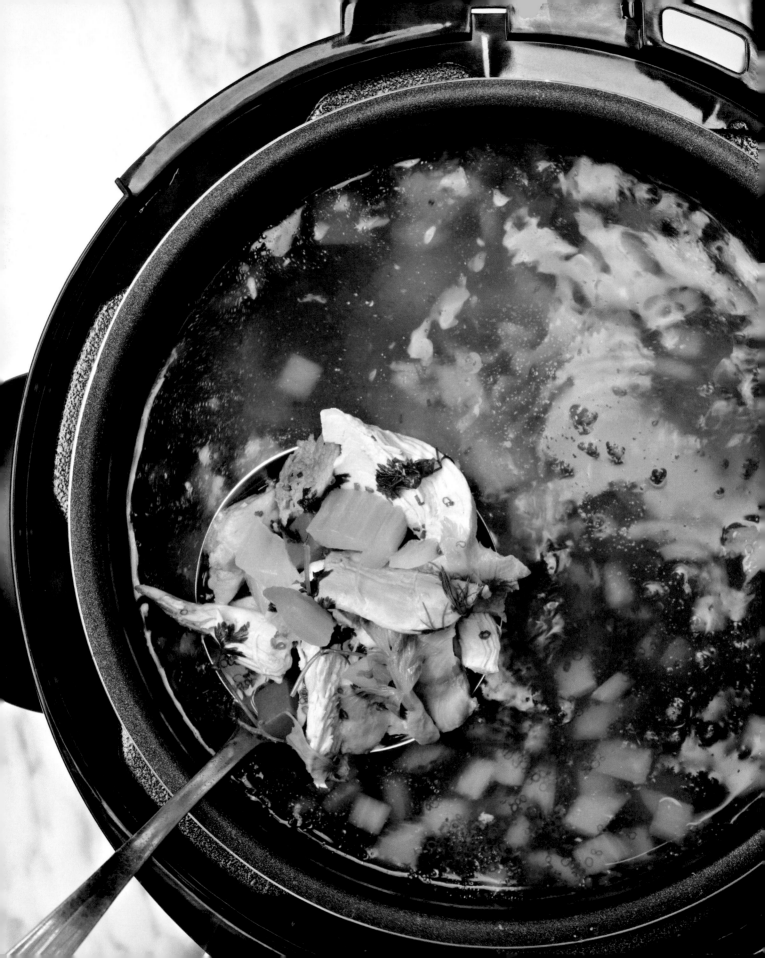

Pressure Cooker Chicken Soup with Parsnips, Carrots, Celery, and Leeks

SERVES 8

You will be amazed by how beautifully flavorful and clear chicken soup broth is when you make it in a pressure cooker. This is definitely a bowl of chicken soup you want to savor slowly, spoonful by spoonful.

1½ pounds skinless chicken pieces

10 cups homemade Chicken Stock (page 271) or good-quality canned low-sodium chicken broth

1 tablespoon kosher salt, plus more as needed

Freshly ground black pepper

3 medium carrots, cut into ½-inch dice

2 medium parsnips, cut into ½-inch dice

2 celery stalks, cut into ½-inch dice

1 medium onion, cut into ½-inch dice

1 large leek, white and light green parts only, quartered lengthwise, thoroughly rinsed under cold running water, and cut into ½-inch pieces

2 tablespoons mixed chopped fresh flat-leaf parsley, fresh chervil leaves, and fresh chives, for garnish

1 tablespoon chopped fresh dill, for garnish

In a pressure cooker, combine the chicken, stock, salt, and pepper to taste. Attach the lid and bring to full pressure, and then cook under pressure for 20 minutes.

Release the pressure. Remove the chicken pieces, leaving the stock in the pressure cooker, and set them aside on a plate or in a bowl to cool slightly.

Add the carrots, parsnips, celery, onion, and leek to the pressure cooker. Attach the lid, bring to full pressure, and then cook under pressure for 5 minutes.

When the chicken pieces are just cool enough to handle, remove and discard the bones and any fat and cartilage. Cut the meat into bite-size pieces. As soon as the vegetables are done, release the pressure, and stir the chicken into the soup. Taste the broth and adjust the seasoning, if necessary.

Ladle the soup into individual heated bowls or soup plates. Garnish each bowl with some of the mixed fresh herbs and dill.

WOLFGANG'S HEALTHY TIPS

→ I like to make this with dark meat from thighs or legs, but you can also use chicken breasts.

→ If you have any chicken bones left over from a roast chicken, or from boning chicken meat before cooking it, save them in a sealable plastic freezer bag and add them to the pressure cooker along with the chicken pieces to contribute even more flavor.

→ Freeze any extra soup in individual-portion containers to reheat for future meals.

→ If you'd like more of a main course, cook some brown rice, farro, quinoa, or another whole grain separately and scoop some into each bowl before ladling in the soup.

→ I find that the flavor of chicken soup benefits greatly from being cooked with some salt. But if you're trying to reduce your sodium intake, by all means cut back on the amount I include here.

Nutrition Facts Per Serving: Calories: 181; Calories from Fat: 38; Total Fat: 4.23g; Saturated Fat: 1.23g; Monounsaturated Fat: 2.07g; Polyunsaturated Fat: 0.93g; Cholesterol: 25mg; Sodium: 581mg; Total Carbohydrate: 21.98g; Dietary Fiber: 2.90g; Sugars: 8.63g; Protein: 12.69g

Tortilla Soup

SERVES 8

Traditional tortilla soups can include rich ingredients that health-conscious eaters shy away from. That won't happen with this version, which gets its rich texture and flavor from pureed fresh corn and corn tortillas and is satisfyingly but sensibly garnished.

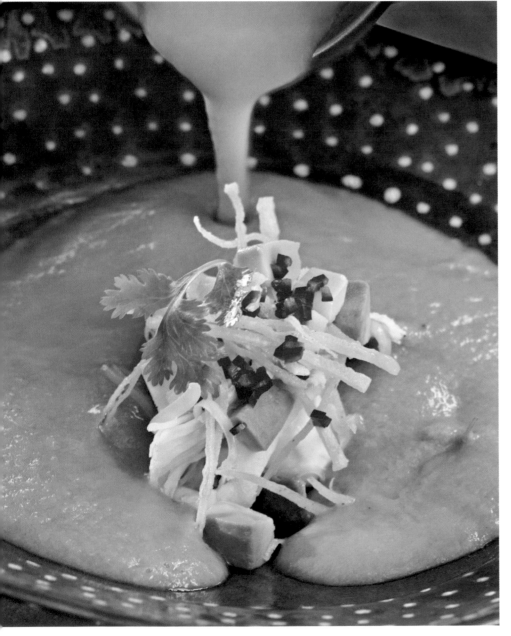

Soup:

2 ears fresh sweet corn

4 large garlic cloves

1 small onion (about 2 ounces), quartered

1 small jalapeño, halved, stemmed, seeded, and deveined

2 tablespoons corn oil

2 corn tortillas, cut into 1-inch squares

2 large ripe tomatoes (about 1 pound), peeled, seeded (see page 288), and coarsely chopped

¼ cup tomato paste

2 teaspoons ground cumin

8 cups homemade Chicken Stock (page 271) or good-quality canned low-sodium chicken broth, heated

Juice of 1 lime

Kosher salt

Freshly ground black pepper

To Assemble:

2 corn tortillas

½ ripe Hass avocado, pitted, peeled, and diced

1 large cooked chicken breast half, skin and bones removed, meat shredded

1 fresh red jalapeño or Fresno chile, halved, stemmed, seeded, deveined, and finely diced (optional)

¼ cup chopped fresh cilantro leaves

½ cup reduced-fat sour cream or ½ cup shredded reduced-fat cheddar

Cut the corn kernels off the cobs: Hold an ear of corn at an angle with one end resting securely on a cutting board. Using a large, sharp knife, carefully cut down along the cob to remove the kernels. Repeat with the other ear of corn. Reserve the cobs.

Working in batches if necessary, in a food processor fitted with the stainless-steel blade, combine the corn, garlic, onion, and jalapeño. Pulse the machine until the mixture is coarsely chopped, stopping once or twice to scrape down the bowl with a rubber spatula. Transfer the mixture to a large bowl and set aside.

In a large stockpot, heat the oil over medium-high heat. Add the tortilla squares, reduce the heat slightly, and cook, stirring occasionally, until they are slightly crisp and beginning to turn golden, 5 to 7 minutes. Add the chopped vegetables and sauté, stirring, just until the vegetables are fragrant and thoroughly blended with the tortillas, 2 to 3 minutes.

Add the tomatoes, tomato paste, and cumin and sauté, stirring occasionally, until the tomatoes have softened and the mixture has begun to thicken, 5 to 7 minutes more. Stir in the stock and add the corncobs. Raise the heat to high, bring the liquid to a boil, and then reduce the heat to maintain a brisk simmer. Simmer, stirring occasionally, until the liquid has reduced by about a third, about 30 minutes.

While the soup is simmering, preheat the oven or a toaster oven to 350°F. Cut the tortillas into thin strips and arrange them on a small baking tray. Bake until the strips are crisp and golden brown, 10 to 15 minutes.

With a slotted spoon, remove the corncobs from the pot and discard them. In a food processor or blender, working in batches to avoid overfilling, and following the manufacturer's instructions for working carefully with hot liquids to avoid spattering, puree the soup; or puree the soup in the pot using an immersion blender. Return the puree to the pot, stir in the lime juice, and season with salt and pepper.

Assemble the dish: Arrange the tortillas, avocado, chicken, chile (if using), and cilantro in the centers of heated serving bowls. Ladle in the hot soup. Pass sour cream or cheese for guests to garnish their bowls to taste.

WOLFGANG'S HEALTHY TIPS

→ Make a lunchtime meal of this if you like, serving larger portions and a simple salad on the side.

→ If you won't be eating all the soup right away, store it in the refrigerator for up to 3 days, or freeze it in individual-serving containers. But be sure to prepare the garnishes fresh before serving.

→ For a vegan version, use vegetable broth instead of chicken broth and leave out the chicken, sour cream, and cheese. If you like, add some cubes of firm tofu and non-dairy sour cream, and soy- or nut-based cheese substitutes.

Nutrition Facts Per Serving: Calories: 217; Calories from Fat: 67; Total Fat: 7.55g; Saturated Fat: 1.96g; Monounsaturated Fat: 3.99g; Polyunsaturated Fat: 1.60g; Cholesterol: 28mg; Sodium: 455mg; Total Carbohydrate: 22.32g; Dietary Fiber: 2.57g; Sugars: 8.01g; Protein: 14.91g

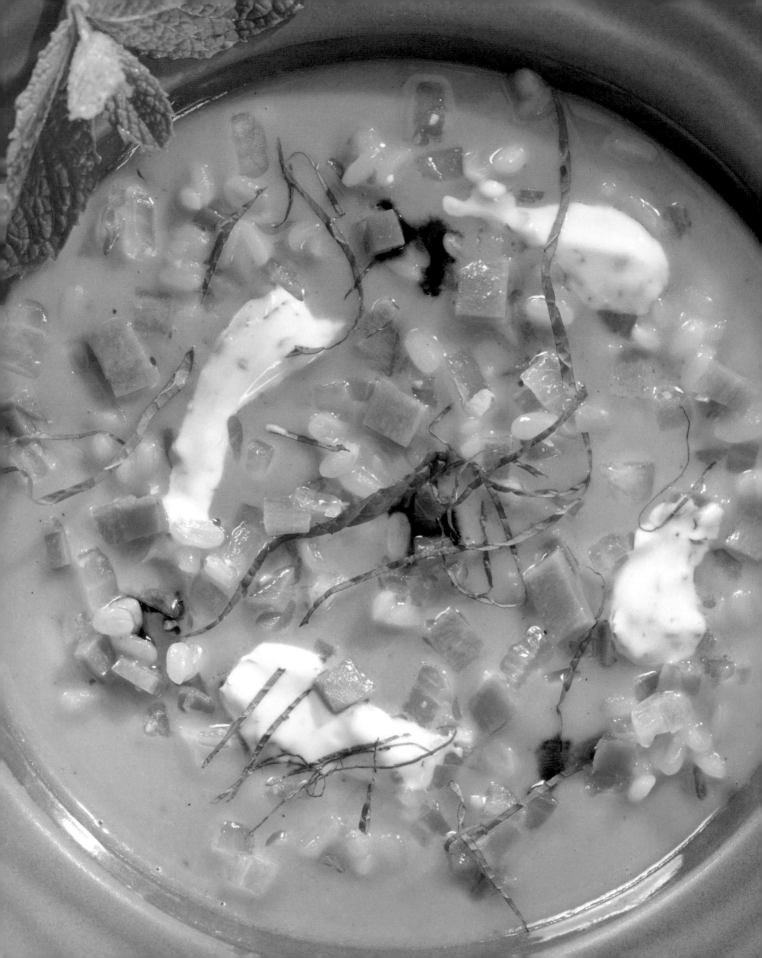

Curried Lentil Soup with Mint-Lemon Yogurt

SERVES 8

In well under an hour, you can have a delicious, healthy soup ready to serve to your family and friends. The flavors and textures are robust and satisfying, perfect for dinner or lunch on a cold day. Have fun changing the seasonings to suit your tastes.

Curried Lentil Soup:

½ celery stalk

1 sprig fresh flat-leaf parsley

1 sprig fresh thyme

3 tablespoons extra-virgin olive oil

1½ cups chopped yellow onion (from about 1 medium onion)

½ cup chopped carrot (from about 1 medium carrot)

5 garlic cloves, minced

2 tablespoons homemade Curry Powder (page 285) or store-bought mild to medium-hot curry powder

1 pound golden lentils (about 2⅓ cups), carefully sorted to remove any stones or other debris, rinsed

10 cups homemade Chicken Stock (page 271), Vegetable Stock (page 274), or good-quality canned low-sodium broth, heated

Kosher salt

Freshly ground black pepper

Juice of ½ lemon

Mint-Lemon Yogurt:

1 cup nonfat plain yogurt

1 tablespoon honey

1 tablespoon chopped fresh mint leaves

½ teaspoon grated lemon zest

To Assemble:

8 teaspoons balsamic vinegar

8 fresh mint leaves, cut into thin julienne strips, plus 8 fresh mint sprigs

Prepare the Curried Lentil Soup: Tie the celery, parsley, and thyme together with kitchen twine to make a bouquet garni.

In a large saucepan, heat the oil over high heat. Add the onion, carrot, garlic, and bouquet garni and sauté, stirring frequently, until the onions are glossy and transparent, about 5 minutes. Stir in the Curry Powder and sauté until fragrant, about 30 seconds. Stir in the lentils and stock, season lightly with salt and pepper, and bring to a boil. Reduce the heat and simmer, skimming any foam that rises to the top as necessary, until the lentils are tender, 25 to 30 minutes.

Remove and discard the bouquet garni. With a ladle, transfer two-thirds of the soup to a blender. Cover the blender with a dry kitchen towel and, leaving the lid slightly ajar to avoid spattering, puree the soup. Stir the puree back into the pan, stir in the lemon juice, and adjust the seasoning to taste. Set the pan over medium-low heat and gently reheat the soup.

Prepare the Mint-Lemon Yogurt: In a small serving bowl, stir together the yogurt, honey, mint, and lemon zest.

Assemble the dish: Ladle the soup into heated bowls. Add a dollop of the yogurt mixture to each portion. Drizzle each with 1 teaspoon of the balsamic vinegar, garnish with mint julienne and sprigs, and serve immediately.

WOLFGANG'S HEALTHY TIPS

→ Instead of serving this as a first course, make it the centerpiece of a light but satisfying meal by adding your favorite salad and warm, crusty whole-grain bread.

→ Nonfat yogurt used for the garnish adds a surprising sense of richness to each serving, and a light drizzle of balsamic vinegar really sparks up the flavor.

→ Make this a completely vegetarian recipe, if you like, by substituting vegetable stock for the chicken stock, and go vegan by using non-dairy yogurt or sour cream, too. No one will believe it's meat-free, because the soup is so hearty and filling.

→ If you won't be eating all the soup right away, store it in the refrigerator for up to 3 days, or freeze it in individual-serving containers. But be sure to prepare the garnishes fresh before serving.

Nutrition Facts Per Serving: Calories: 316; Calories from Fat: 51; Total Fat: 5.67g; Saturated Fat: 0.88g; Monounsaturated Fat: 3.91g; Polyunsaturated Fat: 0.88g; Cholesterol: 0mg; Sodium: 728mg; Total Carbohydrate: 45.61g; Dietary Fiber: 18.43g; Sugars: 8.91g; Protein: 21.06g

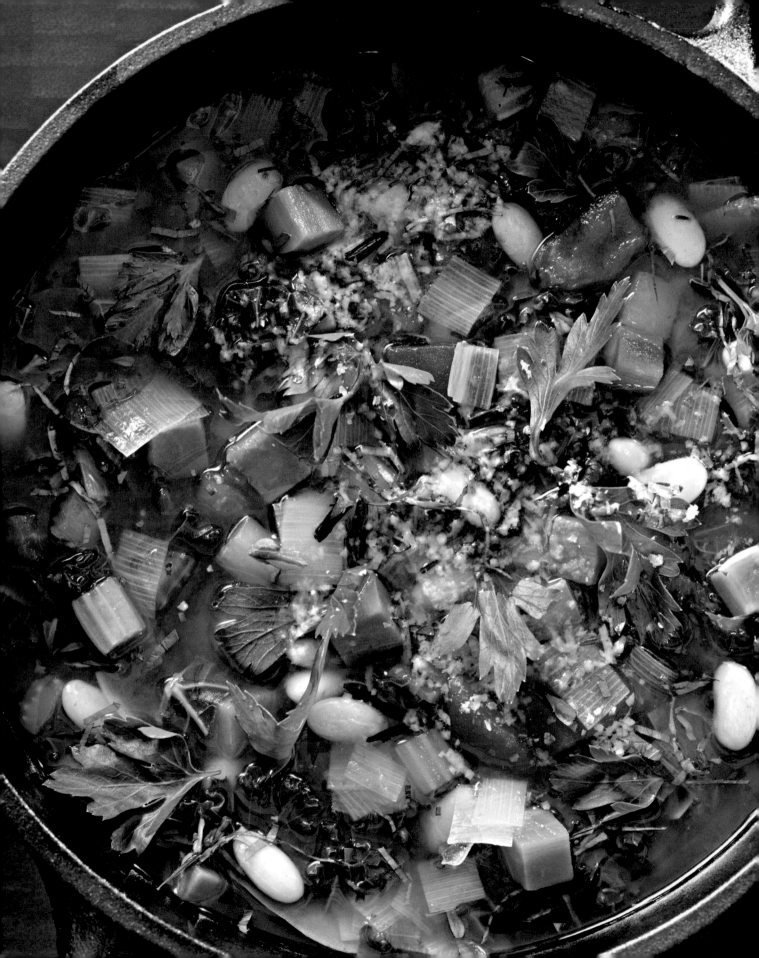

"Ten Thousand Lakes" Minestrone with Wild Rice and White Beans

SERVES 8

With the wild rice that gives it such a nutty, earthy, satisfying flavor and texture (not to mention its name, a reference to Minnesota, where so much of that grain is grown), I like to think of this healthy recipe as a New World take on the Italian classic.

⅓ cup dried cannellini beans or other dried white beans, sorted, rinsed, and soaked overnight in cold water to cover

2 tablespoons extra-virgin olive oil

3 medium leeks, white parts only, halved lengthwise, thoroughly rinsed, and chopped

6 garlic cloves, chopped

2 medium carrots, cut into ½-inch pieces

2 celery stalks, chopped

1 (14-ounce) can crushed tomatoes

1½ cups packed chopped kale leaves

⅓ cup uncooked wild rice

1 large bay leaf

2 teaspoons kosher salt, plus more as needed

½ teaspoon freshly ground black pepper, plus more as needed

1 teaspoon dried thyme

7 cups homemade Vegetable Stock (page 274), Chicken Stock (page 271), or good-quality canned low-sodium broth

Chopped fresh flat-leaf parsley, fresh basil, or fresh chives, for garnish

6 tablespoons freshly grated Parmesan, for garnish (optional)

Drain the soaked cannellini beans, put them in a saucepan, and add enough cold water to cover by 2 inches. Bring to a boil over high heat and cook for 30 minutes. Drain and set aside.

In a large, heavy soup pot, heat the oil over medium heat. Add the leeks and sauté, stirring constantly, until tender, 3 to 5 minutes. Add the garlic and sauté, stirring, until fragrant, about 30 seconds.

Add the carrots, celery, tomatoes, kale, wild rice, drained cannellini beans, bay leaf, salt, pepper, and thyme. Stir together briefly, and then stir in the stock. Bring the liquid to a boil, and then reduce the heat to maintain a simmer. Cover the pot and simmer until the beans and rice are tender, about 1½ hours.

(Alternatively, heat a pressure cooker over medium heat. Add the oil and the leeks and sauté the leeks until fragrant, 1 to 2 minutes. Add the garlic and stir briefly; then, stir in the carrots, celery, tomatoes, kale, wild rice, drained cannellini beans, bay leaf, salt, pepper, thyme, and stock. Bring to a boil, secure the lid, and bring to high pressure, following the manufacturer's instructions. Turn the heat to low and set a timer for 20 minutes. When the cooking time is up, turn off the heat and release the pressure, following the manufacturer's instructions. Continue simmering with the lid off until the soup is thick but still fairly fluid, about 10 minutes more.)

Taste and adjust the seasoning, if necessary. Ladle the soup into heated serving bowls and garnish with parsley, basil, or chives and, if you like, grated Parmesan.

WOLFGANG'S HEALTHY TIPS

→ Whether you make it on the stovetop or in a pressure cooker, this soup is worth preparing in quantity and freezing in individual portions for future quick, healthy meals.

→ Using vegetable stock and leaving out the optional Parmesan garnish makes the recipe completely vegan.

→ Once you've tried it this way, feel free to make healthy ingredient substitutions. Try Swiss chard or collard greens in place of the kale, or any other dried bean variety for the white beans.

→ Speaking of beans, instead of soaking them overnight, you could also "quick soak" them. Put the dried beans in a small saucepan and add 1 cup cold water. Bring to a boil over high heat, then continue boiling for 2 minutes. Remove the pan from the heat and leave the beans to soak for 1 hour before draining them and beginning the recipe as written.

Nutrition Facts Per Serving: Calories: 222; Calories from Fat: 54; Total Fat: 6.06g; Saturated Fat: 1.24g; Monounsaturated Fat: 3.75g; Polyunsaturated Fat: 1.07g; Cholesterol: 6mg; Sodium: 476mg; Total Carbohydrate: 32.83g; Dietary Fiber: 4.92g; Sugars: 8.16g; Protein: 10.72g

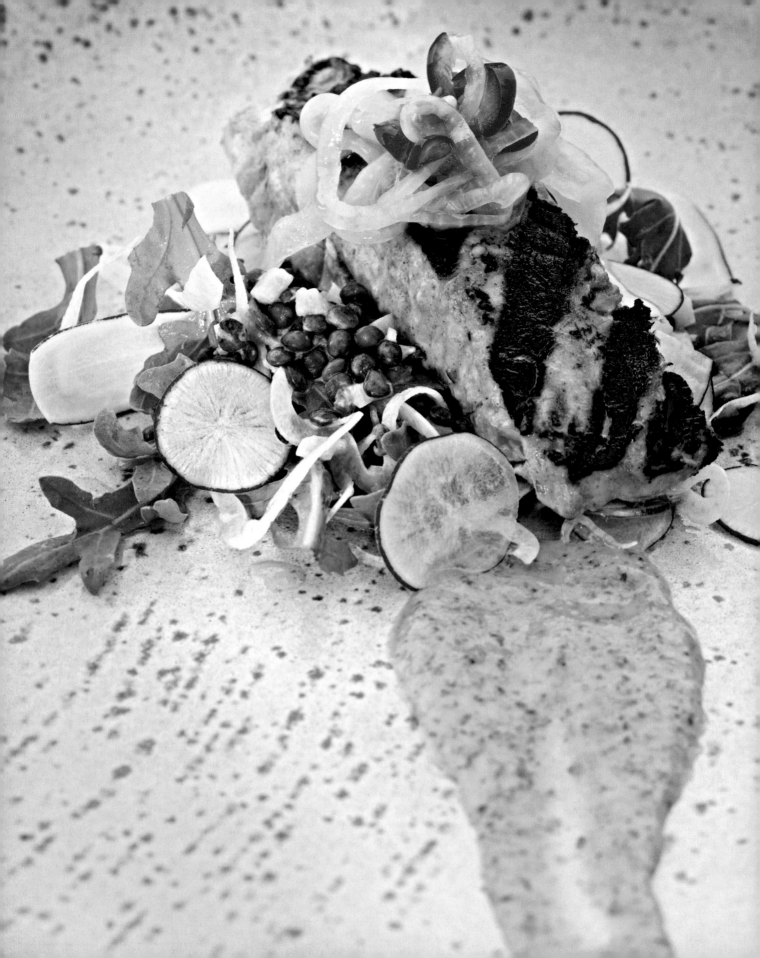

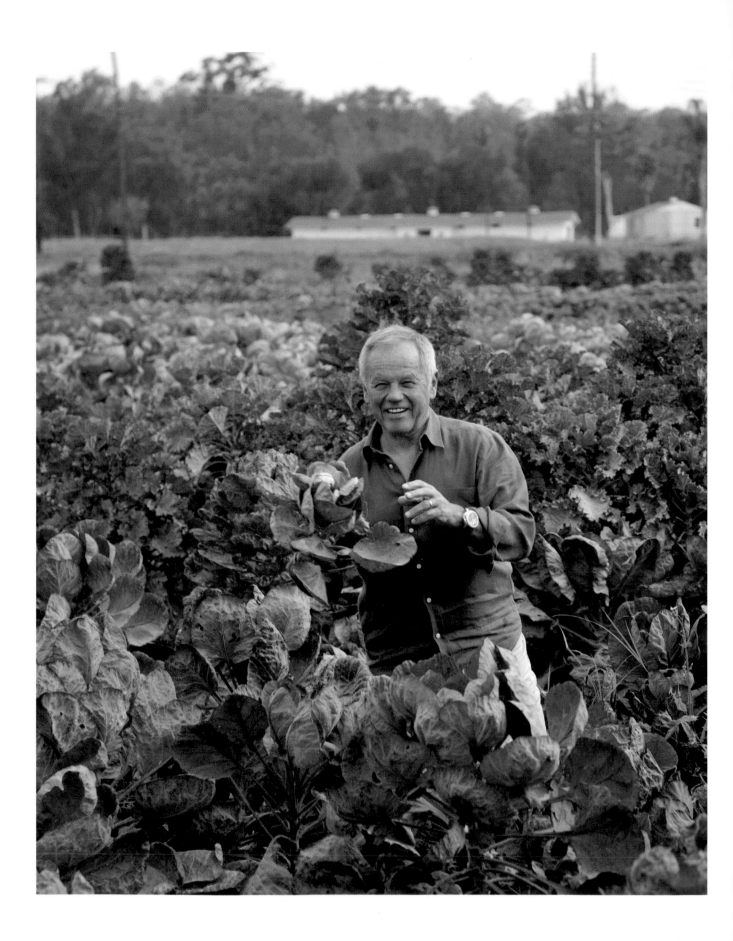

SALADS

Salads have come a long way since I first started cooking in restaurants more than five decades ago. Back then, in the European kitchens where I worked, salads were mostly considered simple appetizers or side dishes, featuring lettuces and a few other vegetables and usually dressed with vinaigrettes or maybe mayonnaise. Yes, there were some grander salads, such as southern France's *salade Niçoise*. And, after I came to America, I learned of standbys like the chef's salad and the Waldorf salad, oversize bowls that were often high in fat and calories even when they were supposed to be health-conscious lunchtime choices.

I've seen all that change in recent years, as more and more people realize—thanks to the wealth of fresh seasonal produce available everywhere and the creative cooking it can inspire—that salads can be incredibly varied, delicious, satisfying, and truly healthy. As the recipes that follow show, they can also be incredibly versatile. You'll find salads here that work perfectly as appetizers, others as sides, and still more as main courses; and many can play multiple roles.

So dig into one or more of these salads soon, and learn how great-tasting fresh food can make you feel great, too.

- → Chino Chopped Vegetable Salad
- → Arugula Salad with Tangerines, Asian Pear, Dried Cranberries, and Toasted Almonds
- → Autumn Greens Salad with Oranges, Raisins, and Warm Goat Cheese Croutons
- → Kale Salad with Pine Nuts and Raisins
- → Baby Beet Salad with Arugula, Goat Cheese, and Hazelnuts
- → Frisée and Apple Salad with Smoked Whitefish Crostini
- → Grilled Ahi Tuna Salade Niçoise
- → Tandoori Salmon Salad with Pickled Cippolini Onions, Cucumber Raita, and Marinated Lentils
- → Thai Grilled Chicken Salad with Mango and Coconut-Lime Vinaigrette
- → Stir-Fried Shrimp Salad with Tomato-Ginger Sauce and Chinois Vinaigrette
- → Chinois Chicken Salad with Chinese Mustard Vinaigrette
- → Chinois Grilled London Broil Salad with Cilantro-Mint-Yogurt Dressing
- → Melon Salad with Prosciutto, Mozzarella, and Ice Wine Dressing

Chino Chopped Vegetable Salad

SERVES 4

Years ago, I named this signature Spago salad after the wonderful organic farm run by the Chino family in northern San Diego County, source of some of our restaurant's finest produce. Use the best farmers' market produce available. For the best texture and most attractive presentation, I cut the vegetables, except the corn kernels, into uniform ¼-inch dice.

1 cup diced carrots

¾ cup fresh corn kernels (from about 1 medium ear)

½ cup diced green beans

½ cup diced red onion

½ cup diced radicchio

½ cup diced celery

1 small vine-ripened tomato, peeled, seeded (see page 288), and cut into ¼-inch dice

2 cups mixed baby salad leaves of your choice, several small leaves reserved for garnish

1 recipe Dijon-Balsamic Vinaigrette (page 275)

4 teaspoons grated Parmesan

Kosher salt

Freshly ground black pepper

8 cherry tomatoes, halved

Bring a pot of salted water to a boil. Fill a bowl with ice cubes and water. Put the carrots, corn, and green beans in a wire sieve, lower it into the boiling water, and cook until the vegetables are tender-crisp, 2 to 3 minutes. Plunge the sieve into the ice water to stop the cooking process. Drain well.

In a large bowl, combine the blanched vegetables, onion, radicchio, celery, and tomato. Put the salad leaves in a separate bowl.

Drizzle about two-thirds of the vinaigrette over the chopped vegetable mixture and toss well. Sprinkle in the Parmesan and toss again. Season to taste with salt and pepper. Drizzle the remaining dressing over the salad leaves and toss well.

Arrange beds of salad leaves on four chilled salad plates. Mound the chopped vegetable salad on top. Top the vegetables with the reserved salad leaves. Arrange cherry tomato halves around the base of the salad. Serve immediately.

WOLFGANG'S HEALTHY TIPS

→ With all its flavor and crunch, this salad is an excellent way to start a healthy meal.

→ Don't be discouraged by the high percentage of calories from fat in this recipe. Look instead at the very low total calorie count and then consider that all of these very nutritious fresh vegetables are rich in nutrients and low in calories, while most of the fat comes from a little heart-healthy olive oil in the dressing.

→ Just as I do, feel free to vary the salad mixture based on what's best at the market. I also like to include such ingredients as blanched diced artichoke hearts, or slivered sugar-snap or snow peas; and diced fresh mushrooms or, for a little splurge, ripe avocado.

Nutrition Facts Per Serving: Calories: 170; Calories from Fat: 94; Total Fat: 10.91g; Saturated Fat: 1.65g; Monounsaturated Fat: 7.65g; Polyunsaturated Fat: 1.61g; Cholesterol: 1mg; Sodium: 93mg; Total Carbohydrate: 16.10g; Dietary Fiber: 3.51g; Sugars: 7.82g; Protein: 3.43g

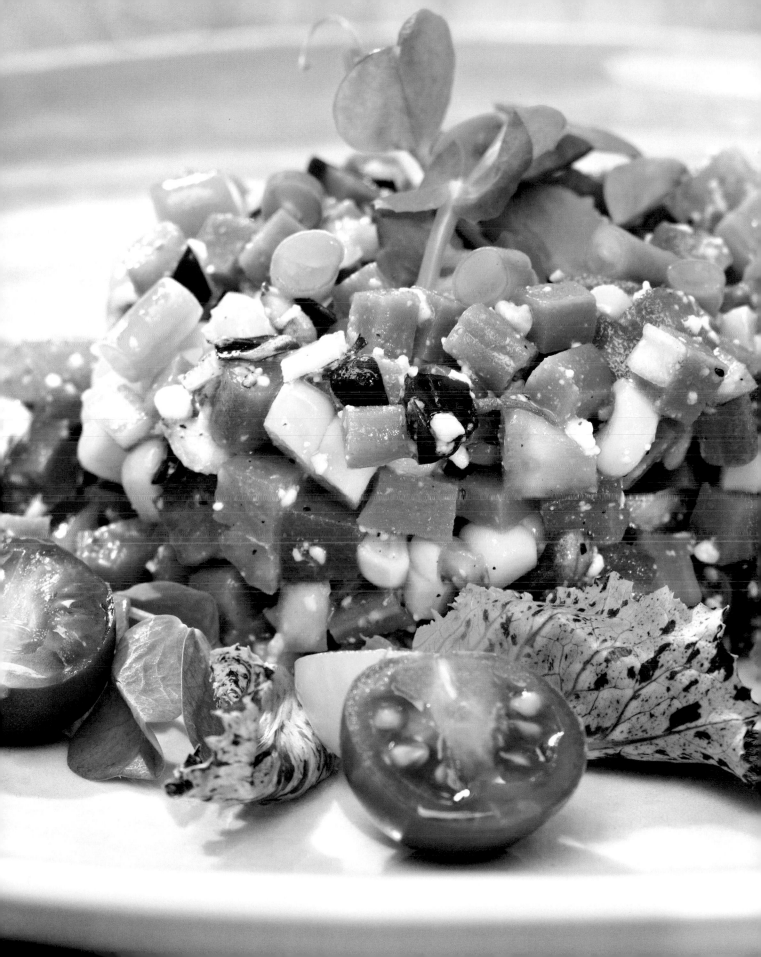

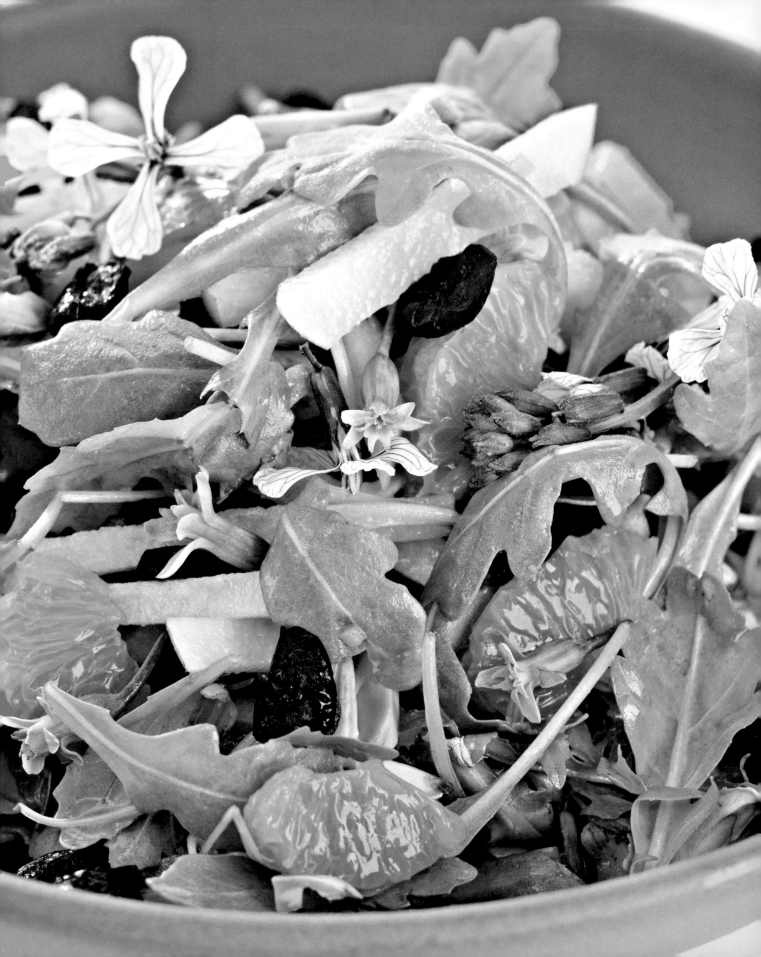

Arugula Salad with Tangerines, Asian Pear, Dried Cranberries, and Toasted Almonds

SERVES 4

Serve this colorful, zesty salad as a first course or buffet dish for a holiday party or on any occasion during the colder months. It also works well as a side dish to grilled, broiled, or roasted meat or poultry.

Citrus-Ginger Vinaigrette:

½ cup fresh orange juice

½ cup fresh lemon juice

2 teaspoons very finely chopped fresh ginger

½ teaspoon powdered mustard

2 tablespoons extra-virgin olive oil

Kosher salt

Freshly ground black pepper

Arugula Salad:

1 pound baby arugula leaves

3 large tangerines or mandarins

2 Asian pears, cored, peeled, and cut into thick matchsticks, about 3 inches by ¼ inch

¼ cup slivered almonds, toasted (see page 289)

½ cup dried cranberries

Kosher salt

Freshly ground black pepper

At least several hours ahead of time, prepare the Citrus-Ginger Vinaigrette: In a small nonreactive saucepan, combine the orange and lemon juices, ginger, and mustard powder. Bring to a boil over medium heat, and then continue boiling until the juice has reduced to ¼ cup, about 10 minutes. Remove from the heat and set aside to cool to room temperature. Pour the cooled juice reduction into a bowl. Whisk the reduction briskly while drizzling in the olive oil. Season to taste with salt and pepper. Transfer the dressing to a covered container and refrigerate until ready to use.

About 2 hours in advance, prepare the Arugula Salad: Fill a large bowl or basin with ice cubes and water. Rinse the arugula leaves under cold running water, and then immerse them in the ice water to make them extra crispy. Leave them to soak for 1 hour. Drain them and pat thoroughly dry with a clean kitchen towel or paper towels. Transfer to a plastic bag or covered container and refrigerate until just before serving time.

Peel the tangerines or mandarins: With the tip of a small, sharp knife, carefully slit the membrane on each of the segments; then, with your fingertips, assisted by the knife if necessary, peel off and discard the membranes. Put the segments in a bowl, cover, and refrigerate.

A few minutes before serving, put the arugula leaves in a large salad bowl. Add half each of the tangerine segments, pear, toasted almonds, and cranberries.

Add the dressing, season to taste with salt and pepper, and toss the salad thoroughly until the leaves are evenly coated. Leave the mixture in the salad bowl or transfer to an attractive serving bowl or individual bowls or plates. Garnish with the remaining tangerines, pears, almonds, and cranberries and serve.

WOLFGANG'S HEALTHY TIPS

→ The nuts and olive oil in this recipe bring its fat content right up to the one-third mark. If you like, cut back on or eliminate the almonds.

→ Use other varieties of firm pear, or crispy apple, in place of the Asian pear.

→ If you can't find dried cranberries, dried cherries or seedless raisins will also work well. So will diced dried apricots.

Nutrition Facts Per Serving: Calories: 326; Calories from Fat: 107; Total Fat: 11.97g; Saturated Fat: 1.48g; Monounsaturated Fat: 8.01g; Polyunsaturated Fat: 2.48g; Cholesterol: 0mg; Sodium: 33mg; Total Carbohydrate: 53.90g; Dietary Fiber: 10.45g; Sugars: 37.82g; Protein: 6.79g

Autumn Greens Salad with Oranges, Raisins, and Warm Goat Cheese Croutons

SERVES 4

I love the robust style of this salad, which has lots of color, flavor, and texture to brighten up cool, overcast days. But that's not to say you can't enjoy it all year round.

Warm Goat Cheese Croutons:

4 long, diagonal slices whole wheat French-style baguette, each about ¼ inch thick

1 garlic clove, halved

¼ pound fresh creamy goat cheese, cut into 4 equal pieces

1½ teaspoons chopped fresh thyme leaves

Freshly ground black pepper

Autumn Greens Salad:

½ pound arugula leaves, rinsed and patted thoroughly dry

1 small head radicchio, leaves separated, rinsed, and patted thoroughly dry

1 small head Belgian endive, leaves separated, rinsed, and patted thoroughly dry

1 seedless orange, segmented (see page 289), each segment cut into 2 or 3 pieces depending on size

2 tablespoons seedless raisins, plumped in warm water to cover for 30 minutes, well drained

1 recipe Dijon-Sherry-Tarragon Vinaigrette (page 275)

Prepare the Warm Goat Cheese Croutons: Preheat the oven to 450°F.

Place the bread on a baking sheet and toast in the oven until light golden, 3 to 4 minutes. Lightly rub the toasted bread on both sides with the cut sides of the garlic clove halves. Gently smear a portion of the goat cheese on top of each slice, sprinkling it with a little fresh thyme and pepper. Return the baking sheet to the oven and continue baking just until the cheese has warmed, about 1 minute more.

Meanwhile, prepare the Autumn Greens Salad: In a large bowl, combine the arugula, radicchio, and endive, tearing the leaves into bite-size pieces if necessary. Add the orange segments and raisins. Toss the salad mixture with enough of the dressing to coat the leaves and fruit lightly.

To serve, divide the salad among four plates. Top each plate, slightly off-center, with a Warm Goat Cheese Crouton.

> **WOLFGANG'S HEALTHY TIPS**
>
> → Although about 40 percent of the calories in this salad come from fat, it's full of healthy ingredients and could fit in nicely with a meal featuring a lower-fat main dish.
>
> → If you want to bring the calories from fat below one-third (32 percent), simply omit the goat cheese from the recipe and serve the salad with garlic toasts.

Nutrition Facts Per Serving: Calories: 321; Calories from Fat: 130; Total Fat: 14.47g; Saturated Fat: 5.47g; Monounsaturated Fat: 6.82g; Polyunsaturated Fat: 2.19g; Cholesterol: 13mg; Sodium: 307mg; Total Carbohydrate: 38.23g; Dietary Fiber: 8.25g; Sugars: 13.97g; Protein: 12.05g

Kale Salad with Pine Nuts and Raisins

SERVES 4

Kale salads seem to be hugely popular everywhere in recent years, and with good reason. The beautiful, dark green, crinkly leaves have a delicious, robust flavor and texture that goes well here with the sweet raisins, crunchy pine nuts, and tangy vinaigrette.

1 bunch kale (about ½ pound)

¼ cup golden raisins, plumped in hot water to cover for 10 minutes, drained well

¼ cup pine nuts, toasted (see page 289)

6 tablespoons Lemon Vinaigrette (page 276)

Kosher salt

Freshly ground black pepper

Freshly shaved Parmesan, for serving (optional)

With a sharp knife, cut out the stems and tough ribs from the kale leaves. In batches, stack the leaves, roll them up lengthwise, and cut them crosswise into strips ½ inch wide. You should have about 8 packed cups of shredded kale.

In a large bowl, combine the kale, raisins, and pine nuts. Drizzle with the Lemon Vinaigrette and season to taste with salt and pepper. Toss lightly but thoroughly.

Transfer the salad to individual chilled serving bowls or plates, taking care to divide the ingredients evenly. Garnish with Parmesan, if you like.

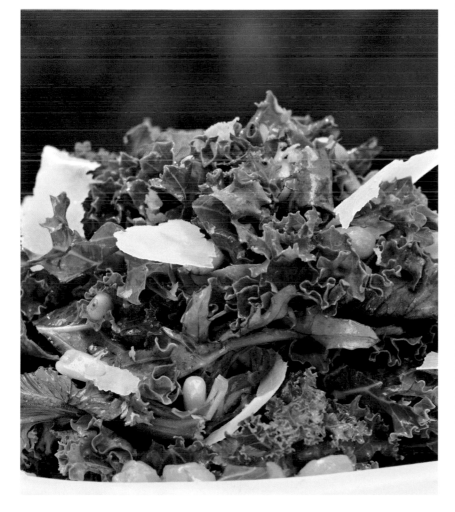

WOLFGANG'S HEALTHY TIPS

→ Yes, about half of the calories in this salad come from fat. But it's mostly heart-healthy fat from the olive oil in the salad dressing. And the kale itself is rich in vitamins, minerals, and other nutrients.

→ Serve this to start a meal featuring a lean main course. Offer it as a side dish with grilled, broiled, or roasted lean protein. Or make a double batch to offer as part of a buffet.

Nutrition Facts Per Serving: Calories: 230; Calories from Fat: 116; Total Fat: 13.00g; Saturated Fat: 1.60g; Monounsaturated Fat: 7.25g; Polyunsaturated Fat: 4.15g; Cholesterol: 0mg; Sodium: 79mg; Total Carbohydrate: 24.93g; Dietary Fiber: 3.57g; Sugars: 8.19g; Protein: 6.01g

Baby Beet Salad with Arugula, Goat Cheese, and Hazelnuts

SERVES 4

Sweet beets and tangy, creamy goat cheese complement each other perfectly in what has become a classic salad combination that pleases the eye as much as it does the mouth.

1½ pounds baby beets, preferably mixed in colors, washed and leaves trimmed

1 recipe Orange Vinaigrette (page 277)

Kosher salt

Freshly ground black pepper

2 cups baby arugula leaves or mixed baby lettuces, rinsed and patted thoroughly dry

2 ounces fresh creamy goat cheese

1 ounce hazelnuts, toasted (page 289) and coarsely chopped

Preheat the oven to 350°F.

Place the beets in a small roasting pan and pour in enough cold water to reach about one-quarter of the way up the sides of the beets. Cover the pan with foil, place it in the oven, and roast until the beets are tender, about 2 hours. To check for doneness, carefully remove the foil from one side of the pan, opening it away from you to avoid the steam, and gently insert a bamboo skewer into a beet: The skewer should slide in easily when the beets are done. With a large spoon, transfer the beets to a heatproof dish and let cool at room temperature until cool enough to handle.

With the help of a small, sharp knife, carefully peel the beets; their skins should slip off easily. Cut any larger beets into bite-size wedges. Put the peeled beets into a large bowl, drizzle with 1 tablespoon of the vinaigrette, and season to taste with salt and pepper. Arrange the beets attractively around the edges of individual serving plates.

Put the arugula leaves in another bowl, drizzle with just enough vinaigrette to coat them lightly, and toss well. Divide the arugula evenly among the plates, mounding the leaves in the center of each plate.

Crumble the goat cheese over the leaves and beets and sprinkle with hazelnuts. Drizzle any remaining vinaigrette over the beets. Serve immediately.

WOLFGANG'S HEALTHY TIPS

→ Yes, the fat calorie percentage is a bit high (47 percent) from the goat cheese and the heart-healthy olive oil in the dressing. But, overall, the salad is fairly low in calories and fat, making it an excellent first course before a lean main dish.

→ Roasting the beets, rather than boiling them as they are often prepared, helps to caramelize their natural sugars and concentrate their flavor, making every bite a more intensely delicious experience.

→ If you like, substitute Warm Goat Cheese Croutons (page 78) for the crumbled goat cheese.

Nutrition Facts Per Serving: Calories: 230; Calories from Fat: 109; Total Fat: 12.20g; Saturated Fat: 3.16g; Monounsaturated Fat: 7.69g; Polyunsaturated Fat: 1.35g; Cholesterol: 6mg; Sodium: 203mg; Total Carbohydrate: 24.00g; Dietary Fiber: 6.30g; Sugars: 16.66g; Protein: 7.47g

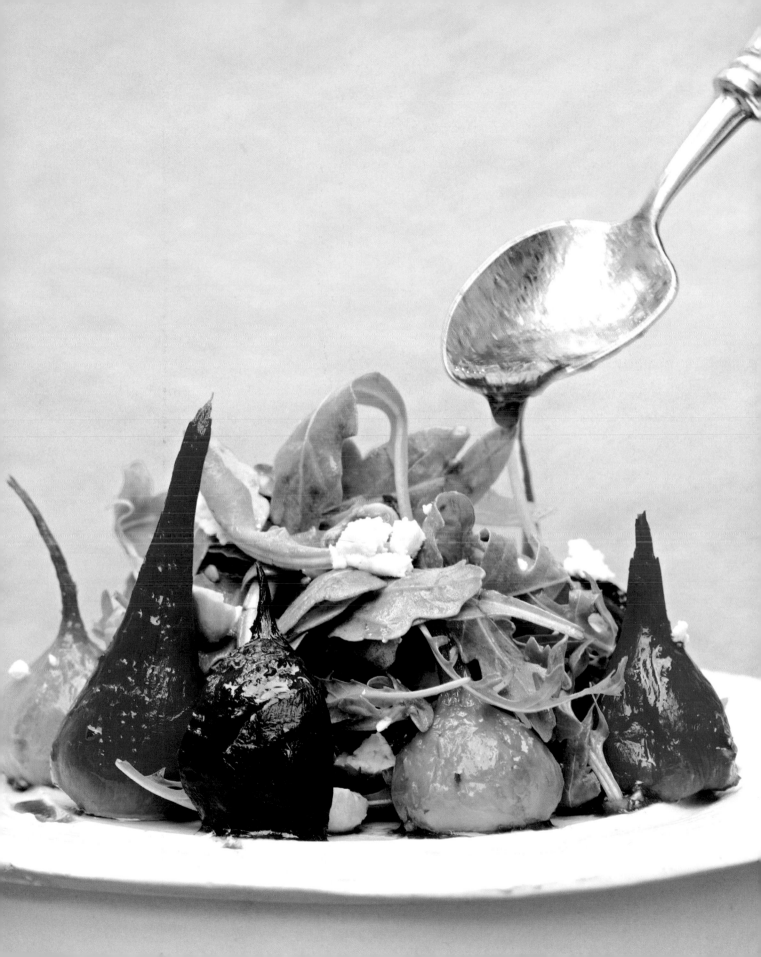

Frisée and Apple Salad with Smoked Whitefish Crostini

SERVES 4

Even the lightest, freshest of salads can be elevated to a dish that delivers deep pleasure when you get the perfect combination of ingredients with complementary colors, shapes, textures, and tastes—a great yin-yang balance of salty and sweet, rich and tangy, crispy and tender.

½ cup Lemon Vinaigrette (page 276)

Smoked Whitefish Crostini:

½ pound smoked whitefish or smoked trout fillets, skinned and any bones removed, flesh flaked

½ cup low-fat sour cream

1 tablespoon prepared horseradish

½ tablespoon fresh lemon juice

1 tablespoon chopped fresh chives

1 tablespoon chopped fresh dill

Kosher salt

Freshly ground black pepper

8 thin slices whole wheat or multigrain bread

Frisée and Apple Salad:

4 small heads frisée (curly endive)

1 cup torn radicchio leaves

1 cup baby arugula leaves

2 large Granny Smith apples

Kosher salt

Freshly ground black pepper

To Assemble:

2 tablespoons chopped fresh chives

Small fresh dill sprigs

At least an hour before preparing the salads, make the Lemon Vinaigrette. Set aside in the refrigerator.

Prepare the Smoked Whitefish Crostini: In a food processor fitted with the stainless-steel blade, combine the flaked smoked fish, sour cream, horseradish, and lemon juice. Pulse until coarsely but evenly pureed. Pulse in the chives, dill, and salt and pepper to taste. Transfer to a bowl and refrigerate.

Shortly before you plan to serve the salad, toast the bread slices until golden brown. Set aside.

Prepare the Frisée and Apple Salad: Remove and discard the coarse darker outer leaves from the frisée. Separate the pale inner leaves and place them in a strainer. Rinse thoroughly under cold running water. Drain well. Spread the leaves on a clean kitchen towel or paper towels, roll them up, and squeeze gently to remove excess water. Unroll the leaves and place them into a large salad bowl, tearing any larger leaves into bite-size pieces if necessary.

Place the radicchio and arugula in a strainer and rinse thoroughly under cold running water. Drain well. Dry thoroughly with paper towels and add the leaves to the frisée. Gently toss all the leaves to combine them.

With a sharp knife, quarter and core the apples. Cut them into very thin slices; or, using the julienne disc on a food processor, cut them into thin julienne strips. Arrange the apples on top of the salad leaves, reserving a few pieces to garnish the crostini.

Drizzle the Lemon Vinaigrette over the salad mixture and sprinkle with a little salt and pepper.

Assemble the dish: Spread the smoked whitefish mixture on the toasted bread slices. Garnish with the reserved apple pieces.

Garnish the crostini with chives and dill and arrange them on a platter to serve alongside the salad. Toss the salad just before serving. Taste, and adjust the seasonings if necessary.

> ## WOLFGANG'S HEALTHY TIPS
>
> → I conceived this salad as a whole dish complete with the crostini garnish, to work either as a first course or a light lunch main dish. You could certainly serve the two parts separately, though, offering the crostini as a delicious hors d'oeuvre in its own right.
>
> → Vary the ingredients as you like, using different salad leaves such as Belgian endive or baby spinach, crispy pears instead of apple, and smoked trout or sturgeon in place of the whitefish.

Nutrition Facts Per Serving: Calories: 544; Calories from Fat: 165; Total Fat: 18.36g; Saturated Fat: 4.86g; Monounsaturated Fat: 9.60g; Polyunsaturated Fat: 3.90g; Cholesterol: 28mg; Sodium: 984mg; Total Carbohydrate: 71.90g; Dietary Fiber: 23.21g; Sugars: 17.44g; Protein: 28.17g

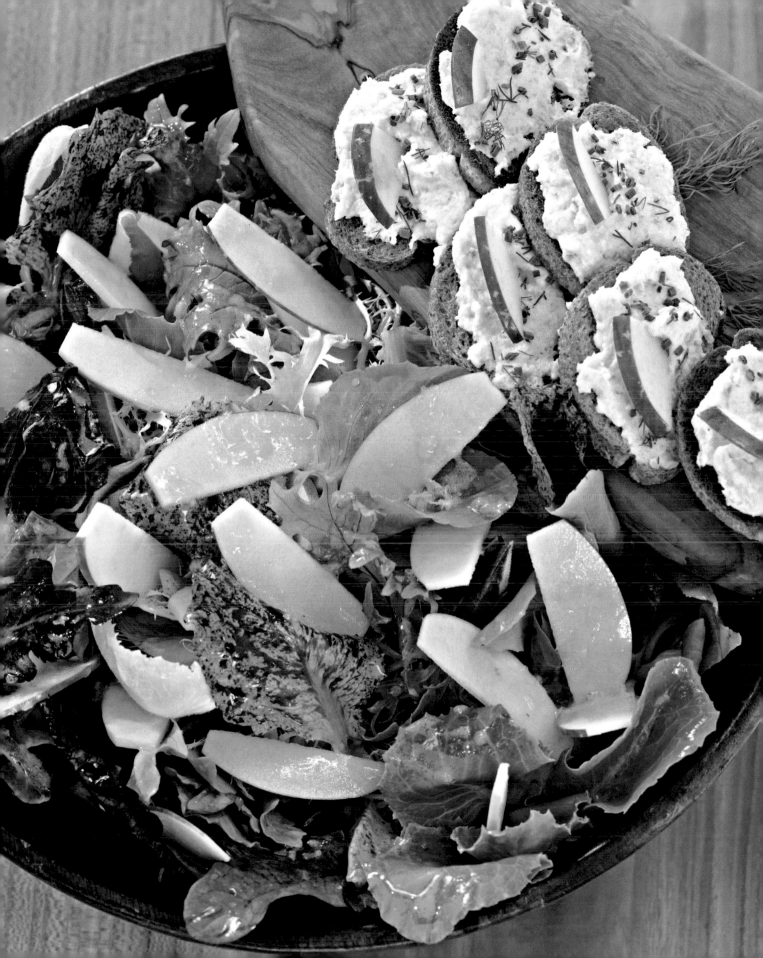

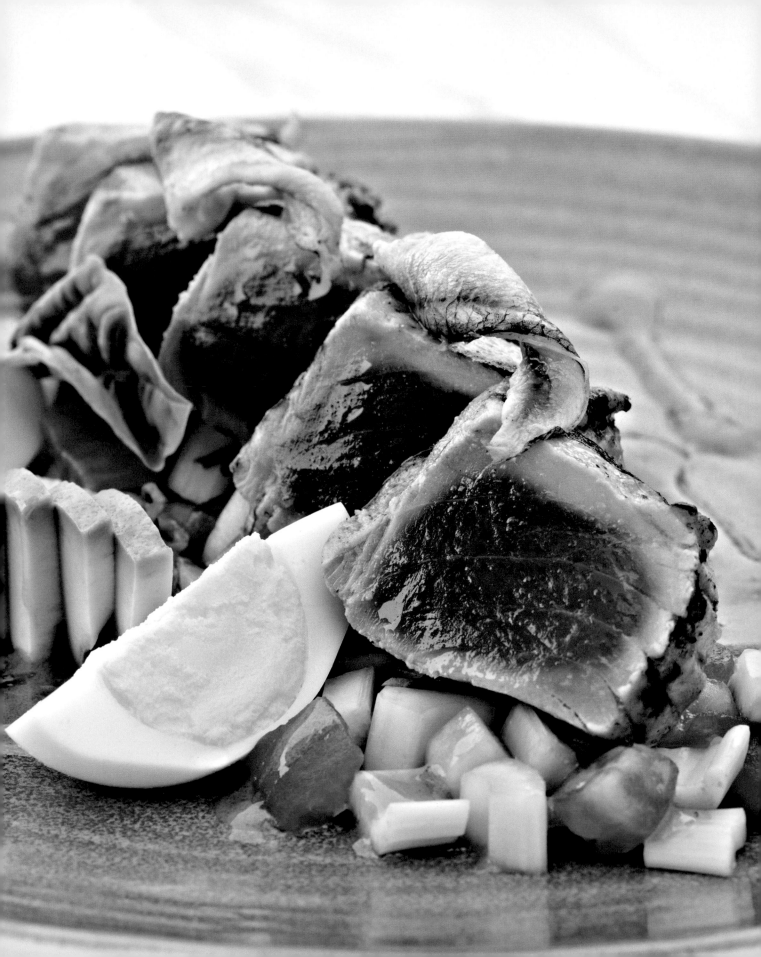

Grilled Ahi Tuna Salade Niçoise

SERVES 4

So many people in restaurants order the famous tuna salad as a light lunch, unaware that the vinaigrette and oil-packed canned tuna traditionally used make it high in fat. This version lightens up the classic by using grilled fresh tuna and less oil in the dressing. Start marinating the fish 1 to 3 hours before grilling.

Tuna:

Juice of 2 limes

1 tablespoon extra-virgin olive oil

1 tablespoon chopped shallot

1 teaspoon finely chopped fresh tarragon leaves

Kosher salt

Freshly ground black pepper

1 pound absolutely fresh ahi tuna fillet

Salad:

2 heads butter lettuce

4 sun-ripened tomatoes, peeled, seeded (see page 288), and cut into ¼-inch dice

1 cucumber, peeled, halved lengthwise, seeded, and cut into ¼-inch dice

Tender inner stalks from 1 head of celery, chopped

½ avocado, pitted, peeled, and thinly sliced

2 hard-boiled eggs, quartered

8 whole oil-packed anchovy fillets, well drained

Mustard Vinaigrette:

3 tablespoons sherry wine vinegar

1 teaspoon Dijon mustard

½ teaspoon minced fresh tarragon leaves

Pinch of kosher salt

Pinch of freshly ground black pepper

3 tablespoons extra-virgin olive oil

Prepare the Tuna: In a nonreactive bowl, stir together the lime juice, olive oil, shallot, tarragon, and salt and pepper to taste.

Cut the tuna fillet into 4 equal pieces. With a small, sharp knife, make shallow crosswise cuts ¼ inch apart along the length of each piece. Add the tuna to the marinade and turn to coat thoroughly. Cover the bowl with plastic wrap and refrigerate for 1 to 3 hours.

Prepare the Salad: Break up the butter lettuces into individual leaves. Rinse them under cold running water and pat dry with clean kitchen towels or paper towels.

In a large salad bowl, combine the lettuce leaves, diced tomatoes, cucumber, and celery. Set the avocado, hard-boiled eggs, and anchovies aside.

Make the Mustard Vinaigrette: In a small bowl, combine the vinegar, mustard, tarragon, salt, and pepper and stir with a whisk. Whisking continuously, slowly trickle in the oil to form a thick dressing.

Preheat an outdoor grill, an indoor countertop grill, a stovetop ridged grill pan, or the broiler. When the grill or broiler is hot, remove the tuna from the marinade and cook until nicely seared but still rare, 1 to 2 minutes per side.

Add a little of the dressing to the vegetable mixture and toss well to coat. On a serving platter or individual serving plates, mound the vegetable mixture and place the avocado and eggs alongside. Drizzle a little more dressing around the vegetables and plate. Cut each tuna fillet piece along the score marks into slices ¼ inch thick and drape them over the vegetables. Place the anchovies on top of the tuna. Serve immediately.

WOLFGANG'S HEALTHY TIPS

→ You'll notice that, though lighter, this recipe gets about 40 percent of its calories from fat. But, overall, it's low in calories, and the fats are healthy ones, including those in the tuna (rich in heart-beneficial omega-3 fatty acids), olive oil, and avocado.

→ If you still want to make this leaner, leaving out the eggs and the avocado will bring the total calories down to about 306 per serving, with about 109 (36 percent) from fat, while dropping the cholesterol to 50mg.

→ If rare fish is not to your liking, feel free to cook the tuna a minute or two longer per side. But try it still pink in the center, for the moistest results.

Nutrition Facts Per Serving: Calories: 370; Calories from Fat: 149; Total Fat: 16.66g; Saturated Fat: 3.09g; Monounsaturated Fat: 11.10g; Polyunsaturated Fat: 2.46g; Cholesterol: 143mg; Sodium: 462mg; Total Carbohydrate: 14.67g; Dietary Fiber: 5.06g; Sugars: 5.93g; Protein: 37.44g

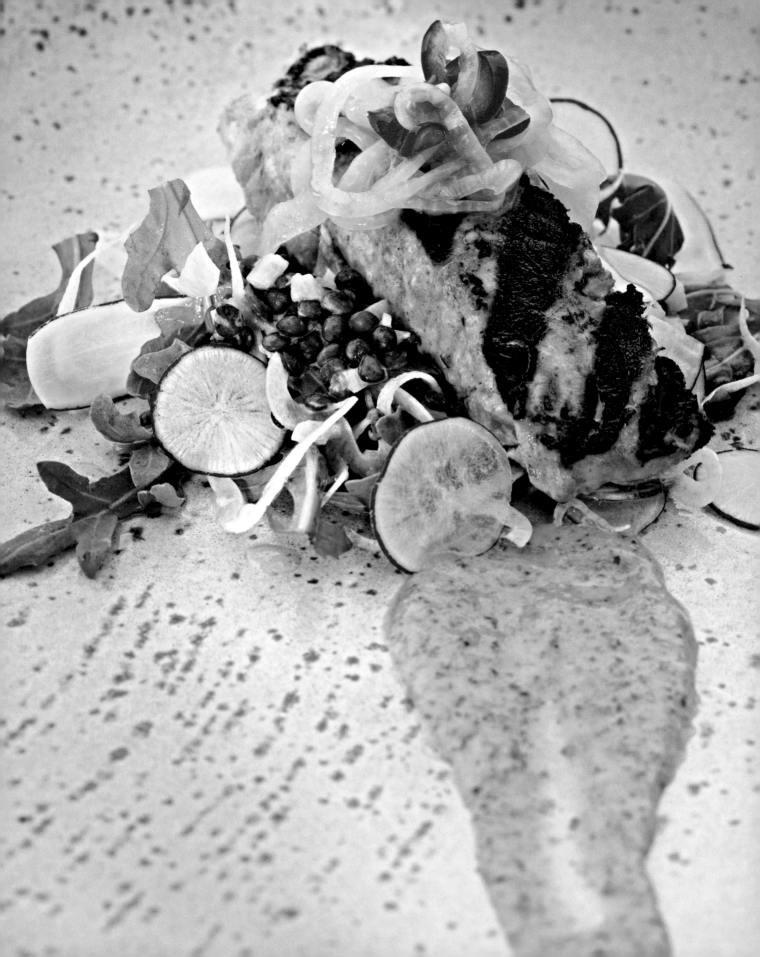

Tandoori Salmon Salad with Pickled Cippolini Onions, Cucumber Raita, and Marinated Lentils

SERVES 4

Yes, the salmon needs to be marinated for 6 hours. And there are lots of parts to this recipe. But each stage on its own is simple, much of the work can be done ahead, and it all adds up to a colorful main-course salad that bursts with color, flavor, texture, and well-balanced nutrition.

Tandoori Seasonings:

3 tablespoons Curry Powder (page 285)

1 teaspoon Kashmiri chile powder or hot paprika

1 teaspoon ground turmeric

1 teaspoon ground coriander

1 teaspoon ground cumin

1 teaspoon sweet paprika

½ teaspoon freshly grated nutmeg

½ teaspoon powdered ginger

¼ teaspoon ground cardamom

Tandoori Salmon:

4 Atlantic salmon fillets, about 4 ounces each, skinned

2 cups nonfat plain yogurt

¼ cup fresh lemon juice

¼ cup fresh lime juice

3 tablespoons chopped fresh cilantro leaves

2 tablespoons minced garlic

2 tablespoons finely grated fresh ginger

2 tablespoons vegetable oil

2 teaspoons ground coriander

2 teaspoons kosher salt

1 teaspoon Kashmiri chile powder or hot paprika

½ teaspoon ground turmeric

Marinated Green Lentil Salad:

1 cup dried green lentils, sorted and rinsed

1 medium yellow onion, cut into large chunks, plus ¼ cup finely chopped yellow onion

1 medium carrot, cut into large chunks

1 celery stalk, cut into large chunks

1 teaspoon plus ½ teaspoon kosher salt

½ cup nonfat plain Greek yogurt

2 tablespoons Champagne vinegar

1 tablespoon honey

½ teaspoon sugar

½ Japanese cucumber, cut into ¼-inch dice

Pickled Cippolini Onions:

½ cup Champagne vinegar

1 slice fresh ginger

4 teaspoons sugar

1 tablespoon kosher salt

1 Fresno chile pepper or other hot or medium-hot fresh chile, thinly sliced crosswise (with seeds)

5 cippolini onions, very thinly sliced crosswise into rings

Cucumber Raita:

1 Japanese cucumber, peeled and cut into chunks

¼ red onion, cut into chunks

2 tablespoons honey

1 teaspoon Curry Powder (page 285)

2 cups fresh cilantro leaves

1 cup fresh mint leaves

1½ cups nonfat plain Greek yogurt

To Assemble:

4 cups packed baby arugula leaves

1 medium fennel bulb, trimmed and thinly shaved

8 red radishes, trimmed and thinly shaved

At least 8 hours before serving or the night before, prepare the Tandoori Seasonings: In a small bowl, stir together the Curry Powder, chile powder or hot paprika, turmeric, coriander, cumin, sweet paprika, nutmeg, ginger, and cardamom.

Prepare the Salmon: Lightly season the salmon fillets with 1½ tablespoons of the Tandoori Seasonings. Put them in a nonreactive bowl, cover, and refrigerate for about 2 hours.

In a separate bowl, stir together the yogurt, lemon juice, lime juice, cilantro, garlic, ginger, oil, coriander, salt, chile powder or paprika, turmeric, and 2 tablespoons more of the Tandoori Seasonings. (Store any remaining Tandoori Seasonings in a small airtight container in the pantry for another use. It will keep for several

CONTINUES

months.) Pour the yogurt mixture over the salmon fillets, turn them to coat, cover the dish, and place in the refrigerator to marinate for at least 6 hours or overnight.

As soon as the salmon is marinating, prepare the Marinated Green Lentil Salad: In a large saucepan, combine the lentils, large chunks of onion, carrot, celery, and 1 teaspoon of the salt. Add cold water to cover by several inches. Bring to a boil over high heat; then, reduce the heat to low and simmer until the lentils are tender, about 45 minutes. Drain thoroughly. Pick out and discard the onion, carrot, and celery chunks. Transfer the lentils to a medium bowl.

In a small bowl, stir together the yogurt, vinegar, honey, the remaining ½ teaspoon salt, and sugar. Fold in the diced cucumber and finely chopped onion. Stir the mixture into the lentils. Cover and refrigerate until serving time.

At least 3 hours before serving time, or up to the night before, prepare the Pickled Cippolini Onions: In a small nonreactive saucepan, combine the vinegar, ginger, sugar, salt, chile, and ¼ cup water. Bring to a boil and cook, stirring, until the sugar and salt have dissolved.

Place the onions in a nonreactive bowl. Stir in the vinegar mixture. Set aside until the liquid has cooled to room temperature, then cover and refrigerate. Leave the onions marinating in the liquid until serving time.

Up to 1 hour before cooking the salmon, prepare the Cucumber Raita: In a blender, combine the cucumber, onion, honey, and Curry Powder. Blend until smoothly pureed. Add the cilantro and mint and pulse until smoothly blended. Add the yogurt and pulse 2 or 3 times, just until blended. Transfer to a bowl, cover, and refrigerate.

Cook the Salmon: Preheat an outdoor grill, a nonstick stovetop ridged grill pan, a countertop electric ridged grill, or the broiler. Grill or broil the salmon until nicely browned on both sides but still moist inside, 5 to 7 minutes total.

Assemble the dish: While the salmon is cooking, in a large bowl, toss together the arugula, fennel, and radishes. Arrange beds of this salad on individual serving plates. Spread a bed of the Marinated Lentils on top of the salad on each plate. Place a grilled salmon fillet on top of each bed of lentils. Garnish each plate with some Cucumber Raita, passing the rest at the table. Drain the Pickled Cippolini Onions and scatter them on top of the salmon. Serve immediately.

WOLFGANG'S HEALTHY TIPS

→ The variety of lively seasonings in this recipe alone helps to make you stop and savor every bite.

→ The Marinated Green Lentil Salad is one of the most filling parts of the dish. Prepare it on its own as a side salad to go with other grilled or broiled foods. Or make double the quantity for a great buffet dish.

→ Make the Cucumber Raita by itself, too, to serve as a low-fat sauce for any grilled seafood, meat, or poultry.

Nutrition Facts Per Serving: Calories: 498; Calories from Fat: 45; Total Fat: 5.05g; Saturated Fat: 1.20g; Monounsaturated Fat: 1.75g; Polyunsaturated Fat: 2.10g; Cholesterol: 19mg; Sodium: 296mg; Total Carbohydrate: 82.98g; Dietary Fiber: 24.27g; Sugars: 35.27g; Protein: 34.52g

Thai Grilled Chicken Salad with Mango and Coconut-Lime Vinaigrette

SERVES 4

So many people enjoy Chinese chicken salads that I thought I'd try a Southeast Asian version. This result mixes savory, sweet, salty, and spicy flavors; crispy, chewy, soft, and crunchy textures; and a rainbow of colors.

Thai Grilled Chicken:

¾ cup low-sodium soy sauce

¼ cup chopped garlic

¼ cup chopped scallion, white parts only (reserve green parts for salad)

¼ cup chopped fresh ginger

Juice of 1 lime

1 lime, thinly sliced

4 boneless skinless chicken breast halves (about 1 pound total)

Salad:

1 medium head Napa cabbage, leaves separated, trimmed, rinsed, and patted dry

1 large ripe but firm mango (about 12 ounces)

1 cup finely shredded carrot

½ cup very thinly sliced white onion

½ cup very thinly sliced scallion, green parts only (reserved from above)

2 red radishes, very thinly sliced

Kosher salt

To Assemble:

½ cup Coconut-Lime Vinaigrette (page 278)

¼ cup cashews, toasted (see page 289) and coarsely crushed

½ cup fresh cilantro leaves

1 lime, cut into 8 wedges

Prepare the Thai Grilled Chicken: Start marinating the chicken 2 hours ahead. In a shallow, nonreactive dish, stir together the soy sauce, garlic, scallion, ginger, lime juice, and sliced lime. Add the chicken breasts and turn to coat evenly in the marinade. Cover with plastic wrap and refrigerate for 2 hours, turning the chicken occasionally.

Preheat an outdoor grill, an indoor countertop grill, a ridged stovetop grill pan, or the broiler.

Meanwhile, prepare the Salad: Reserve 12 medium cabbage leaves. Stack the remaining leaves, cut them crosswise into thin strips, and put the strips in a bowl.

Peel the mango and cut off the fruit in thin slices parallel to and around the pit. Stack the slices, cut them crosswise into thin strips, and add to the bowl with the cabbage. Add the carrot, onion, scallion, and radishes to the cabbage and mango. Sprinkle lightly with salt and set aside.

Cook the Thai Grilled Chicken: When the grill or broiler is hot, remove the chicken breasts from the marinade, discarding the marinade. Grill or broil the chicken until just cooked through, 4 to 5 minutes per side. (Carefully cut into the center of one breast to check for doneness.) Transfer to a plate and cover with foil. Set aside to rest for a few minutes.

Assemble the dish: Arrange 3 of the reserved cabbage leaves like spokes on each of four large serving plates. Drizzle about 6 tablespoons of the vinaigrette over the salad ingredients in the bowl and toss lightly but thoroughly. Mound the salad mixture in the center of each plate.

Transfer the grilled chicken breasts to a clean cutting board. With a sharp knife, cut each breast crosswise into thin slices. Arrange one sliced breast on top of each salad. Garnish each serving with 1 tablespoon of the cashews and 2 tablespoons of the cilantro.

Lightly drizzle the remaining vinaigrette over the chicken. Place 2 lime wedges on each plate for guests to squeeze over their salads. Serve immediately.

> **WOLFGANG'S HEALTHY TIPS**
>
> → You won't leave the table hungry after sitting down to this lean but incredibly flavorful main-dish salad. Notice how its wide variety of flavors and textures helps to satisfy you.
>
> → You could substitute boneless and skinless dark-meat chicken or lean pork tenderloin for the chicken breasts.

Nutrition Facts Per Serving: Calories: 514; Calories from Fat: 130; Total Fat: 14.53g; Saturated Fat: 4.80; Monounsaturated Fat: 6.46g; Polyunsaturated Fat: 3.28g; Cholesterol: 151mg; Sodium: 607mg; Total Carbohydrate: 34.96g; Dietary Fiber: 8.16g; Sugars: 18.39g; Protein: 56.75g

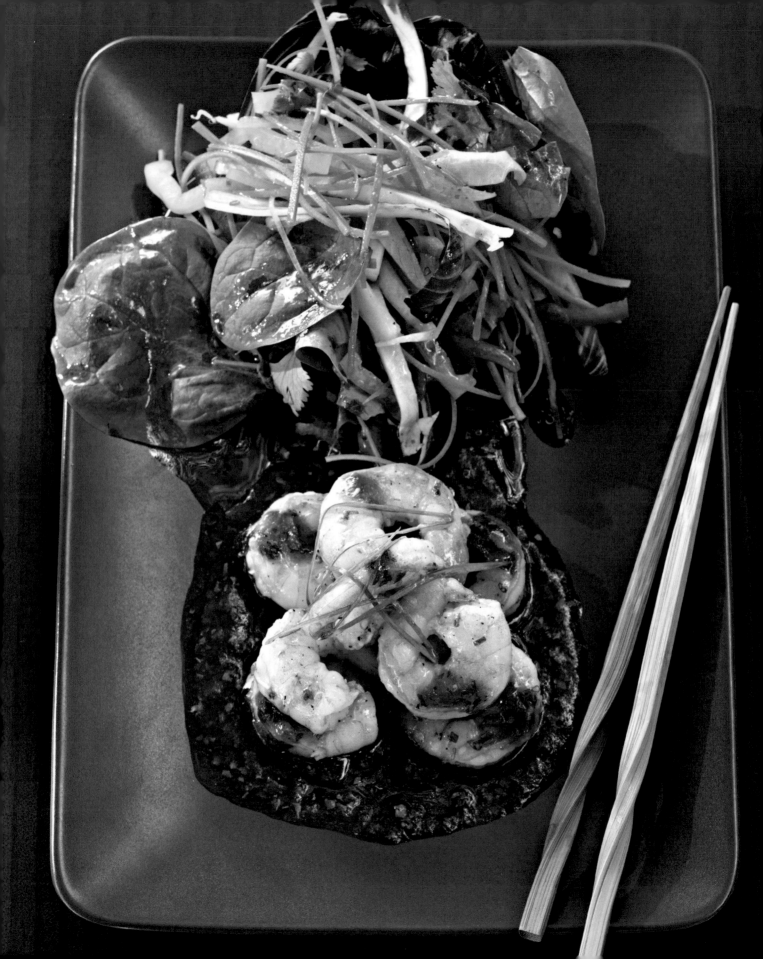

Stir-Fried Shrimp Salad with Tomato-Ginger Sauce and Chinois Vinaigrette

SERVES 4

With this main-dish salad's satisfying textures and bright flavors reminiscent of a classic Asian stir-fry, you'll hardly notice that it is mostly vegetables. The fresh, crispy mixture tossed with a zesty dressing and the spicy fresh tomato sauce are served at room temperature alongside stir-fried shrimp.

Tomato-Ginger Sauce:

1 pound Italian plum tomatoes, cored and cut into chunks

2 jalapeños, halved, stemmed, seeded, and deveined

2 garlic cloves

2 teaspoons minced fresh ginger

1 teaspoon tomato paste

½ bunch finely chopped fresh cilantro leaves

2 tablespoons fresh lime juice

1 tablespoon honey

Kosher salt

Freshly ground black pepper

Chinois Vinaigrette:

2 tablespoons rice wine vinegar

1 tablespoon peanut oil

1 tablespoon low-sodium soy sauce

1 tablespoon fresh lemon juice

1 teaspoon toasted Asian-style sesame oil

Kosher salt

Freshly ground black pepper

Stir-Fried Shrimp Salad:

4 large radicchio leaves

1 head Belgian endive, leaves separated

3 cups baby spinach

1 large carrot, cut into thin julienne strips

1 red or yellow bell pepper, halved, stemmed, seeded, deveined, and cut into thin julienne strips

1½ pounds extra-large shrimp (16 to 20 per pound), peeled and deveined

Kosher salt

Freshly ground black pepper

1 tablespoon peanut oil

To Assemble:

1 small scallion, dark green part only, cut diagonally into very thin slices

Prepare the Tomato-Ginger Sauce: In a blender or a food processor fitted with the stainless-steel blade, combine the tomatoes, jalapeños, garlic, ginger, and tomato paste. Pulse until coarsely chopped, then process until pureed. Pour the puree through a fine-mesh strainer set over a bowl, pressing it through with a rubber spatula; discard the solids left in the strainer. Stir the cilantro, lime juice, and honey into the sauce. Season to taste with salt and pepper. Set aside.

Prepare the Chinois Vinaigrette: In a small bowl, combine the rice vinegar, peanut oil, soy sauce, lemon juice, and sesame oil and whisk thoroughly. Season to taste with salt and pepper.

Prepare the Stir-Fried Shrimp Salad: Place a radicchio leaf and an endive leaf on one side of each serving plate. In a salad bowl, combine the spinach, carrot, and bell pepper, add the vinaigrette, and toss thoroughly. Mound the salad on top of the radicchio and endive. Set aside.

Season the shrimp lightly with salt and pepper. In a large nonstick skillet or wok, heat the peanut oil over high heat. Working in batches, if necessary, to avoid crowding the pan, stir-fry the shrimp just until they are uniformly pink, about 3 minutes.

Assemble the dish: Spoon some Tomato-Ginger Sauce next to the salad on each plate, reserving a few spoonfuls. Arrange the shrimp on top of the sauce, drizzle with the remaining sauce, and garnish with scallions. Serve immediately.

WOLFGANG'S HEALTHY TIPS

→ Most of the fat in this dish comes from small touches of oils that pack big flavor punches in the Asian kitchen—peanut oil and dark amber-colored toasted sesame oil.

→ If you like, add even more vegetables to the salad, such as julienned Japanese or Persian cucumber, thinly sliced fresh mushrooms, or some Caramelized Onions (page 282).

Nutrition Facts Per Serving: Calories: 189; Calories from Fat: 59; Total Fat: 6.63g; Saturated Fat: 1.24g; Monounsaturated Fat: 2.89g; Polyunsaturated Fat: 2.49g; Cholesterol: 71mg; Sodium: 523mg; Total Carbohydrate: 21.74g; Dietary Fiber: 7.73g; Sugars: 10.76g; Protein: 12.27g

Chinois Chicken Salad with Chinese Mustard Vinaigrette

SERVES 4 AS A MAIN COURSE, 8 AS AN APPETIZER

With a few minor adjustments to the dressing and extra vegetables, one of the all-time favorite recipes at my Chinois restaurant in Santa Monica becomes a healthy main course or appetizer. I bet anyone who has had the original would enjoy this version equally.

Chinese Mustard Vinaigrette:

¼ cup rice vinegar

2 tablespoons honey

1 tablespoon low-sodium soy sauce

2 teaspoons sesame oil

2 teaspoons dry Chinese or English mustard (such as Colman's)

Kosher salt

Freshly ground black pepper

2 tablespoons peanut oil

Chicken Salad:

4 cups shredded cooked skinless breast chicken meat (from a leftover or store-bought roast or rotisserie chicken or other recipe)

4 cups shredded Napa cabbage

2 cups shredded iceberg or romaine lettuce

1 cup julienned snow peas

1 cup shredded carrot

¼ cup thinly sliced pickled sushi ginger, drained and cut into thin julienne strips

To Assemble:

1 tablespoon black or white sesame seeds

1 scallion, trimmed and cut diagonally into thin slices

Prepare the Chinese Mustard Vinaigrette: In a blender or a food processor fitted with the stainless-steel blade, combine the rice vinegar, honey, soy sauce, sesame oil, dry mustard, and a little salt and pepper. Blend or process until smooth. With the machine running, drizzle in the peanut oil to form a thick, smooth dressing. Taste the vinaigrette and adjust the seasonings, if necessary. Transfer the vinaigrette to a bowl and set aside.

Prepare the Chicken Salad: In a large bowl, combine the chicken, cabbage, lettuce, snow peas, carrot, and ginger. Toss with enough of the vinaigrette to coat all the ingredients well.

Assemble the dish: If using white sesame seeds, in a dry pan, toast them over low heat, stirring continuously, until golden, about 1 minute.

Mound the salad mixture on chilled serving plates. Garnish with sesame seeds and scallions and serve immediately.

WOLFGANG'S HEALTHY TIPS

→ The mustard powder and honey in the dressing give it plenty of creamy body without the need for too much oil. And its lively seasonings have a big impact on every bite, making the salad very satisfying.

→ All of the good raw vegetables help to make you eat the salad slowly, so your hunger will be completely gone by the time you're finished.

→ Add other vegetables if you like, such as strips of red, orange, or yellow bell pepper, shredded scallion, or matchsticks of jicama.

→ If you can find little cardboard Chinese takeout boxes, perhaps in a restaurant supply store (or ask to buy some from your favorite Chinese restaurant), try serving individual appetizer or main-course portions in them, providing chopsticks for eating the salad straight from the box.

Nutrition Facts Per Serving (based on 4 servings): Calories: 421; Calories from Fat: 134; Total Fat: 14.97g; Saturated Fat: 3.19g; Monounsaturated Fat: 6.64g; Polyunsaturated Fat: 5.14g; Cholesterol: 119mg; Sodium: 394mg; Total Carbohydrate: 22.79g; Dietary Fiber: 4.57g; Sugars: 13.91g; Protein: 46.80g

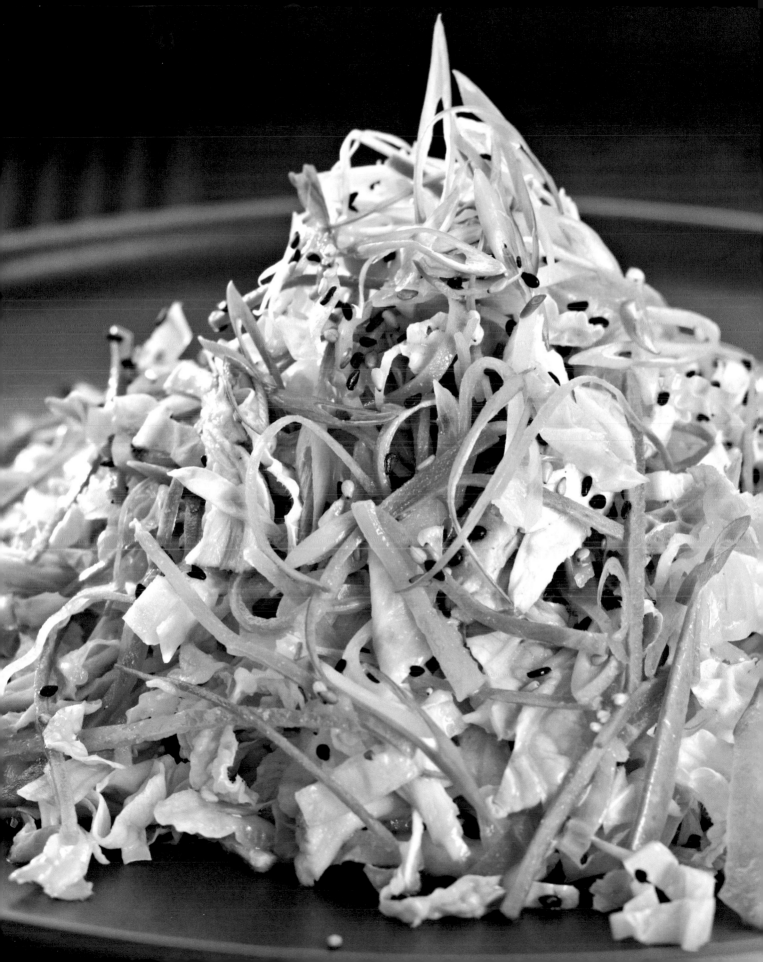

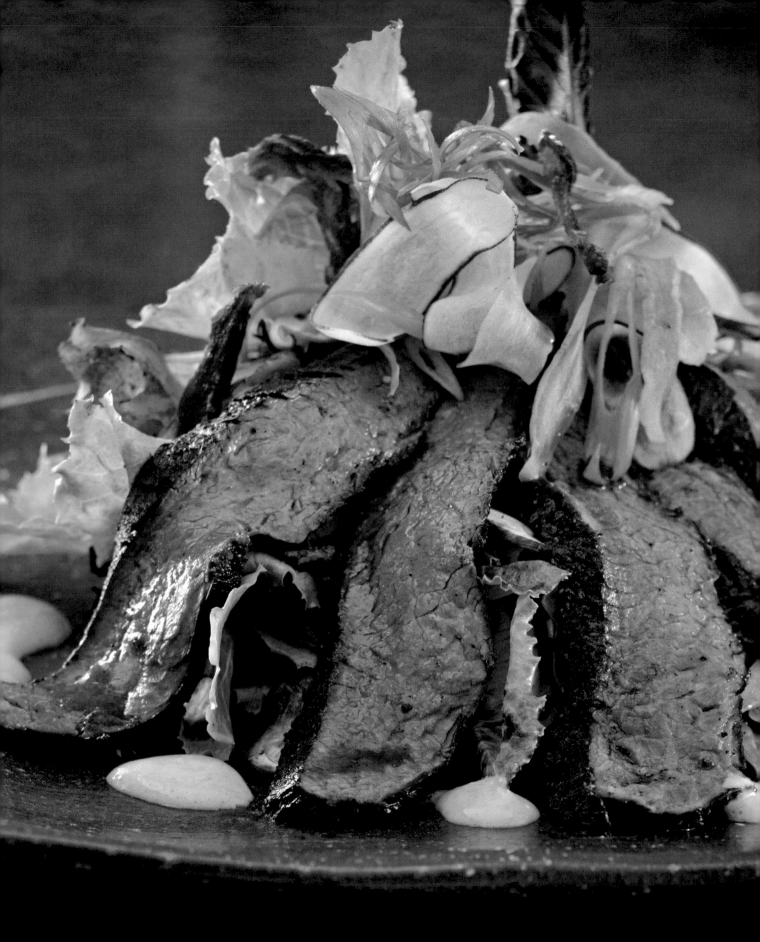

Chinois Grilled London Broil Salad with Cilantro-Mint-Yogurt Dressing

SERVES 4

Asian flavors make an already rich-tasting cut of lean meat even livelier, while the bed of salad vegetables adds even more taste and texture while filling you up.

1½ pounds flank steak

½ cup low-sodium soy sauce

¼ cup mirin (Japanese rice cooking wine)

½ cup chopped scallions, plus 2 scallions, cut diagonally into thin slices, for serving

1 tablespoon minced fresh ginger

1 teaspoon red pepper flakes

1 garlic clove, minced

Freshly ground black pepper

10 ounces baby spinach leaves

1 small head radicchio, cut crosswise into chiffonade strips

4 dates, pitted and cut lengthwise into thin strips

1 large carrot, cut lengthwise into very thin slices

1 large or 2 medium radishes, cut lengthwise into very thin slices

1 cup Cilantro-Mint-Yogurt Dressing (page 280)

Thoroughly trim the flank steak of connective tissue and excess fat; put the steak in a shallow, flat, nonreactive dish large enough to hold it flat. In a mixing bowl, stir together the soy sauce, mirin, chopped scallions, ginger, red pepper flakes, and garlic. Pour the mixture over the steak, cover with plastic wrap, and place in the refrigerator to marinate for 1 to 2 hours.

Prepare a fire in an outdoor grill or preheat a broiler, stovetop ridged grill pan, countertop grill, or broiler.

Remove the steak from the marinade. Discard the marinade. Pat the steak dry with paper towels and season on both sides with black pepper. Grill or broil until medium rare, about 5 minutes per side. Remove the steak from the grill and let rest in a warm place, covered with foil, for about 10 minutes.

Meanwhile, in a large bowl, combine the spinach and radicchio and toss well. Arrange beds of the salad mixture on four serving plates.

Carve the steak diagonally across the grain into thin slices. Arrange the steak slices on top of the beds of salad and garnish with the dates, carrot, radishes, and diagonally sliced scallions. Drizzle the salad or dot the plate surrounding it with some of the Cilantro-Mint-Yogurt Dressing. Pass the remaining dressing at the table.

WOLFGANG'S HEALTHY TIPS

→ A lean and flavorful cut of beef, flank steak (which is sometimes referred to as London broil on menus and in butcher shops) can be tough. But cooking it quickly on the grill and then slicing it thinly across the grain makes every bite tender.

→ I like the way the slivers of date add unexpected touches of sweetness as you eat the salad, complementing both the meat and its tangy-sweet dressing. If you don't have dates on hand, try other dried fruit such as apricots or just a few spoonfuls of seedless raisins.

→ Add any other vegetables you like to the salad mixture, such as thinly sliced mushrooms or bell peppers, or different kinds of salad leaves.

Nutrition Facts Per Serving: Calories: 338; Calories from Fat: 84; Total Fat: 9.42g; Saturated Fat: 4.56g; Monounsaturated Fat: 4.26g; Polyunsaturated Fat: 0.60g; Cholesterol: 117mg; Sodium: 331mg; Total Carbohydrate: 17.18g; Dietary Fiber: 3.52g; Sugars: 10.82g; Protein: 42.04g

Melon Salad with Prosciutto, Mozzarella, and Ice Wine Dressing

SERVES 4

Serve this salad as a refreshing start to an elegant warm-weather dinner party. Or enjoy it as a light lunchtime main dish.

½ ripe cantaloupe, seeded

½ ripe honeydew melon, seeded

2 tablespoons ice wine (Eiswein) or other sweet white dessert wine

1 tablespoon extra-virgin olive oil

2 teaspoons balsamic vinegar, preferably aged

Kosher salt

Freshly ground black pepper

½ pound low-fat mozzarella cheese, cut into ¾-inch cubes

4 thin slices prosciutto, trimmed of excess fat, cut lengthwise into strips about ¾ inch wide

2 cups loosely packed baby arugula leaves (about 1½ ounces)

Cut each melon half into wedges about ¾ inch thick. With a paring knife, carefully and neatly cut the rind and any hard, dark green flesh from each slice, leaving just the ripe fruit. Cut the fruit into ¾-inch dice. Arrange the melon in a large, shallow, nonreactive dish or pan.

In a small mixing bowl, stir together the ice wine, olive oil, and balsamic vinegar. Season to taste with salt and pepper.

Drizzle 1½ tablespoons of the ice wine dressing over the melon cubes and turn to coat them evenly. Arrange the cubes attractively on individual chilled serving plates. Reserve the dish with the dressing. (Alternatively, cover and refrigerate the melon for no more than an hour before arranging the cubes on the plates.)

Place cubes of mozzarella among the melon cubes on each plate. Drape the prosciutto among the cubes of melon and cheese. Put the arugula in the shallow dish in which you dressed the melon and add the remaining ice wine dressing. Toss until the arugula is evenly coated. Mound the arugula attractively on top of the melon in the center of each plate. Serve immediately.

WOLFGANG'S HEALTHY TIPS

→ Looking at the Nutrition Facts, you'll notice that this is somewhat higher in fat than many recipes in this book, with about 39 percent of calories coming from fat in the mozzarella and prosciutto. You can reduce the fat by using nonfat mozzarella and taking special care to trim all visible fat from the prosciutto, or by leaving out the cheese and/or prosciutto completely and serving this as a very refreshing and delicious low-fat melon and arugula salad.

→ Alternatively, simply pair this dish with one of the very low-fat main courses and desserts in this book for a complete meal that meets your healthy eating goals.

→ Try the recipe with other melons, too, such as Crenshaws or Persian melons. You can make it with just one kind of melon, if you like. The recipe also works well with ripe peaches or nectarines, or juicy pears.

Nutrition Facts Per Serving: Calories: 311; Calories from Fat: 120; Total Fat: 13.37g; Saturated Fat: 6.94g; Monounsaturated Fat: 5.51g; Polyunsaturated Fat: 0.92g; Cholesterol: 34mg; Sodium: 506mg; Total Carbohydrate: 24.70g; Dietary Fiber: 2.22g; Sugars: 20.14g; Protein: 18.00g

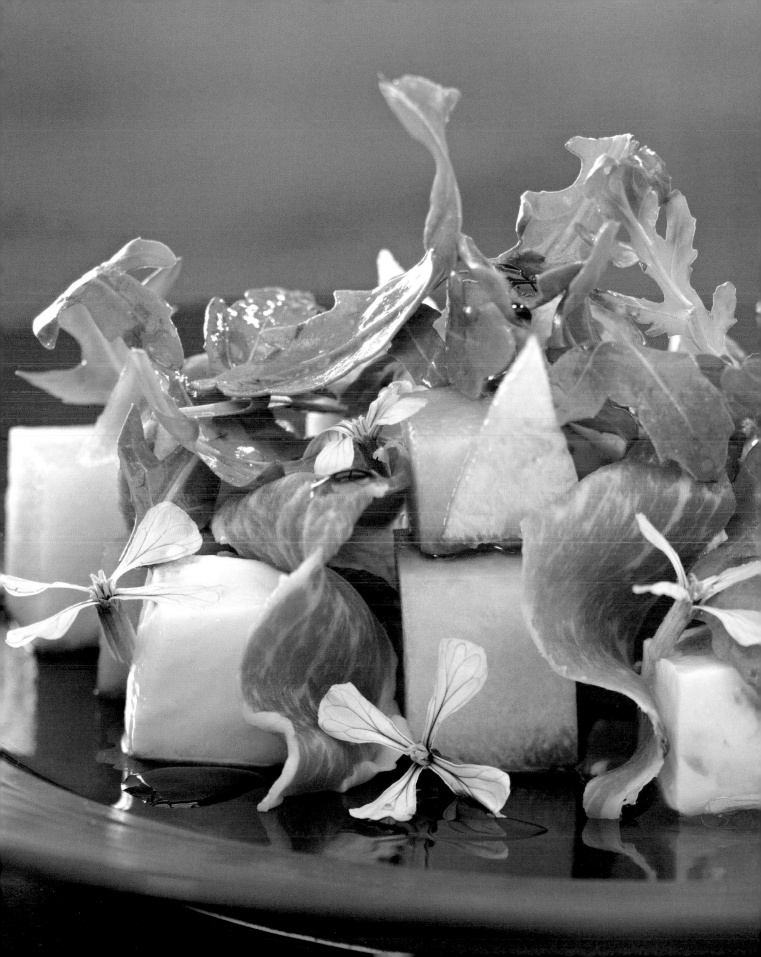

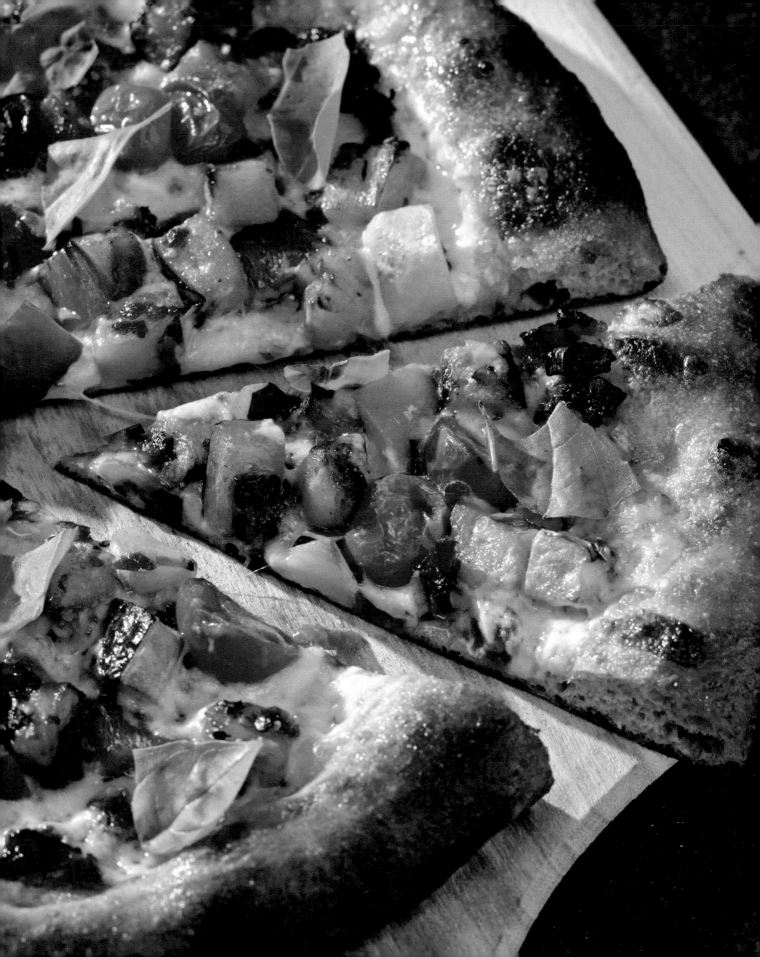

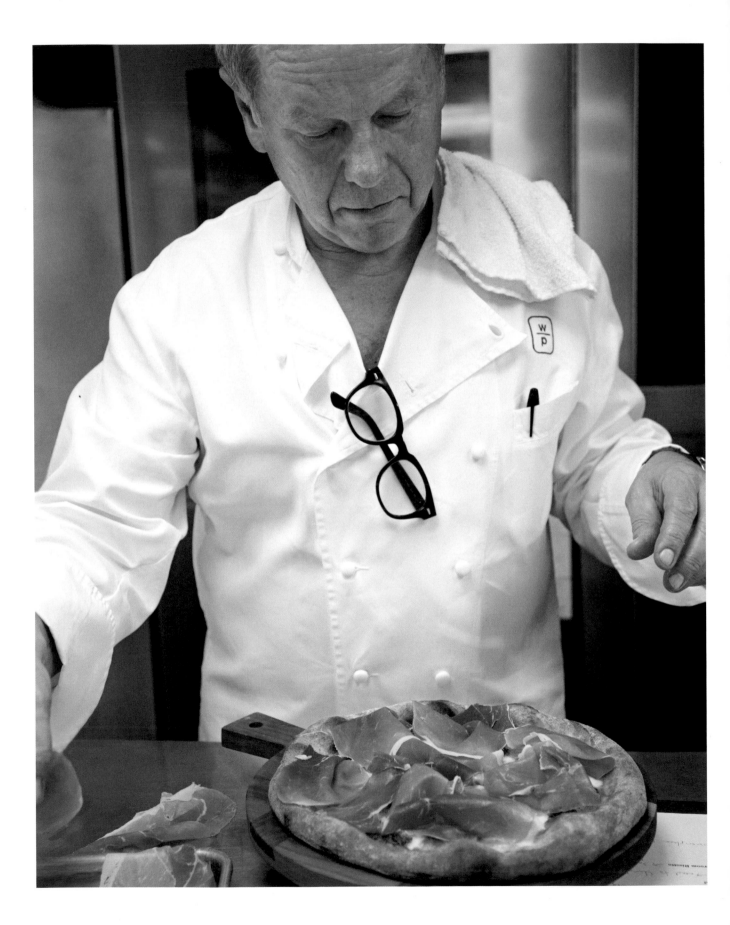

PASTA AND PIZZA

So many people love pasta and pizza. And so many people who are trying to eat more healthfully worry that consuming too many carbs from these popular dishes will prevent them from losing weight, or make them gain weight. But if you think that way, you are missing out on some of dining's greatest pleasures.

I believe that you can make pasta and pizza a regular part of your healthy eating plan by observing a few simple rules, which I've tried to follow in the recipes in this chapter. First, try as much as possible to serve moderate portions of high-fiber, nutrient-rich whole-grain pasta varieties, whether whole wheat or made from other grains such as brown rice or spelt. You'll find more and more good-tasting choices like these today in the pasta aisles of well-stocked supermarkets. And make your pizza with a higher-fiber whole wheat dough like the recipe I provide (page 287).

Just as important, of course, is what you combine with them. The recipes that follow feature an abundance of fresh vegetables and other healthy ingredients, while cutting down on high-fat dairy products and oil. You'll find that there are many other ways to pack your pasta and pizza with flavor, making every bite a health-filled pleasure.

→ Pasta with Fresh Tomatoes, Basil, and Garlic

→ Pasta with Fresh Tomatoes, Black Olives, and Anchovies

→ Bow Ties with Spring Vegetables and Roasted Garlic

→ Pasta with Wild Mushrooms, Fava Beans, Onion and Garlic Soubise, and Fresh Thyme

→ Pasta with Broccoli Rabe, Goat Cheese, Sun-Dried Tomatoes, and Toasted Pine Nuts

→ Sweet Potato Gnocchi with Onion-Garlic-Raisin Sauce, Sautéed Wild Mushrooms, and Peas

→ Chicken Pad Thai

→ Mandarin Noodles with Sautéed Pork Tenderloin and Vegetables

→ Healthier Pizzas

   ★ Summer Vegetable Pizza

   ★ Prosciutto Pizza

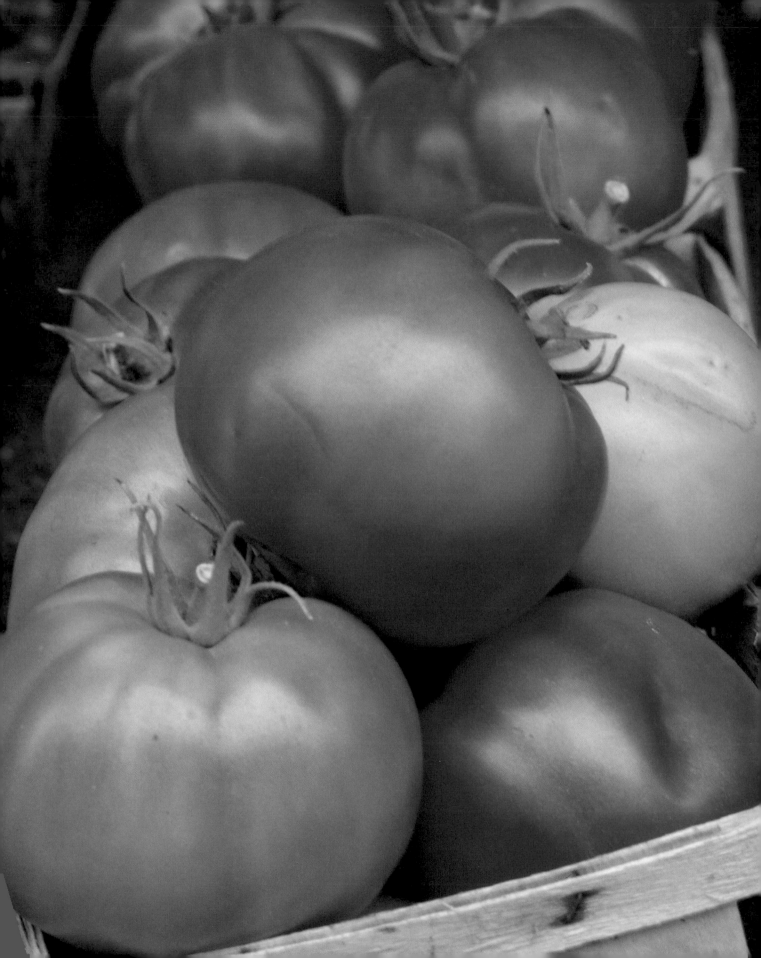

Pasta with Fresh Tomatoes, Basil, and Garlic

SERVES 4

When fresh produce is in season and at its peak, the simplest preparations are the most spectacularly delicious. This classic pasta featuring sun-ripened summer tomatoes is a perfect example.

2 tablespoons extra-virgin olive oil

1 tablespoon chopped garlic

2 teaspoons chopped shallot

2 pounds whole sun-ripened tomatoes, peeled, seeded (see page 288), and coarsely chopped

2 teaspoons tomato paste

1 teaspoon kosher salt

¼ cup Light Sun-Dried Tomato Pesto (page 281)

12 ounces thin whole wheat spaghettini or other thin whole grain pasta strands

1 teaspoon chopped fresh thyme leaves

¼ cup chopped fresh basil leaves

Freshly grated Parmesan, for serving (optional)

Bring a large pot of water to a boil.

In a 12-inch skillet, heat the olive oil over medium heat. Sauté the garlic and shallot just until they begin to color, about 5 minutes. Add the tomatoes, tomato paste, and salt and cook, stirring occasionally, until a thick but still fluid sauce forms, about 15 minutes. Stir in the Light Sun-Dried Tomato Pesto.

As soon as the pot of water comes to a boil, salt the water. Add the pasta and cook until al dente—tender but still slightly chewy—following the manufacturer's suggested cooking time.

Drain the pasta and add it, still slightly dripping, to the tomato sauce along with the thyme. Gently stir to coat the pasta with the sauce.

To serve, divide the pasta and sauce evenly among four large, warm plates or bowls. Garnish with basil and, if desired, Parmesan.

WOLFGANG'S HEALTHY TIPS

→ A spoonful of Light Sun-Dried Tomato Pesto (page 281) per serving further amps up the taste of the tomatoes. But if the produce you start with is spectacularly flavorful, you can leave out the pesto.

→ Serve this pasta as an appetizer, a light main course, or even as a side for simply grilled seafood, poultry, or meat.

Nutrition Facts Per Serving: Calories: 276; Calories from Fat: 81; Total Fat: 9.05g; Saturated Fat: 1.35g; Monounsaturated Fat: 6.32g, Polyunsaturated Fat: 1.37g, Cholesterol: 0mg; Sodium: 88mg; Total Carbohydrate: 43.82g; Dietary Fiber: 3.35g; Sugars: 6.96g; Protein: 9.04g

Pasta with Fresh Tomatoes, Black Olives, and Anchovies

SERVES 4

Enjoy this rustic Italian pasta dish as a casual main course—or as smaller appetizer servings—only when the best summer sun-ripened tomatoes are available. They are the foundation for the uncooked sauce, which is warmed only by the still-hot, just-drained pasta stirred into it.

2 tablespoons extra-virgin olive oil

½ cup plus 1 tablespoon chopped fresh flat-leaf parsley leaves

2 garlic cloves

2 anchovy fillets, patted dry with paper towels

¼ teaspoon red pepper flakes

1 pound red or mixed red and yellow cherry tomatoes, some left whole, some halved

¾ pound large sun-ripened tomatoes, peeled, seeded (see page 288), and coarsely chopped

¼ cup pitted, coarsely chopped cured black olives

¼ cup well-drained sun-dried tomatoes, cut into thin strips

½ tablespoon sugar

½ teaspoon kosher salt

¼ teaspoon freshly ground black pepper

¾ pound bite-size whole wheat pasta, such as fusilli, bow ties, or medium shells

Freshly grated Parmesan, for serving (optional)

Bring a large pot of water to a boil.

In a food processor fitted with the stainless-steel blade, combine the olive oil, ½ cup of the parsley, garlic, anchovies, and red pepper flakes. Process until uniformly pureed.

Pour the puree into a large bowl. Add the cherry tomatoes, chopped tomatoes, olives, and sun-dried tomatoes. Season with the sugar, salt, and black pepper. Set aside.

As soon as the pot of water comes to a boil, salt the water. Add the pasta and cook until al dente—tender but still slightly chewy—following the manufacturer's suggested cooking time. Drain the pasta and immediately add it to the bowl with the tomato mixture. Add the remaining 1 tablespoon parsley and toss well.

Spoon the pasta into individual large, shallow serving bowls. Serve immediately, passing Parmesan for guests who want it.

WOLFGANG'S HEALTHY TIPS

→ The anchovies don't really contribute a noticeable flavor to the dish but, instead, subtly season it with their brininess. If you like anchovies, feel free to increase the quantity.

→ For a vegan dish, leave out the anchovies and the optional Parmesan. You'll probably want to add some salt to replace the saltiness of the anchovies.

→ Try substituting fresh basil leaves for some or all of the parsley.

Nutrition Facts Per Serving: Calories: 290; Calories from Fat: 83; Total Fat: 9.29g; Saturated Fat: 1.42g; Monounsaturated Fat: 6.44g; Polyunsaturated Fat: 1.43g; Cholesterol: 1mg; Sodium: 207mg; Total Carbohydrate: 46.23g; Dietary Fiber: 7.44g; Sugars: 7.96g; Protein: 9.72g

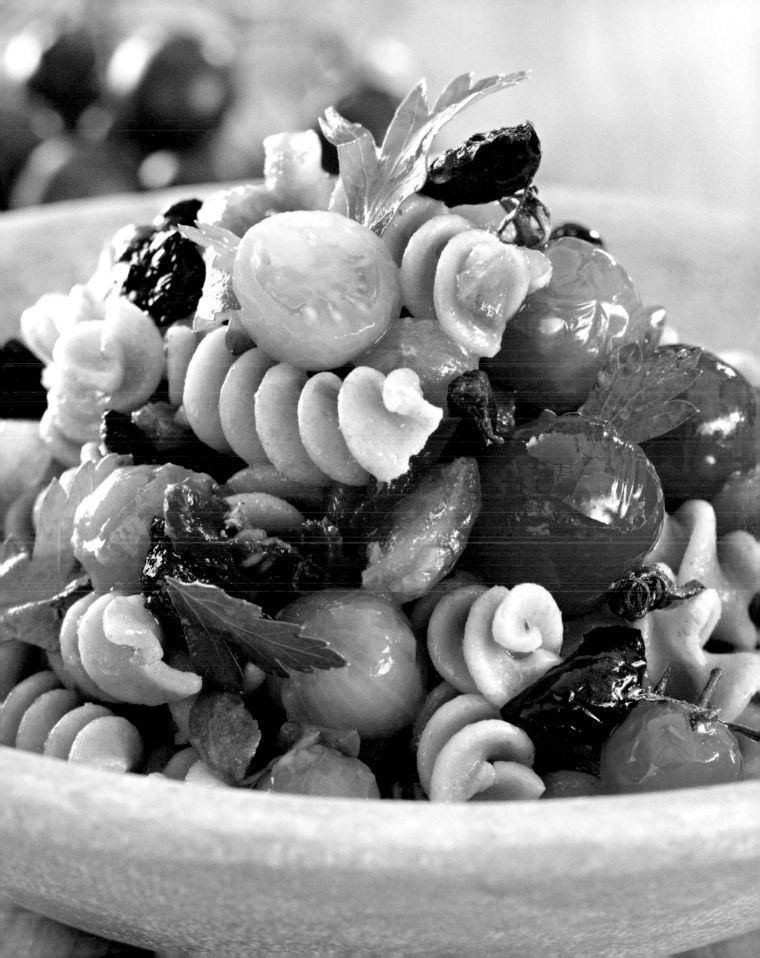

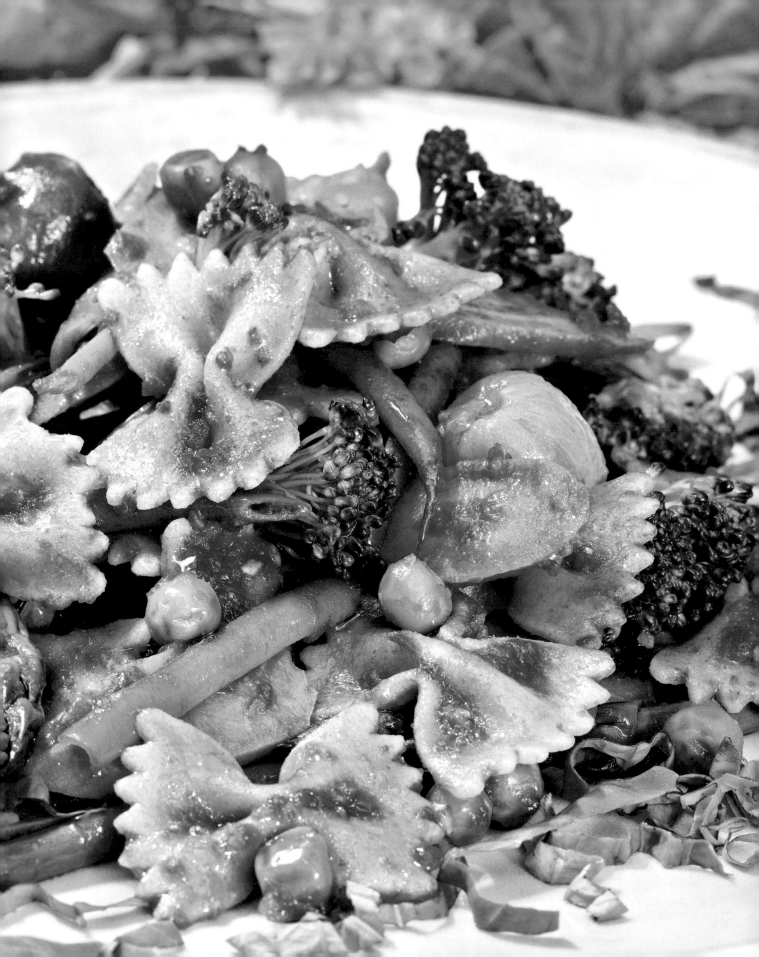

Bow Ties with Spring Vegetables and Roasted Garlic

SERVES 4

When fresh new produce fills the farmers' market, try this beautiful pasta dish. It has the power to make you forget that you're not having meat with your meal.

2 cups homemade Chicken Stock (page 271), Vegetable Stock (page 274), or good-quality canned low-sodium broth

2 tablespoons chopped drained sun-dried tomatoes

¼ cup packed finely shredded fresh basil leaves

1 tablespoon Roasted Garlic (page 284)

¼ cup chopped fresh flat-leaf parsley

1 sprig fresh sage

Kosher salt

Freshly ground black pepper

1 cup green beans cut into 1-inch pieces

1 cup thinly sliced carrots

12 spears pencil thin asparagus, trimmed and cut into 2-inch pieces

1 cup small broccoli florets

1 cup fresh or frozen peas

12 ounces dried whole wheat bow tie pasta or other bite-size whole-grain pasta shapes

¼ cup freshly grated Parmesan (optional)

Bring a large pot of water and a medium saucepan of lightly salted water to a boil.

In a blender, combine 1 cup of the stock with the sun-dried tomatoes, 2 tablespoons of the basil, the Roasted Garlic, and the parsley. Blend until pureed. Transfer the mixture to a saucepan with the remaining 1 cup stock, the sage, and salt and pepper to taste. Bring to a boil over high heat, then reduce the heat to medium and simmer briskly until the liquid reduces and thickens slightly.

While the sauce reduces, in separate batches, boil each of the vegetables for 1 minute in the saucepan of salted water. As each vegetable is done, remove it with a wire skimmer, rinse under cold running water until cool, drain well, and transfer to a bowl.

Remove the sage sprig from the sauce. Add all the vegetables to the sauce and stir well to heat them through. Keep warm.

As soon as the large pot of water comes to a boil, salt the water. Add the pasta and cook until al dente—tender but still slightly chewy—following the manufacturer's suggested cooking time.

Drain the pasta and stir it, still slightly dripping, into the sauce until well coated. Remove the pan from the heat and stir in the Parmesan, if using.

To serve, divide the pasta and vegetables among four large warmed plates or pasta bowls. Sprinkle each plate with some of the remaining 2 tablespoons basil. Serve immediately.

WOLFGANG'S HEALTHY TIPS

→ You'll be delighted by how big the flavors are in this light pasta-and-vegetable main dish, thanks to the powerful impact of a little Roasted Garlic (page 284), sun-dried tomatoes, fresh basil, and a medley of springtime produce.

→ If you like, stir other vegetables into the sauce, briefly blanching or sautéing those that need a little precooking or, for cherry tomato halves, simply adding them raw to the sauce.

→ Make the dish vegetarian by using vegetable stock, or vegan by eliminating the optional Parmesan as well.

Nutrition Facts Per Serving: Calories: 348; Calories from Fat: 52; Total Fat: 5.92g; Saturated Fat: 1.63g; Monounsaturated Fat: 3.29g; Polyunsaturated Fat: 1.01g; Cholesterol: 4mg; Sodium: 405mg; Total Carbohydrate: 61.73g; Dietary Fiber: 9.69g; Sugars: 6.37g; Protein: 17.29g

Pasta with Wild Mushrooms, Fava Beans, Onion and Garlic Soubise, and Fresh Thyme

SERVES 4

Even devoted meat eaters will love how robust and satisfying this pasta tastes. Use any kind of wild mushrooms available in your supermarket—or even regular cultivated white mushrooms.

1½ cups homemade Chicken Stock (page 271), Vegetable Stock (page 274), or good-quality canned low-sodium broth

½ pound assorted fresh wild mushrooms such as chanterelles, shiitakes, or porcini, wiped clean with a damp paper towel, trimmed

2 tablespoons extra-virgin olive oil

2 tablespoons minced shallot

1 tablespoon minced garlic

¼ cup Onion and Garlic Soubise (page 283)

Kosher salt

Freshly ground black pepper

1 tablespoon minced fresh thyme leaves

12 ounces whole wheat spaghetti or other whole-grain pasta strands

½ pound shelled fava beans, blanched and peeled (see page 288)

2 heaping tablespoons coarsely chopped fresh flat-leaf parsley

¼ cup freshly shaved Parmesan, for serving (optional)

Bring a large pot of water to a boil.

In a saucepan, bring the stock to a boil over medium-high heat, and then reduce the heat to very low and keep warm.

Cut the mushrooms into bite-size pieces.

In a large nonstick skillet or sauté pan, heat the olive oil over high heat. Add the shallot, garlic, and mushrooms and sauté, stirring continuously, until fragrant, about 2 minutes. Add the hot stock and stir and scrape with a wooden spoon to deglaze the pan. Stir in the Onion and Garlic Soubise and continue to cook for 2 minutes more. Season to taste with salt and pepper.

Stir in the chopped thyme. Continue cooking until the liquid has reduced by half, about 10 minutes.

As soon as the pot of water comes to a boil, salt the water. Add the pasta and cook until al dente—tender but still slightly chewy—following the manufacturer's suggested cooking time.

A few minutes before the pasta is done, add the fava beans to the sauce to cook briefly.

Drain the pasta and add it, still dripping, to the sauce, tossing to mix it well. Stir in the parsley and remove the pan from the heat.

To serve, divide the pasta among four large heated plates or bowls, taking care to distribute the mushrooms, fava beans, and sauce equally among the servings. Serve immediately, passing Parmesan at the table, if desired.

WOLFGANG'S HEALTHY TIPS

→ Instead of the fava beans, use ½ pound of any other vegetable you like, such as small snow peas, 1-inch pieces of asparagus, or coarsely chopped broccoli, blanching them and adding them toward the end of cooking the sauce.

→ Use vegetable stock for a vegetarian version, and also leave out the optional Parmesan for a vegan version.

→ If, on the other hand, you'd like a slightly meatier taste without adding too much fat, include a few slices of Canadian bacon, cut into thin strips and sautéed along with the mushrooms.

Nutrition Facts Per Serving: Calories: 462; Calories from Fat: 74; Total Fat: 8.33g; Saturated Fat: 1.29g; Monounsaturated Fat: 5.63g; Polyunsaturated Fat: 1.42g; Cholesterol: 0mg; Sodium: 229mg; Total Carbohydrate: 75.27g; Dietary Fiber: 17.31g; Sugars: 6.49g; Protein: 24.82g

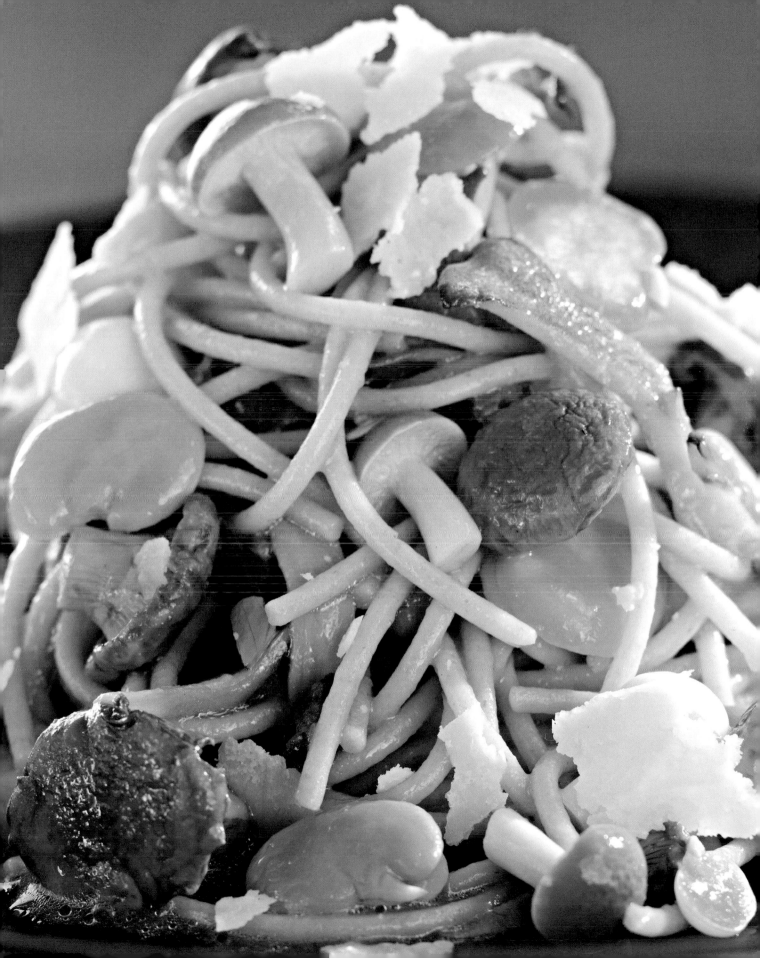

Pasta with Broccoli Rabe, Goat Cheese, Sun-Dried Tomatoes, and Toasted Pine Nuts

SERVES 4

A little bit of something rich and flavorful can go a long way, as the fresh, creamy goat cheese proves in this robust pasta dish.

1 tablespoon extra-virgin olive oil

3 cups broccoli rabe, cut into 1- to 1½-inch pieces

4 garlic cloves, minced

¼ to ½ teaspoon red pepper flakes

Kosher salt

Freshly ground black pepper

1½ cups homemade Chicken Stock (page 271) or good-quality canned low-sodium broth

1 teaspoon chopped fresh thyme leaves

4 ounces fresh, creamy goat cheese, crumbled

¾ pound dried whole wheat bow tie pasta or other bite-size whole-grain pasta shapes

¼ cup thinly sliced sun-dried tomatoes

2 tablespoons pine nuts, toasted (see page 289)

Bring a large pot of water to a boil.

In a nonstick sauté pan, heat the olive oil over medium-high heat. Add the broccoli rabe, garlic, and red pepper flakes and sauté, stirring frequently, until the broccoli rabe is bright green and just beginning to turn tender, 3 to 5 minutes. Season lightly with salt and pepper, transfer to a bowl, and set aside.

Still over medium-high heat, add the stock to the pan and stir and scrape to deglaze the pan. Add the thyme. Bring the liquid to a brisk simmer. Add about three-quarters of the goat cheese and stir until it melts and the liquid has a creamy coating consistency. Cover and keep warm.

As soon as the pot of water comes to a boil, salt the water. Add the pasta and cook until al dente—tender but still chewy—following the manufacturer's suggested cooking time.

Drain the pasta and immediately add it to the pan of sauce along with the broccoli rabe and sun-dried tomatoes. Cook over medium-low heat, stirring gently, until all the ingredients are heated through, about 2 minutes. Season to taste with salt and pepper.

Divide the pasta among four heated serving plates or shallow pasta bowls. Sprinkle with the remaining goat cheese and toasted pine nuts. Serve immediately.

WOLFGANG'S HEALTHY TIPS

→ If you can't find the long, skinny stalks of broccoli rabe, feel free to use regular broccoli or broccolini instead. Or try other robust vegetables such as cauliflower, asparagus, or ribbons of kale leaves with their tough ribs removed.

→ For a vegan version of the pasta, eliminate the goat cheese and use vegetable stock, starting with 2 cups and reducing it a bit longer to give it a little more body.

Nutrition Facts Per Serving: Calories: 316; Calories from Fat: 103; Total Fat: 11.51g; Saturated Fat: 4.97g; Monounsaturated Fat: 4.91g; Polyunsaturated Fat: 1.63g; Cholesterol: 13mg; Sodium: 356mg; Total Carbohydrate: 40.20g; Dietary Fiber: 5.92g; Sugars: 1.76g; Protein: 15.50g

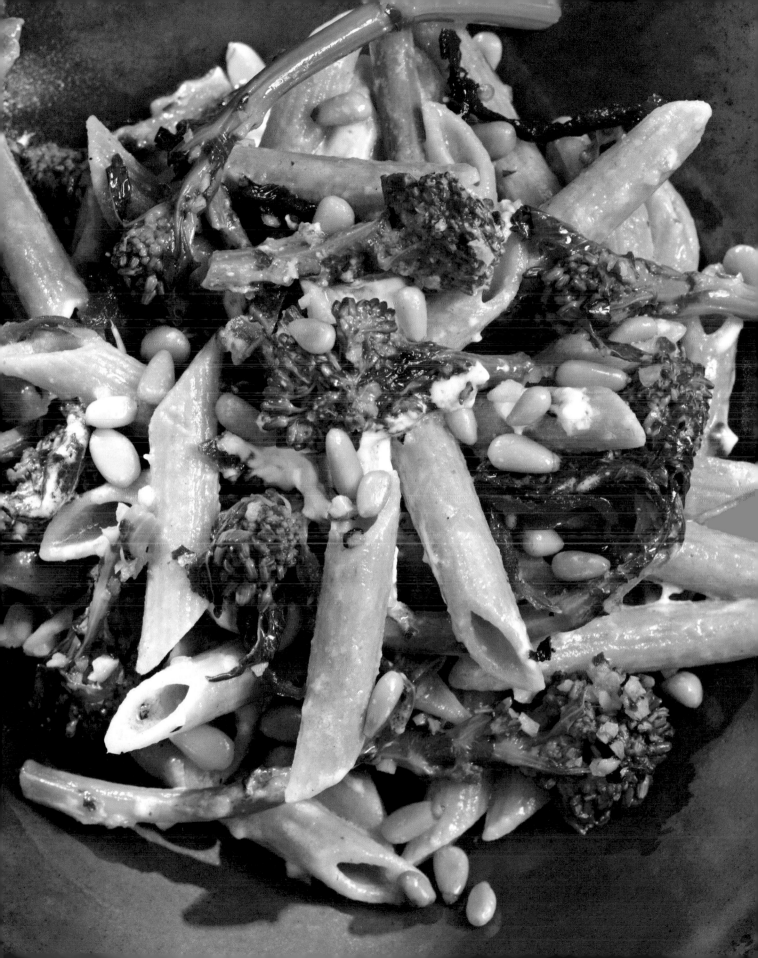

Sweet Potato Gnocchi with Onion-Garlic-Raisin Sauce, Sautéed Wild Mushrooms, and Peas

SERVES 8

Enjoy this autumn-colored, deeply flavorful, luxuriously textured pasta as an appetizer, as a side for roast chicken or pork or your Thanksgiving turkey, or in double portions as a main dish.

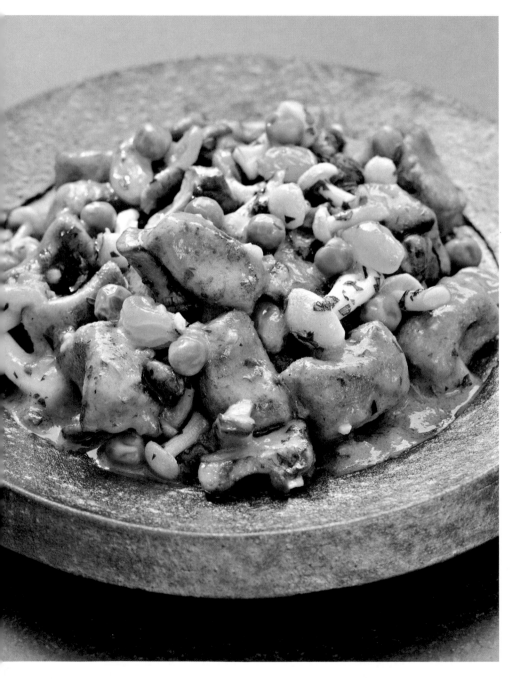

Sweet Potato Gnocchi:

1½ pounds sweet potatoes, peeled and quartered

½ to ⅔ cup whole wheat flour, plus more for dusting

2 tablespoons freshly grated Parmesan

½ large lightly beaten egg

Kosher salt

Freshly ground white pepper

Onion-Garlic-Raisin Sauce:

1 tablespoon extra-virgin olive oil

1 large shallot, minced

3 garlic cloves, minced

1 cup dry white wine

2 cups homemade Chicken Stock (page 271) or good-quality canned low-sodium broth

¼ cup packed seedless raisins

¼ cup Onion Soubise (page 283)

½ teaspoon minced fresh rosemary leaves

Kosher salt

Freshly ground white pepper

Sautéed Wild Mushrooms and Peas:

1 tablespoon extra-virgin olive oil

½ pound mixed wild mushrooms, such as shiitakes, porcini, and chanterelles, cleaned, trimmed, and cut into bite-size slices

½ cup fresh peas, blanched (see page 288), or frozen baby peas

1 large shallot, minced

2 garlic cloves, minced

Kosher salt

Freshly ground black pepper

To Assemble:

2 teaspoons chopped fresh flat-leaf parsley leaves

2 teaspoons minced fresh chives

½ cup freshly grated Parmesan, for serving (optional)

Prepare the Sweet Potato Gnocchi: Put the sweet potatoes in a pan of salted water. Bring to a boil over high heat, then reduce the heat to maintain a brisk simmer and cook until fork-tender, 25 to 30 minutes. Drain well. Press the sweet potatoes through a ricer into a bowl. Set aside to cool to room temperature.

Lightly dust a clean work surface with flour. Transfer the cooled riced sweet potatoes to the dusted surface. Sprinkle ½ cup of the flour over the potatoes. Sprinkle on the Parmesan. Make a well in the center and place the beaten egg in the well along with salt and pepper to taste. From the edges of the well, using a fork, start stirring the sweet potatoes into the egg, continuing until the mixture forms a ball, taking care not to overwork the dough. If the dough seems wet and hard to handle, sprinkle and work in the remaining flour.

To test for texture, bring a small sauce-pan of salted water to a boil. Shape a couple of gnocchi from the dough, each about ¼ inch in diameter and 1 inch long. Place the gnocchi in the boiling water and cook until they rise to the surface, 1 to 2 minutes, and then remove with a slotted spoon. If the gnocchi fall apart during boiling, work a little more flour into the remaining dough, but only a small amount at a time.

Line a baking sheet with parchment paper, lightly dust with flour. Divide the gnocchi dough into 8 portions. On a lightly floured surface, roll each portion into a long rope about ¼ inch in diameter and 15 inches long. Cut into 1-inch pieces and arrange the pieces in one layer on the prepared baking sheet. Set aside at room temperature until ready to use, up to 2 hours.

Prepare the Onion-Garlic-Raisin Sauce: In a medium saucepan, heat the olive oil over medium heat. Add the shallot and garlic and sauté until translucent, 3 to 5 minutes. Add the wine and stir and scrape with a wooden spoon to deglaze the pan. Boil the wine until it has reduced to about 1/4 cup, 7 to 10 minutes. Pour in the stock, bring to a boil, and continue boiling until the liquid has reduced by half, about 15 minutes.

While the sauce is reducing, bring a pot of salted water to a boil.

When the sauce is almost done reducing, stir the raisins, Onion Soubise, and rosemary into the sauce, season to taste with salt and pepper, cover, and keep warm.

Prepare the Sautéed Wild Mushrooms and Peas: Heat a large nonstick sauté pan over high heat. Add the olive oil and, when it is hot, add the mushrooms and sauté, stirring continuously, until tender-crisp, about 5 minutes. Stir in the peas, shallot, and garlic and sauté 2 to 3 minutes more. Season to taste with salt and pepper. Stir the sautéed mushrooms into the sauce.

Assemble the dish: Place the gnocchi in the boiling water and cook until they rise to the surface, 1 to 2 minutes. Drain well, then add the gnocchi to the pan of sauce. Stir gently to coat and combine. Serve immediately, spooning the gnocchi, sauce, and mushrooms onto heated plates or serving bowls. Garnish with parsley and chives and pass Parmesan at the table, if desired.

WOLFGANG'S HEALTHY TIPS

→ Gnocchi are usually made with regular potatoes, white flour, and often a generous amount of cheese. Using sweet potatoes and whole wheat flour, and only lightly seasoning them with Parmesan, turns them into a stream-lined recipe that you might even find more flavorful than the original.

→ Many gnocchi recipes feature sauces rich in butter, cream, or cheese. Here, a hearty mushroom sauce gives extra appeal without all that fat.

→ For a vegetarian version, use vegetable stock in place of the chicken stock.

→ It's not difficult to prepare the gnocchi from scratch. But since you're already making the effort to do it, I've given quantities that yield 8 servings. Save any gnocchi you don't want to cook right away by freezing them on a tray and then packing them in airtight freezer bags. Cook frozen gnocchi for a couple of extra minutes, testing one to make sure it's done.

Nutrition Facts Per Serving: Calories: 243; Calories from Fat: 46; Total Fat: 5.09g; Saturated Fat: 1.08g; Monounsaturated Fat: 3.28g; Polyunsaturated Fat: 0.73g; Cholesterol: 14mg; Sodium: 169mg; Total Carbohydrate: 39.36g; Dietary Fiber: 5.68g; Sugars: 10.88g; Protein: 7.01g

Chicken Pad Thai

SERVES 4 TO 8

With its generous amounts of vegetables and its lively flavors, the popular Thai noodle dish makes an admirably healthy main-course pasta, especially when you add lean chicken breast and tofu for protein.

Lime-Tamarind Sauce:

1¼ cups light brown sugar

6 tablespoons fresh lime juice

6 tablespoons tamarind paste

2 teaspoons kosher salt

1 teaspoon paprika

Garlic-Chile Sauce:

6 tablespoons Asian fish sauce

2 tablespoons rice vinegar

2 tablespoons sugar

2 tablespoons minced fresh cilantro leaves

4 teaspoons minced garlic

4 teaspoons minced Thai green chiles or small fresh green Mexican chiles

Stir-Fried Noodles:

8 ounces dried rice noodles, linguine size

2 eggs

2 teaspoons nonfat milk

Nonstick cooking spray

1 tablespoon peanut oil

2 teaspoons minced green chile

2 teaspoons chopped shallot

2 teaspoons minced fresh ginger

1 teaspoon minced lemongrass

2 Kaffir lime leaves, or 2 (2-by-½-inch) strips lime zest

2 tablespoons chopped fresh cilantro leaves, plus sprigs for garnish

1 pound boneless skinless chicken breast, cut into ¼-inch-thick strips

4 ounces firm tofu, well drained on paper towels, cut into ½-inch cubes

1 cup julienned cucumber

1 cup julienned carrot

2 cups bean sprouts

To Assemble:

½ cup thinly sliced green onion, for serving

1 lime, cut into 4 wedges, for serving

First, prepare the Lime-Tamarind Sauce: In a small saucepan, combine the sugar, lime juice, tamarind, salt, and paprika. Bring to a boil over medium-high heat, stirring frequently. Continue boiling and stirring just until the sauce has reduced and thickened slightly, 2 to 3 minutes. Set aside to cool.

Prepare the Garlic-Chile Sauce: In a small nonreactive bowl, stir together the fish sauce, rice vinegar, sugar, cilantro, garlic, chiles, and 2 tablespoons water. Set aside.

Prepare the Stir-Fried Noodles: Put the rice noodles in a bowl with 2 quarts of cold water and leave them just until softened, no more than a few minutes. Drain and set aside. (This can be done several hours ahead and covered.)

In a small bowl, beat together the eggs and milk. Heat a small skillet over medium heat. Coat with nonstick cooking spray. Add the egg mixture and cook until it forms soft, moist curds. Transfer to a plate and set aside to cool. Chop coarsely.

Heat a large nonstick wok over high heat. Add the peanut oil. When it's almost smoking-hot, add the chile, shallot, ginger, lemongrass, Kaffir lime, chopped cilantro, and chicken; stir-fry until the chicken loses its pink color, about 2 minutes. Add the noodles, tofu, cucumber, carrots, half of the bean sprouts, the scrambled egg, and both sauces. Continue stir-frying until the noodles have separated, heated through, and are glazed with the sauce and mixed with the other ingredients, 1 to 2 minutes more.

Assemble the dish: Transfer the noodles to a serving platter or individual serving plates, forming a mound. Arrange the remaining bean sprouts on top and garnish with cilantro sprigs and green onions. Serve with lime wedges to squeeze over the noodles.

Nutrition Facts Per Serving (based on 4 servings): Calories: 826; Calories from Fat: 134; Total Fat: 14.94g; Saturated Fat: 3.61g; Monounsaturated Fat: 5.59g; Polyunsaturated Fat: 5.74g; Cholesterol: 244mg; Sodium: 825mg; Total Carbohydrate: 103.04g; Dietary Fiber: 3.74g; Sugars: 67.12g; Protein: 65.66g

---

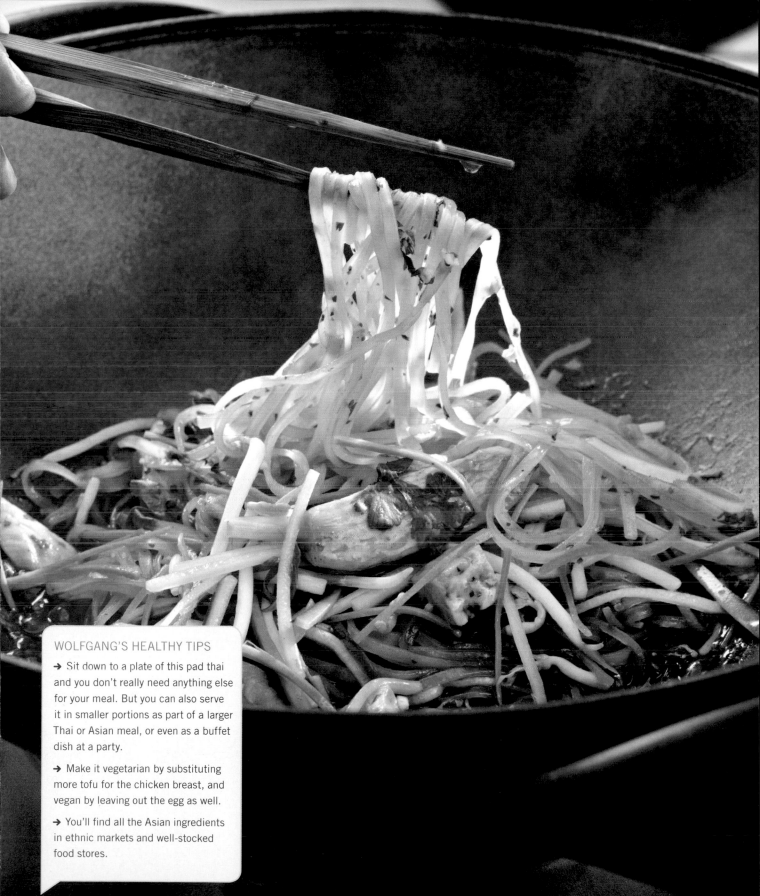

WOLFGANG'S HEALTHY TIPS

→ Sit down to a plate of this pad thai and you don't really need anything else for your meal. But you can also serve it in smaller portions as part of a larger Thai or Asian meal, or even as a buffet dish at a party.

→ Make it vegetarian by substituting more tofu for the chicken breast, and vegan by leaving out the egg as well.

→ You'll find all the Asian ingredients in ethnic markets and well-stocked food stores.

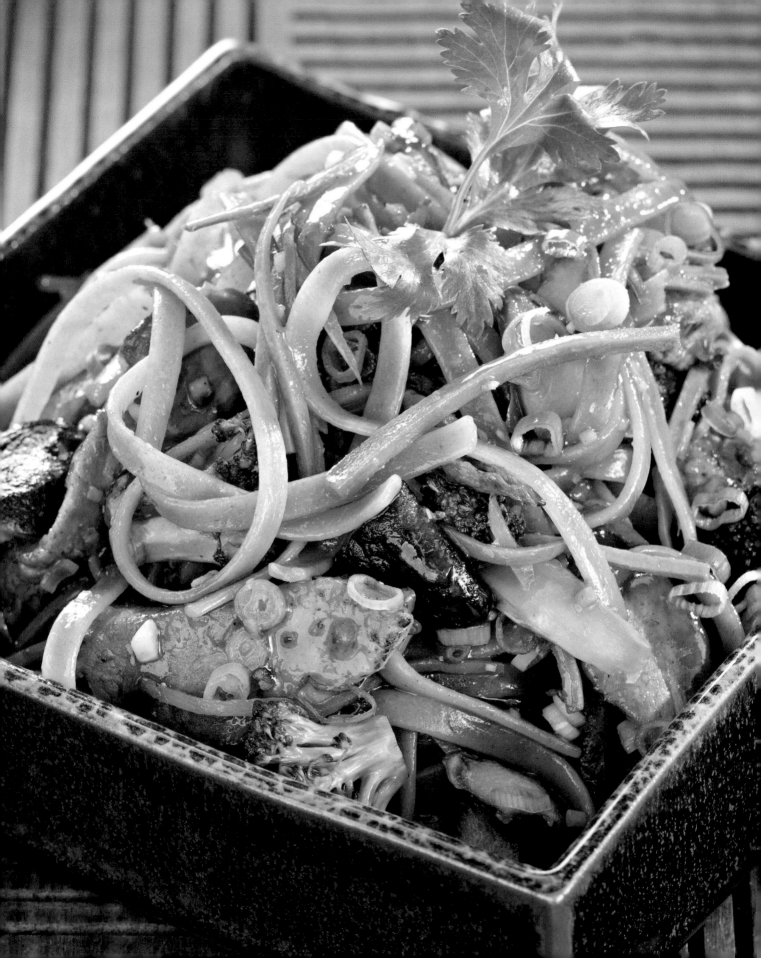

Mandarin Noodles with Sautéed Pork Tenderloin and Vegetables

SERVES 4

At the Chinese New Year, noodles are traditionally served as symbols of long life. Cook whole-grain noodles with minimal fat, lean meat, and lots of vegetables, and you could certainly have a healthier year ahead!

½ pound dried whole wheat pasta strands such as spaghetti or linguine

½ tablespoon peanut oil or vegetable oil

¾ pound pork tenderloin, trimmed of excess fat, cut into thin strips

½ pound fresh shiitake mushrooms, stems removed, caps quartered

¼ pound carrots, cut into thin julienne strips

¼ pound asparagus, trimmed and cut diagonally into thin slices

¼ pound broccoli, crowns cut into small florets, stems cut diagonally into thin slices

1½ tablespoons thinly sliced scallions

½ tablespoon finely chopped ginger

½ tablespoon finely chopped garlic

Kosher salt

Freshly ground black pepper

4 teaspoons Chinese plum wine

¾ cup homemade Chicken Stock (page 271), Vegetable Stock (page 274), or good-quality canned low-sodium broth

1 tablespoon rice wine vinegar (or fresh lime juice)

¼ cup hoisin sauce

Fresh cilantro leaves, for serving

Bring a pot of lightly salted water to a boil. Add the pasta and cook until al dente—tender but still chewy—following the manufacturer's instructions. Drain and set aside.

In a large nonstick wok or skillet, heat the oil over high heat. Add the pork tenderloin strips and stir-fry them, stirring continuously with a wooden or metal spatula, until lightly seared on all sides, about 3 minutes. Add the mushrooms, carrots, asparagus, broccoli, 1 tablespoon of the scallions, and the ginger and garlic, stir-fry for 3 minutes more. Season to taste with salt and pepper. Remove the meat and vegetables from the pan and set aside.

Add the plum wine and deglaze the pan with a wooden spoon, stirring and scraping to dissolve the pan deposits. Bring to a boil over high heat and cook until the liquid has reduced by half, about 1 minute. Add the stock and continue to boil until the liquid has thickened slightly, 2 to 3 minutes more. Add the cooked pasta and the reserved meat and vegetables. Stir in the rice wine vinegar and hoisin and cook briefly, just until heated through. Correct the seasonings, if necessary, with more salt and pepper.

Mound the meat, vegetables, noodles, and sauce in individual plates or bowls or a large serving bowl. Garnish with the remaining chopped scallions and cilantro leaves. Serve immediately.

WOLFGANG'S HEALTHY TIPS

→ Using a nonstick wok or skillet makes it easier to stir-fry without using too much fat. But a little peanut oil helps the ingredients to brown and keeps them from sticking, and it also adds to the authentic flavor.

→ Substitute fresh peeled and deveined shrimp or strips of boneless skinless chicken breast for the pork, and feel free to add more of any kinds of vegetable you like in small pieces that will stir-fry quickly.

→ For a vegetarian or vegan version, replace the meat with cubes of well-drained firm tofu and use vegetable stock.

Nutrition Facts Per Serving: Calories: 362; Calories from Fat: 66; Total Fat: 7.38g; Saturated Fat: 2.29g; Monounsaturated Fat: 3.44g; Polyunsaturated Fat: 1.65g; Cholesterol: 51mg; Sodium: 407mg; Total Carbohydrate: 42.94g; Dietary Fiber: 4.33g; Sugars: 10.28g; Protein: 27.36g

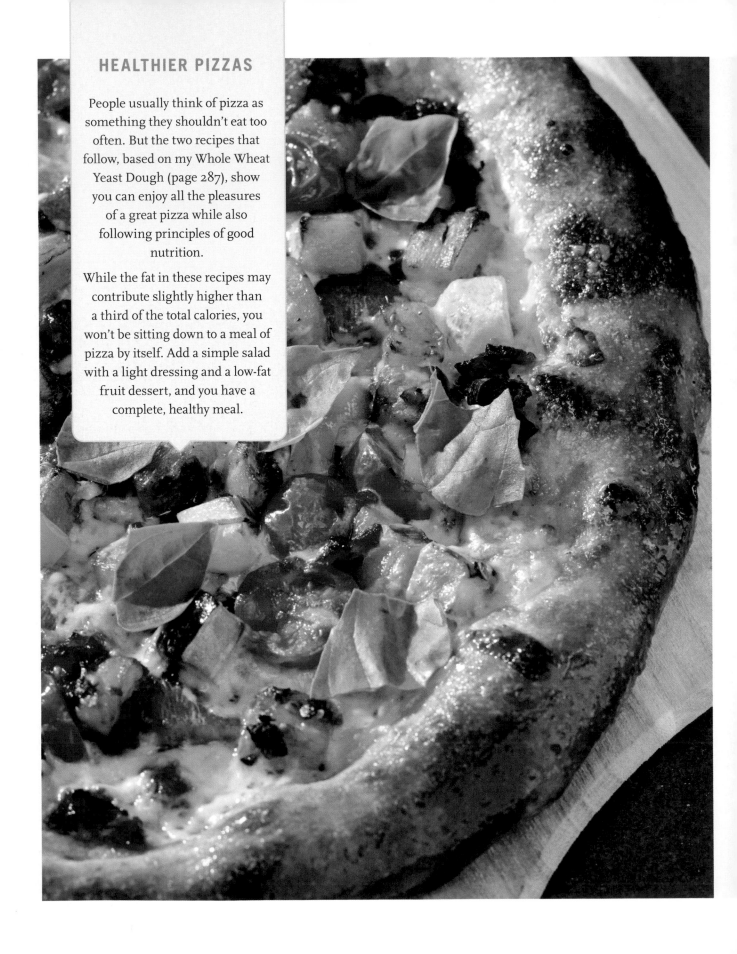

HEALTHIER PIZZAS

People usually think of pizza as something they shouldn't eat too often. But the two recipes that follow, based on my Whole Wheat Yeast Dough (page 287), show you can enjoy all the pleasures of a great pizza while also following principles of good nutrition.

While the fat in these recipes may contribute slightly higher than a third of the total calories, you won't be sitting down to a meal of pizza by itself. Add a simple salad with a light dressing and a low-fat fruit dessert, and you have a complete, healthy meal.

Summer Vegetable Pizza

SERVES 8

What a great way to eat a lot of vegetables! Feel free to vary the vegetable toppings with whatever looks great at the farmers' market.

Nonstick cooking spray

1 tablespoon extra-virgin olive oil

2 cups Asian eggplant cut into ½-inch dice

2 cups zucchini cut into ½-inch dice

2 cups yellow summer squash cut into ½-inch dice

1 cup red bell pepper cut into ½-inch dice

1 cup yellow bell pepper cut into ½-inch dice

3 cups halved cherry tomatoes

1 cup chopped thoroughly drained sun-dried tomatoes

4 teaspoons sugar

Kosher salt

Freshly ground black pepper

1 to 2 teaspoons red pepper flakes (optional)

Whole Wheat Yeast Dough, formed into 4 equal balls (page 287)

2 cups shredded low-fat mozzarella cheese

¼ cup freshly grated Parmesan

8 large fresh basil leaves, torn into small pieces, for serving

Place a pizza stone or baker's tiles on the middle rack of the oven and preheat the oven to 500°F.

Heat a large, heavy skillet over medium heat. Spray with nonstick cooking spray and add the olive oil. Add the eggplant, zucchini, squash, and bell peppers and sauté, stirring frequently, until the vegetables begin to turn tender, 5 to 7 minutes. Stir in the cherry tomatoes and sun-dried tomatoes. Season with the sugar and salt and pepper to taste. Add the red pepper flakes, if you like. Raise the heat to medium high and continue sautéing, stirring frequently, until the tomatoes soften, about 2 minutes more. Transfer to a bowl and set aside to cool.

To prepare each pizza, dip a ball of dough into flour and shake off the excess. Place the ball on a clean, lightly floured surface, and start to stretch it out, pressing down on the center and spreading the dough into an 8-inch circle with a slightly thicker rim. (If you find this difficult, use a small rolling pin to help, and then pinch up the rim.)

Evenly top the 4 circles of dough with the mozzarella. Evenly distribute the vegetable mixture over the cheese.

Using a floured pizza paddle or rimless baking sheet, transfer the pizzas to the stone or tiles, working in batches if necessary. Bake until the crust is nicely browned, 8 to 10 minutes.

Sprinkle each pizza with Parmesan and garnish with basil. Transfer to a cutting board and cut into slices. Serve immediately.

WOLFGANG'S HEALTHY TIPS

→ If you like, just before serving, you could also top each pizza with 1 to 2 cups of a simple salad like baby arugula or spinach leaves tossed with a light vinaigrette (pages 275–278).

→ For another variation, try slicing and grilling the vegetables first. Then, cut them into chunks and arrange them on top of a thin spreading of my Light Pesto (page 281) before topping with the cheese.

Nutrition Facts Per Serving: Calories: 471; Calories from Fat: 160; Total Fat: 17.87g; Saturated Fat: 5.41g; Monounsaturated Fat: 10.35g; Polyunsaturated Fat: 2.11g; Cholesterol: 17mg; Sodium: 426mg; Total Carbohydrate: 58.61g; Dietary Fiber: 8.26g; Sugars: 10.97g; Protein: 17.94g

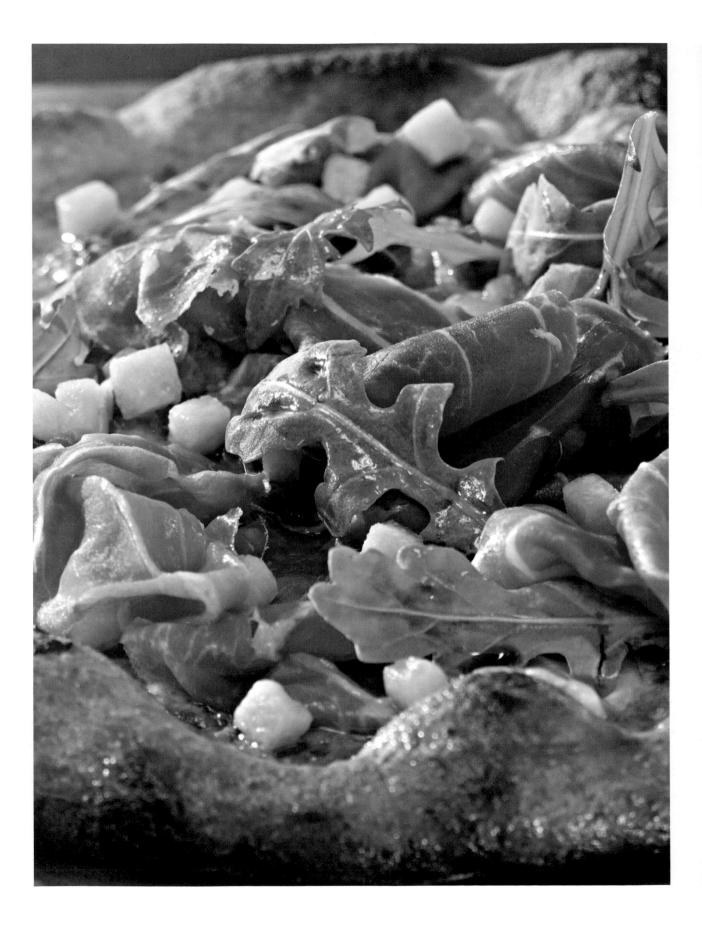

Prosciutto Pizza

SERVES 8

I especially like the simplicity of this pizza. You can even cut each one into thinner slices to serve as an hors d'oeuvre with cocktails or as part of a buffet. The optional melon re-creates, in pizza form, the classic melon-and-prosciutto appetizer.

Whole Wheat Yeast Dough, formed into 4 equal balls (page 287)

½ cup Light Sun-Dried Tomato Pesto (page 281)

1 pound fresh mozzarella cheese, drained and thinly sliced

4 ounces thinly sliced prosciutto

½ cup melon cut into ¼-inch dice (optional)

½ cup packed baby arugula leaves

2 tablespoons aged balsamic vinegar

Place a pizza stone or baker's tiles on the middle rack of the oven and preheat the oven to 500°F.

To prepare each pizza, dip a ball of dough into flour and shake off excess. Place the ball on a clean, lightly floured surface, and start to stretch it out, pressing down on the center and spreading the dough into an 8-inch circle with a slightly thicker rim. (If you find this difficult, use a small rolling pin to help, and then pinch up the rim.)

Brush each circle with the Light Sun-Dried Tomato Pesto, staying within the rim. Evenly distribute the fresh mozzarella slices on top.

Using a floured pizza paddle or rimless baking sheet, transfer the pizzas to the stone or tiles. Bake until the cheese is melted and bubbly and the crust is nicely browned, 8 to 10 minutes. Remove from the oven and drape the prosciutto on top. If you like, dot the prosciutto with the melon cubes. Scatter the arugula leaves on top. Drizzle with balsamic vinegar.

Transfer to a cutting board and cut into slices. Serve immediately.

> ## WOLFGANG'S HEALTHY TIPS
>
> → In place of prosciutto, feel free to substitute very thinly sliced lean ham of any kind, or any other lean cold cut you prefer.
>
> → This is another pizza that is excellent topped with a salad of baby arugula or spinach leaves tossed with a little light vinaigrette (pages 275–278).

Nutrition Facts Per Serving: Calories: 496; Calories from Fat: 191; Total Fat: 21.32g; Saturated Fat: 8.18g; Monounsaturated Fat. 11.15g; Polyunsaturated Fat: 1.99g; Cholesterol. 37mg; Sodium: 709mg; Total Carbohydrate: 46.93g; Dietary Fiber: 4.27g; Sugars: 3.32g; Protein: 24.55g

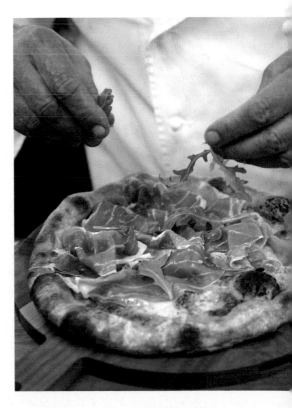

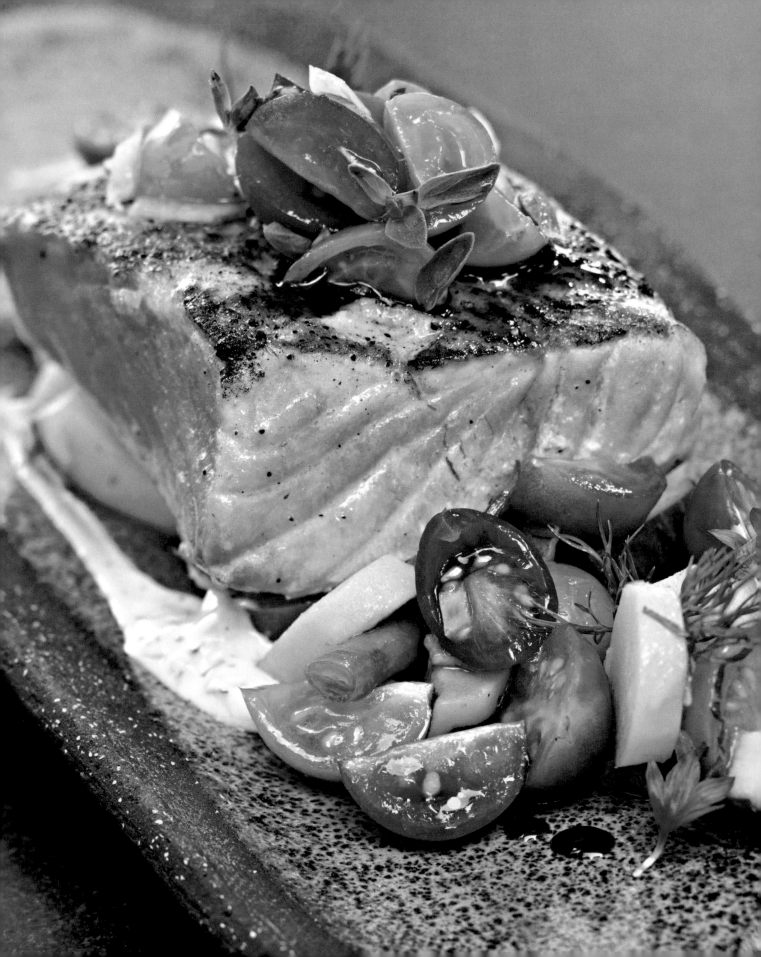

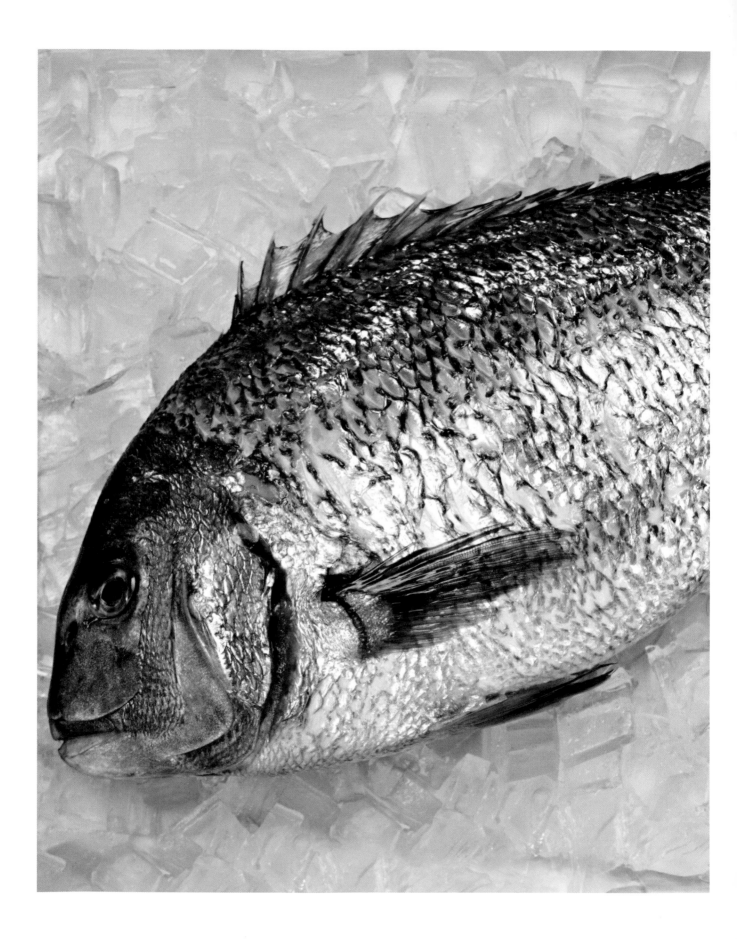

SEAFOOD MAIN DISHES

Not so long ago, it sometimes seemed to me that people who actually chose to eat seafood as a main dish, whether at home or in a restaurant, stood a good chance of being on a diet. How ironic that these dishes were often served with rich butter or cream sauces. And when they asked for something "plain grilled" or with "sauce on the side," they sounded like they were doing some sort of penance rather than enjoying a good meal.

With the fish and shellfish dishes in this chapter, though, you need never feel like you're suffering—or inadvertently cheating. I've created each of the recipes that follow to complement and amplify the flavor and texture of the wonderful fresh seafood you can find more and more often in specialty seafood shops and well-stocked supermarkets alike everywhere.

One of the best things about cooking seafood, by the way, is the flexibility of such recipes. Can't find good halibut, for example? It's no problem. Feel free to substitute any other mild, firm, white-fleshed fish, and there are so many good choices these days.

So please join me in celebrating how wonderful seafood main courses can be!

→ Asian-Style Steamed Snapper with Baby Bok Choy and Brown Rice

→ Thai Steamed Red Snapper Fillets with Brown Rice and Thai Sauce

→ Sea Bass en Papillote with Spicy Tomato Sauce, Fennel, Olives, and Capers

→ Citrus-Glazed Halibut with Braised Daikon and Pea Shoots

→ Tuna Tataki with Ginger-Soy-Lime Vinaigrette and Brown Sushi Rice

→ Broiled Miso Salmon with Spago Cucumber Salad

→ Seared Ahi Tuna with Grilled Pineapple–Mango Salsa

→ Grilled Loup de Mer with Tomatillo-Avocado Vinaigrette and Cherry Tomato Salsa

→ Grilled Salmon with Cucumber-Yogurt Sauce and Warm Potato-Vegetable Salad

→ Grilled Shrimp on Rosemary Skewers with Grilled Limes and Quinoa and Grilled Vegetable Pilaf

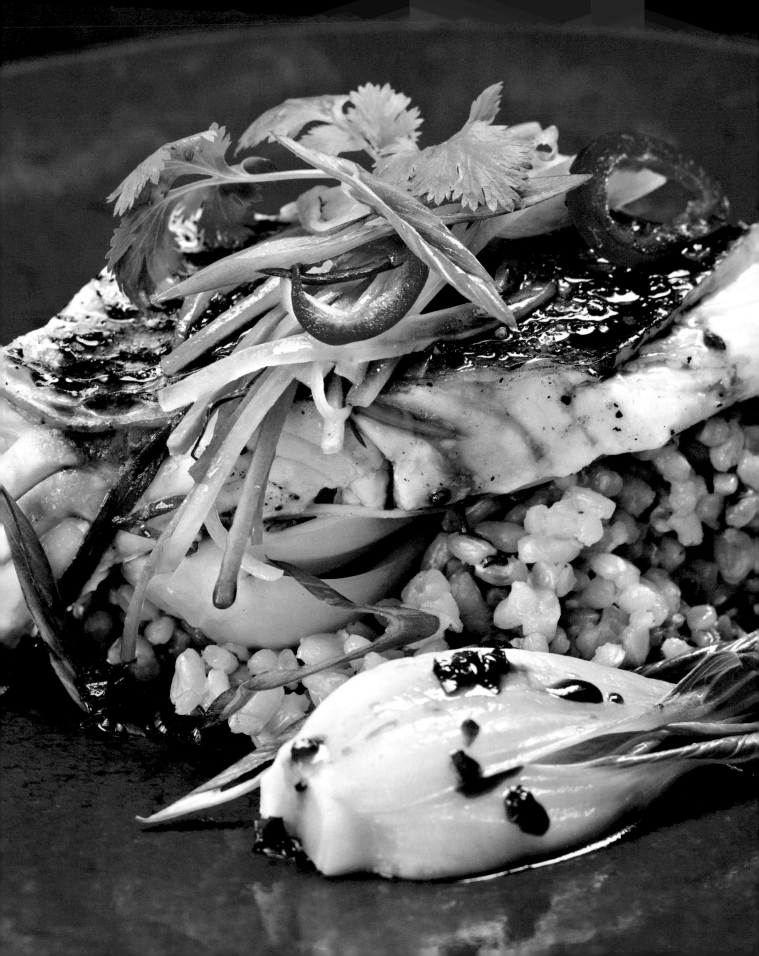

Asian-Style Steamed Snapper with Baby Bok Choy and Brown Rice

SERVES 4

Many people think of steamed food as bland, but this recipe proves that idea wrong. The Asian aromatics in the steaming liquid first scent the fish, and then go on to flavor the quickly made sauce that accompanies it.

Steamed Snapper and Bok Choy:

1 cup white wine

1 teaspoon peanut oil

4 sprigs fresh cilantro, plus more for garnish

3 scallions, cut into 1-inch pieces

1 (3-inch) piece ginger, thinly sliced

1 jalapeno, cut into 3 or 4 pieces

1 stalk fresh lemongrass, outer leaves only, cut into 1-inch pieces (reserve inner leaves for another use), or zest of 1 lemon, cut into long strips

Kosher salt

4 skin-on red snapper fillets, each about 4 ounces, or fillets of grouper or fresh cod

Freshly ground black pepper

4 large Napa cabbage leaves

1 large leek, thoroughly washed, cut into thin julienne strips

1 large carrot, cut into thin julienne strips

1 large celery stalk, cut into thin julienne strips

6 baby bok choy, halved lengthwise

Sauce:

1 tablespoon peanut oil

2 garlic cloves, thinly sliced

½ jalapeño, thinly sliced

1 tablespoon chopped fresh ginger

2½ tablespoons low-sodium soy sauce

1 tablespoon sugar

1 tablespoon unsalted butter, cut into small pieces

2 scallions, thinly sliced on the bias, white and green parts kept separate

To Assemble:

4 cups steamed brown rice or Brown Sushi Rice (page 200)

1 red or green jalapeño, cut into thin rings and seeded, for serving (optional)

Prepare the Steamed Snapper and Bok Choy: Put 4 cups water in the bottom pan of a steamer or in a saucepan large enough for a steamer basket to rest on top. Bring the water to a boil over high heat. Add the wine, oil, cilantro, scallions, ginger, jalapeño, and lemongrass or lemon zest. Season well with salt. Bring back to a boil, then reduce the heat and simmer for 10 minutes to allow the flavors to develop.

Season the fish fillets on both sides with salt and pepper. Line the steamer basket with the cabbage leaves, making sure that the surface is not completely covered so that steam can get through. Place the fish fillets, skin side up, on top of the cabbage leaves. In a small bowl, toss together the leek, carrot, and celery, and scatter the mixture on top of the fish fillets. Place the steamer basket over the saucepan. Cover and steam for 1 minute.

Carefully uncover the basket and arrange the baby bok choy halves around the fish. Cover again and continue steaming until the fish is cooked through, tender enough for the tines of a small fork to slide into the flesh easily without resistance, and the bok choy is tender but still slightly crisp, about 5 minutes more. Remove the vegetable-topped fish and bok choy from the steamer and cover and keep warm while you make the sauce. Reserve ½ cup of the steaming liquid.

CONTINUES

Prepare the Sauce: In a medium sauté pan, heat the peanut oil over medium-high heat. When the oil is hot, add the garlic, jalapeño, and ginger and sauté until the garlic is translucent, about 2 minutes, taking care not to let them brown. Stir in the reserved steaming liquid and the soy sauce and boil for 2 minutes. Stir in the sugar and boil until it has completely dissolved, about 1 minute. Reduce the heat to low and whisk in the butter. Add the scallion whites, stir briefly, and remove from the heat.

Assemble the dish: On each of four heated serving plates, mound about 1 cup of steamed rice. Arrange the steamed bok choy on top, and top it with the snapper fillet, skin side up. Spoon the sauce over the fish and bok choy and garnish with scallion greens, cilantro sprigs, and, if you like, some jalapeño rings.

WOLFGANG'S HEALTHY TIPS

➜ Notice how the aromatics in the steaming water gently but distinctively season the fish in this fat-free cooking method.

➜ Just a touch of butter adds subtle richness to the sauce without contributing too many calories or too much fat.

➜ Try this recipe with any other fish fillets you might prefer.

Nutrition Facts Per Serving: Calories: 379; Calories from Fat: 73; Total Fat: 8.20g; Saturated Fat: 2.91g; Monounsaturated Fat: 3.13g; Polyunsaturated Fat: 2.15g; Cholesterol: 21mg; Sodium: 410mg; Total Carbohydrate: 57.92g; Dietary Fiber: 5.39g; Sugars: 6.16g; Protein: 14.29g

Thai Steamed Red Snapper Fillets with Brown Rice and Thai Sauce

SERVES 4

You won't believe how delicious and big in flavor such a simple steamed dish can be, thanks to a quickly stirred-together sauce made from ingredients found in Asian markets or well-stocked supermarkets. At the Governors Ball following the 2013 Academy Awards, Ang Lee ate two portions of this shortly after receiving his Best Director Oscar for *Life of Pi*.

Thai Dipping Sauce:

1 cup Thai sweet chili sauce

¼ cup fish sauce

¼ cup fresh lime juice

2 tablespoons low-sodium soy sauce

2 tablespoons rice vinegar

3 scallions, chopped

2 tablespoons chopped garlic

2 tablespoons chopped shallot

2 tablespoons chopped ginger

1 sprig fresh cilantro

1 sprig fresh mint

1 Kaffir lime leaf, or 1 long strip fresh lime zest

Steamed Red Snapper:

4 (6-ounce) skinless red snapper fillets

To Assemble:

4 cups steamed brown rice or Brown Sushi Rice (page 200)

Prepare the Thai Dipping Sauce: About 24 hours before serving, in a nonreactive bowl, combine the Thai sweet chili sauce, fish sauce, lime juice, soy sauce, rice vinegar, scallions, garlic, shallot, and ginger. With the side of a heavy knife or a clean meat pounder, press down on the cilantro, mint, and Kaffir lime leaf to crush them slightly; then wrap them in a piece of clean cheesecloth, tie shut with kitchen string, and add to the bowl. Stir well. Cover and refrigerate.

Prepare the Steamed Red Snapper: Put 3 inches of water in the bottom pan of a steamer or in a saucepan large enough for a steamer basket to rest on top. Bring the water to a boil. Arrange the snapper fillets side by side in the steamer. Cover, set over the boiling water, and steam until the fish is cooked through, 3 to 5 minutes.

Assemble the dish: Remove the dipping sauce from the refrigerator and remove and discard the wrapped herbs. Transfer the sauce to small individual bowls. Arrange beds of brown rice on individual heated serving plates. With a spatula, carefully transfer the snapper fillets to rest on top of the rice. Serve the sauce on the side, to be spooned over individual portions to taste.

WOLFGANG'S HEALTHY TIPS

→ For the best flavor, the recipe suggests making the sauce the night before and leaving it to steep in the refrigerator. But don't let that stop you. Even an hour of steeping will produce a delicious sauce.

→ Make this with any other kind of fresh fish fillets you like, whether mild varieties like cod, tilapia, or grouper, or something richer-tasting like salmon or trout, adjusting steaming times according to the thickness of the fillets.

→ The sauce is also excellent with steamed, broiled, or grilled chicken breasts or turkey cutlets. You'll also like it spooned over the last of the rice!

Nutrition Facts Per Serving: Calories: 320; Calories from Fat: 21; Total Fat: 2.44g; Saturated Fat: 0.56g; Monounsaturated Fat: 0.78g; Polyunsaturated Fat: 1.10g; Cholesterol: 20mg; Sodium: 835mg; Total Carbohydrate: 55.50g; Dietary Fiber: 4.58g; Sugars: 2.63g; Protein: 18.10g

Sea Bass en Papillote with Spicy Tomato Sauce, Fennel, Olives, and Capers

SERVES 4

I love surprising people with a main course of seafood cooked *en papillote*—a French term meaning "in a paper pouch" that seals in all the moisture and flavor of the ingredients. Here, Italian-style seasonings might also make it appropriate to use that cuisine's term, *al cartoccio*.

4 (6-ounce) skinless sea bass fillets

Kosher salt

Freshly ground black pepper

Nonstick cooking spray, preferably olive oil flavored

1½ cups bottled arrabbiata sauce or other spicy tomato pasta sauce

¼ cup oil-packed sun-dried tomatoes, well drained and patted dry, cut into ¼-inch-wide strips

2 tablespoons drained small capers

24 pitted Kalamata olives, halved lengthwise

1 small fennel bulb, trimmed, halved, and sliced crosswise into thin shavings

8 fresh basil leaves

Adjust the oven shelf to the middle position and preheat the oven to 450°F.

Tear 4 sheets of aluminum foil, each large enough to fold over and comfortably enclose one of the sea bass fillets. Lightly season each fillet on both sides with salt and pepper. Lightly spray one side of each foil sheet with nonstick cooking spray and center a fillet on one half of each sheet.

Spoon 6 tablespoons of arrabbiata sauce over each fillet. Dot each fillet evenly with sun-dried tomatoes, capers, and olives. Arrange the fennel shavings over the fish and place 2 basil leaves on top of each fillet.

Fold the foil over each fillet. Double-pleat the edges of the foil tightly to create an airtight seal on the packets and carefully transfer the packets to a baking sheet. Bake for about 15 minutes.

Carefully transfer each foil packet to a dinner plate. Warn your guests in advance to watch out for and keep clear of the steam inside. Then, with the tip of a sharp knife, puncture each packet to let out some of the steam and let everyone carefully open their packets to eat the fish and toppings.

WOLFGANG'S HEALTHY TIPS

→ Dishes cooked *en papillote* are traditionally enclosed in parchment paper. But heavy-duty aluminum foil is more convenient and easier to seal.

→ Nonstick cooking spray helps keep the food from sticking to the foil, without adding any significant fat or calories.

→ The sea bass includes a good amount of heart-healthy omega-3 fatty acids. But feel free to substitute any other fish you like, including those even richer in omega-3s, such as halibut, tuna, or salmon.

→ Bottled pasta sauce makes this recipe especially easy. But be sure to read the Nutrition Facts label on the brand you buy and select one that isn't too high in fat. If you're watching your sodium intake, be sure to check that on the label, too.

→ Feel free to add even more vegetables to the packets, especially aromatic ones like carrots or sweet onions, all thinly sliced so they will cook in the brief time in the oven.

→ To soak up all the flavorful juices, serve with a healthy grain side dish such as couscous or simple steamed brown rice.

Nutrition Facts Per Serving: Calories: 202; Calories from Fat: 62; Total Fat: 6.92g; Saturated Fat: 1.48g; Monounsaturated Fat: 3.49g; Polyunsaturated Fat: 1.96g; Cholesterol: 24mg; Sodium: 437mg; Total Carbohydrate: 21g; Dietary Fiber: 5.7g; Sugars: 8.54g; Protein: 13.56g

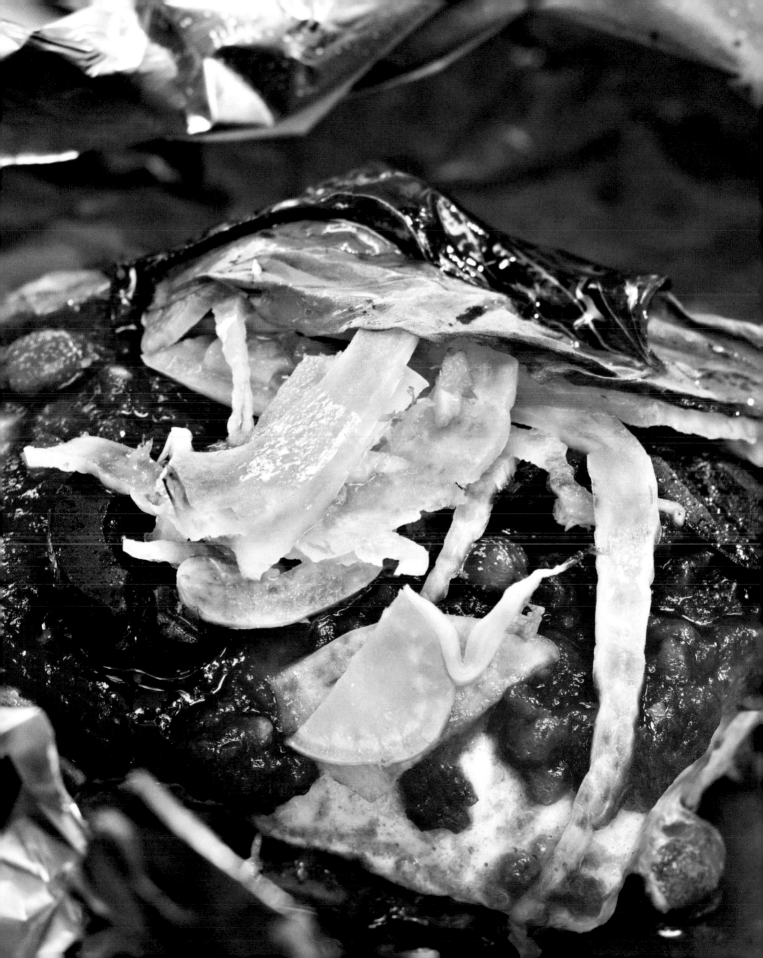

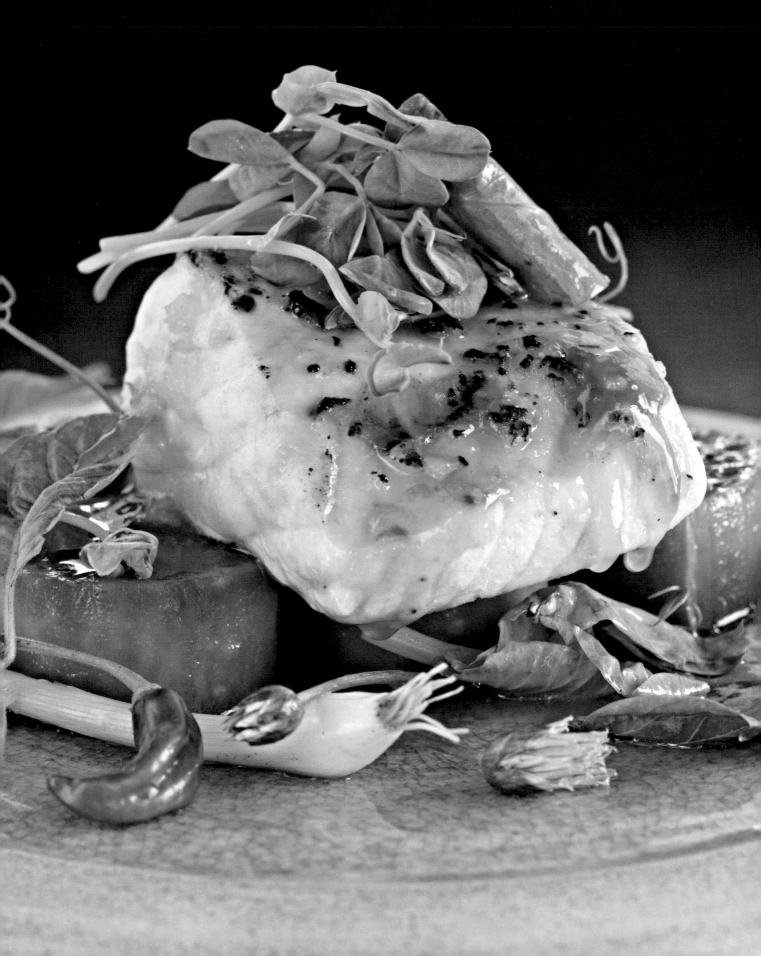

Citrus-Glazed Halibut with Braised Daikon and Pea Shoots

SERVES 4

An easily made, Asian-inspired marinade becomes a glaze that adds a zesty punch of flavor to each bite of lean seafood. I've added even more excitement with simply braised Japanese radish and a fresh salad garnish.

Citrus-Glazed Halibut:

4 (6-ounce) halibut fillets, each about 1 inch thick

Freshly ground black pepper

¼ cup rice vinegar

¼ cup fresh orange juice

¼ cup fresh lemon juice

Grated zest of ½ lemon

¼ cup thin-shred orange or tangerine marmalade

1 teaspoon minced fresh ginger

1 teaspoon minced garlic

1 teaspoon minced fresh chile pepper (optional)

½ teaspoon freshly ground white pepper

Kosher salt

2 tablespoons peanut oil or vegetable oil

Braised Daikon:

1 (8-inch) piece daikon (Japanese white radish), peeled and cut into 1-inch pieces; or 8 red radishes, each about 1 inch long, trimmed

½ cup homemade Vegetable Stock (page 274), Fish Stock (page 273), or good-quality canned low-sodium broth

½ cup low-sodium soy sauce

Pea Shoots:

2 cups pea shoots or small watercress sprigs

1 tablespoon rice vinegar

Pinch of kosher salt

Pinch of freshly ground white pepper

Pinch of sugar

Prepare the Citrus-Glazed Halibut: Put the fish fillets in a dish large enough to hold them side by side. Grind a little black pepper over both sides of the fillets. Cover with plastic wrap and refrigerate until ready to use.

In a nonreactive saucepan, stir together the vinegar, orange juice, lemon juice, lemon zest, marmalade, ginger, garlic, chile pepper (if you'd like a spicier flavor), white pepper, and salt to taste. Bring the mixture to a boil over medium-high heat; reduce the heat slightly and continue boiling until the mixture has reduced to about ½ cup, 5 to 7 minutes. Remove from the heat and let cool. Whisk in the oil. Set aside 2 tablespoons of this glaze. Spoon the rest over the fish fillets and turn to coat the fillets in glaze. Cover again with plastic wrap and refrigerate until ready to cook.

Prepare the Daikon: Put the daikon pieces in a small nonreactive saucepan and add the stock, soy sauce, and reserved 2 tablespoons citrus glaze. Bring to a boil, then reduce the heat to low and simmer gently until the radish pieces are tender when probed with the tip of a sharp knife, about 20 minutes, turning them occasionally so they'll cook evenly and be evenly glazed as the liquid reduces.

While the daikon is simmering, broil the fish: Preheat the broiler.

Transfer the fish fillets to a broiler pan or baking dish large enough to hold them in a single layer. Spoon the citrus glaze from the dish over them. Place under the broiler and cook until nicely browned and

CONTINUES

barely cooked through in the center, 3 to 4 minutes per side depending on thickness, turning them carefully with a spatula.

While the fish is broiling, prepare the Pea Shoots: Place the pea shoots in a bowl and sprinkle them with the vinegar, salt, white pepper, and sugar. Toss well. Set aside.

Assemble the dish: As soon as the fish is done, use a spoon to place 2 pieces of braised radish about 2 inches apart in the center of each heated serving plate, spooning all but a few spoonfuls of the braising liquid over them. With a spatula, place a fish fillet on top of each pair of radishes. Stir any glaze left in the broiler pan into the remaining braising liquid, and spoon that mixture over the fish. Mound the pea shoots on top. Serve immediately.

WOLFGANG'S HEALTHY TIPS

→ Notice how briefly boiling the marinade/glaze mixture concentrates its flavors, which in turn makes the mild, lean fish fillets deeply satisfying.

→ You'll find the crispy, sweet little fresh pea shoots in the produce section of more and more supermarkets, and in farmers' markets. If not, sprigs of watercress will do nicely, as will any baby salad leaves you might like.

→ The recipe will also work great with any other fish fillets you might prefer.

Nutrition Facts Per Serving: Calories: 211; Calories from Fat: 64; Total Fat: 7.16g; Saturated Fat: 1.35g; Monounsaturated Fat: 3.41g; Polyunsaturated Fat: 2.39g; Cholesterol: 27mg; Sodium: 1,242mg; Total Carbohydrate: 23.36g; Dietary Fiber: 2.14g; Sugars: 16.66g; Protein: 13.79g

Tuna Tataki with Ginger-Soy-Lime Vinaigrette and Brown Sushi Rice

SERVES 4 AS A MAIN COURSE, 8 AS AN APPETIZER

The popular Japanese searing method known as *tataki,* usually used to prepare sushi-grade ahi tuna, produces a wonderful, intensely satisfying flavor for this light and refreshing seafood dish. Adding an extra base of Brown Sushi Rice (page 200) makes it even healthier and turns it into a complete main dish. Half portions also make an excellent appetizer.

Ginger-Soy-Lime Vinaigrette:

½ cup low-sodium soy sauce

½ cup fresh lime juice (from about 4 medium limes)

1 teaspoon finely grated fresh ginger

2 small shallots, minced

Freshly ground black pepper

¼ cup extra-virgin olive oil

Tuna Tataki:

1 pound very fresh, sushi-grade ahi tuna fillets

6 tablespoons minced fresh ginger

6 tablespoons sesame seeds

2 tablespoons cracked black pepper

Kosher salt

1 tablespoon peanut oil

¼ cup fresh lime juice (from about 2 medium limes)

To Assemble:

4 cups mixed baby greens

1 recipe Brown Sushi Rice (page 200)

2 medium Japanese cucumbers, cut into small dice

24 thin slices red onion

24 cherry tomatoes, halved

Prepare the Ginger-Soy-Lime Vinaigrette: In a small bowl, stir together the soy sauce, lime juice, ginger, shallots, and a few grinds of pepper. Whisking continuously, drizzle in the olive oil. Set aside.

Prepare the Tuna Tataki: Use a sharp knife to cut notches ½ inch deep at regular ¼-inch intervals perpendicular to the length of the tuna fillets, to make the tuna easier to slice after searing. On a shallow plate, stir together the ginger, sesame seeds, and cracked black pepper. Season the tuna all over with salt and roll the fillets in the ginger mixture, pressing down lightly to make the coating adhere on all sides.

Heat a small nonstick sauté pan over medium-high heat. Add the peanut oil, swirl it around, and then add the tuna and sear on all sides, 30 seconds to 1 minute per side, turning the fillets carefully with tongs. Remove the tuna from the pan and set aside on a plate. Add the lime juice to the pan and quickly stir and scrape with a wooden spoon to deglaze the pan. Immediately drizzle the deglazing liquid over the tuna.

Assemble the dish: Whisk the vinaigrette thoroughly to recombine its ingredients. Put the salad greens in a bowl and toss them with just enough of the vinaigrette to coat them lightly.

Mound the greens on four individual serving plates. Divide the Brown Sushi Rice evenly among the plates, mounding it neatly on top of the greens.

Cut the tuna crosswise at the notches into uniform slices and drape them on top of the rice, dividing them evenly among the plates. Garnish with cucumber, red onion, and cherry tomatoes. Drizzle more of the dressing over each serving. Serve immediately.

> ## WOLFGANG'S HEALTHY TIPS
>
> → If you like, add other salad vegetables such as shredded carrots, baby spinach leaves, or thinly sliced snow peas, to make an even larger salad main course.
>
> → Try the preparation with yellowtail, salmon, or albacore, too.
>
> → The dressing in this recipe has so much bright flavor that it needs very little oil—just enough to help it cling to the salad leaves. Try it with side salads or any other kind of salad to which you want to give Asian flair.

Nutrition Facts Per Serving (based on 4 servings, including Brown Sushi Rice): Calories: 424; Calories from Fat: 116; Total Fat: 13.04g; Saturated Fat: 2.11g; Monounsaturated Fat: 7.56g; Polyunsaturated Fat: 3.37g; Cholesterol: 22mg; Sodium: 706mg; Total Carbohydrate: 56.25g; Dietary Fiber: 4.89g; Sugars: 10.42g; Protein: 21.24g

Broiled Miso Salmon with Spago Cucumber Salad

SERVES 4

Japanese cuisine presents many examples of how you can make light, healthy foods intensely flavorful and satisfying. In this dish, miso paste, made from fermented soybeans, enhances the already rich taste of fresh salmon, which is cooked and then served along with a cucumber salad—inspired by the classic Japanese vinegar-marinated salads called *sunomono*—that has become very popular among customers at Spago.

Miso Salmon:

4 (4-ounce) salmon fillets

½ cup mirin (Japanese rice cooking wine)

¼ cup white miso paste

2 tablespoons dark brown sugar

1 tablespoon low-sodium soy sauce

1 teaspoon minced garlic

1 teaspoon minced fresh ginger

Spago Cucumber Salad:

2 cups thinly sliced Japanese cucumbers

1 teaspoon kosher salt

¼ cup rice vinegar

1 tablespoon sugar

½ teaspoon low-sodium soy sauce

2 teaspoons toasted sesame seeds

To Assemble:

2 tablespoons thinly sliced scallions

Marinate the Miso Salmon: Put the salmon fillets in a shallow nonreactive dish large enough to hold them in a single layer. In a small bowl, stir together the mirin, miso, sugar, soy sauce, garlic, and ginger. Add this marinade to the salmon fillets, turning them to coat on both sides. Cover the dish with plastic wrap and marinate in the refrigerator for at least 3 hours or up to overnight.

Prepare the Spago Cucumber Salad: In a bowl, combine the sliced cucumbers and salt and toss well. Add the rice vinegar, sugar, and soy sauce and toss well. Sprinkle with sesame seeds and toss again. Cover the bowl with plastic wrap and refrigerate until serving time, about 20 minutes.

Meanwhile, broil the Miso Salmon: Preheat the broiler.

Transfer the salmon fillets to a broiler pan or baking dish large enough to hold them in a single layer. Place under the broiler and cook until nicely browned and barely cooked through in the center, 3 to 4 minutes per side depending on thickness, turning them carefully with a spatula.

Assemble the dish: Place a salmon fillet on each of four serving plates. Spoon the cucumber salad around the salmon. Garnish with scallions and serve immediately.

> ## WOLFGANG'S HEALTHY TIPS
>
> → As well as being light, this dish may help your health because salmon is rich in the omega-3 fatty acids that have been found to benefit the cardiovascular system. Try the recipe with other rich cold-water fish like tuna, trout, or mackerel.
>
> → Try marinating other proteins in the miso mixture, such as skinless chicken, lean pork, or even well-drained slices of firm tofu, before broiling or grilling.
>
> → The cucumber salad makes a great, light, refreshing side dish for any broiled, grilled, or sautéed meat, poultry, or seafood.
>
> → Round out your main course with a side of simple steamed brown rice.

Nutrition Facts Per Serving: Calories: 167; Calories from Fat: 29; Total Fat: 3.23g; Saturated Fat: 0.71g; Monounsaturated Fat: 1.11g; Polyunsaturated Fat: 1.41g; Cholesterol: 16mg; Sodium: 886mg; Total Carbohydrate: 17.72g; Dietary Fiber: 1.55g; Sugars: 11.95g; Protein: 10.99g

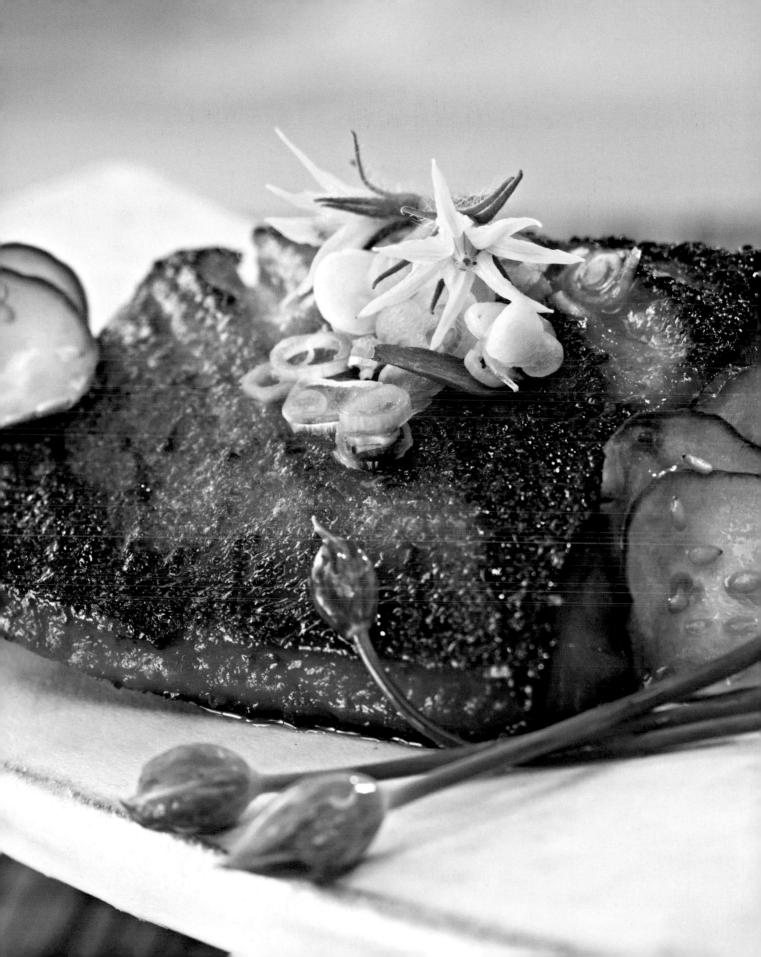

Seared Ahi Tuna with Grilled Pineapple–Mango Salsa

SERVES 4

Most people think of eating tropical fruit for breakfast or in desserts. I do, too, but I also like to make a healthy, sweet-and-spicy salsa with it to serve with grilled fish like the seared ahi tuna in this recipe.

Grilled Pineapple–Mango Salsa:

1 small ripe pineapple

2 teaspoons Asian-style chili oil

Kosher salt

½ cup rice wine vinegar

¼ cup plus 2 tablespoons lime juice (from about 3 limes)

1 tablespoon peanut oil

1 tablespoon Asian-style toasted sesame oil

1 mango, peeled, pitted, and cut into ½-inch dice

1 red bell pepper, stemmed, seeded, deveined, and cut into ¼-inch dice

2 jalapeños, stemmed, seeded, deveined, and finely diced

½ cup diced red onion

3 tablespoons chopped fresh mint leaves

1 tablespoon chopped fresh Thai basil leaves or regular basil leaves

1 teaspoon sugar

½ teaspoon freshly ground white pepper

Seared Ahi Tuna:

1 pound sushi-grade ahi tuna fillet, in one piece

Peanut oil, for drizzling

Kosher salt

2 tablespoons coarsely ground black pepper

2 tablespoons grated fresh ginger

To Assemble:

4 cups mixed baby salad greens

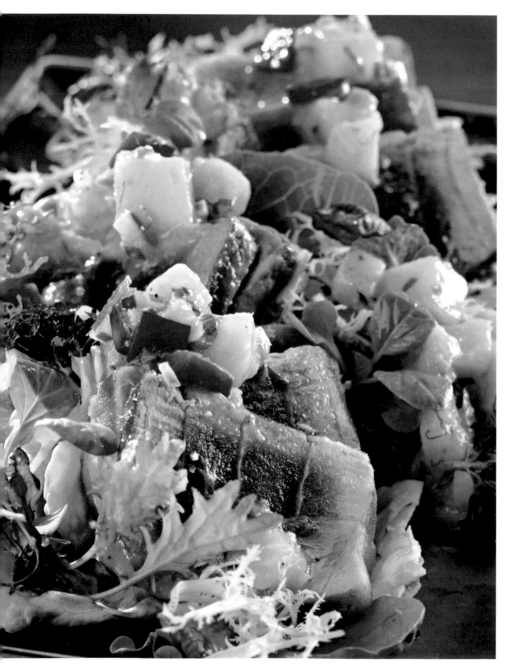

Preheat a hot fire in an outdoor grill or preheat an indoor countertop grill, ridged stovetop grill pan, or broiler.

Prepare the Grilled Pineapple–Mango Salsa: Use a sharp knife to cut off the leaf and stem ends of the pineapple. Then, stand the pineapple upright and cut off the peel in downward vertical slices. Use a small, sharp knife to cut out any tough "eyes" remaining in the fruit. Lay the fruit on its side and cut the pineapple crosswise into 1-inch round slices.

When the grill is hot, rub the pineapple slices all over with the chili oil and season lightly on both sides with salt. Grill or broil the slices until they soften slightly and are nicely browned, 2 to 3 minutes per side. Remove them from the grill and set aside to cool. Then, cut the fruit away from the hard central core on each slice, discarding the core. Coarsely chop the fruit and measure out ¾ cup, reserving the remainder for another use.

In a nonreactive bowl, whisk together the vinegar and lime juice. Whisking continuously, slowly drizzle in the peanut oil and sesame oil. Add the grilled pineapple, mango, red bell pepper, jalapeños, and onion; stir well. Stir in the mint, Thai basil, sugar, and white pepper.

Transfer about one-fourth of the salsa mixture to a food processor fitted with the stainless-steel blade. Process until pureed. Stir the puree back into the salsa. Cover the bowl with plastic wrap and refrigerate until serving time. (The salsa will keep well for up to 24 hours.)

Prepare the Seared Ahi Tuna: Use a sharp knife to lightly score one side of the tuna fillet crosswise at ¼-inch intervals, to make it easier to slice after cooking. Very lightly drizzle the tuna fillet all over with peanut oil. Season all over with salt. On a plate, stir together the black pepper and ginger. Turn the tuna in the mixture, pressing down firmly to coat it on all sides.

Place the tuna on the hot grill or under the broiler and sear it on each side for 30 seconds to 1 minute, until its surface has good brown grill marks. The inside should remain rare.

Remove the tuna from the grill to a cutting board. With a sharp knife, cut the tuna fillet crosswise at the score marks into slices ¼ inch thick.

Assemble the dish: Arrange a bed of baby salad greens on a serving platter or individual plates. Arrange the tuna slices overlapping on top and spoon the salsa over and around them.

WOLFGANG'S HEALTHY TIPS

→ For a complete main dish, add Brown Sushi Rice (page 200) or another grain dish or pilaf (pages 196–204).

→ The tuna and salsa on their own also make 6 to 8 appetizer servings.

→ Try the salsa with other grilled proteins such as salmon, chicken breast, or lean pork, lamb, or beef.

Nutrition Facts Per Serving: Calories: 337; Calories from Fat: 100; Total Fat: 11.22g; Saturated Fat: 2.09g; Monounsaturated Fat: 5.03g; Polyunsaturated Fat: 4.10g; Cholesterol: 44mg; Sodium: 64mg; Total Carbohydrate: 28.25g; Dietary Fiber: 4.81g; Sugars: 18.98g; Protein: 30.27g

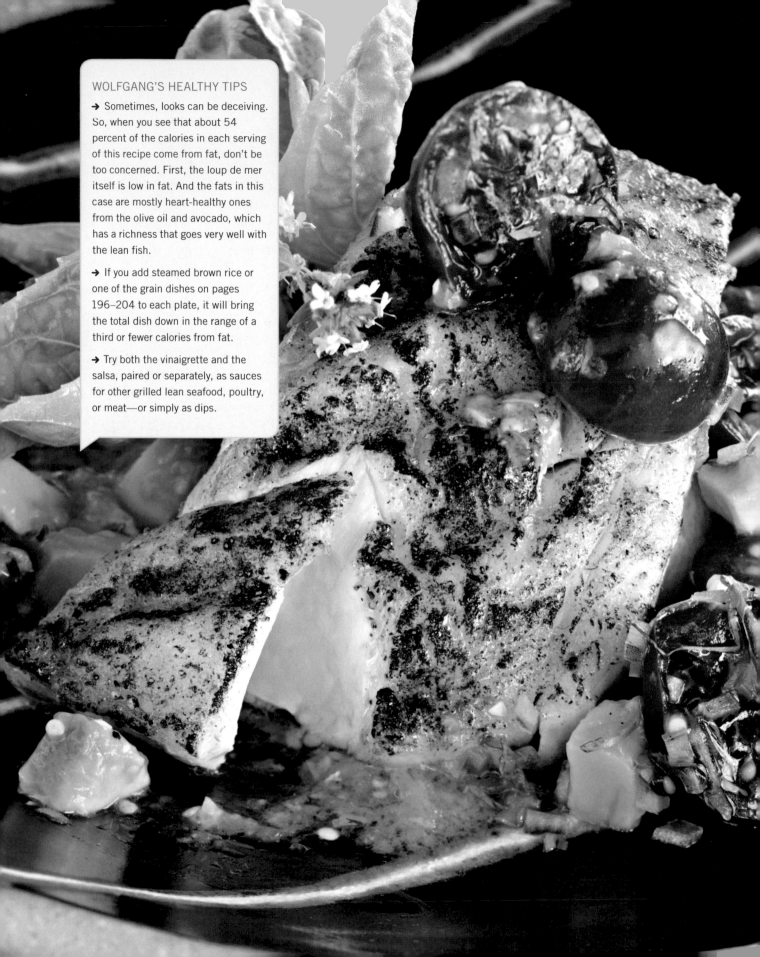

WOLFGANG'S HEALTHY TIPS

→ Sometimes, looks can be deceiving. So, when you see that about 54 percent of the calories in each serving of this recipe come from fat, don't be too concerned. First, the loup de mer itself is low in fat. And the fats in this case are mostly heart-healthy ones from the olive oil and avocado, which has a richness that goes very well with the lean fish.

→ If you add steamed brown rice or one of the grain dishes on pages 196–204 to each plate, it will bring the total dish down in the range of a third or fewer calories from fat.

→ Try both the vinaigrette and the salsa, paired or separately, as sauces for other grilled lean seafood, poultry, or meat—or simply as dips.

Grilled Loup de Mer with Tomatillo-Avocado Vinaigrette and Cherry Tomato Salsa

SERVES 4

When summer grill season approaches and you're craving bright, lively, fresh flavors, try this easy dish made with loup de mer, also known as European sea bass, or any other lean, tender, white-fleshed fish. Two cool yet well-spiced, contrasting yet complementary sauces beautifully highlight the mild-tasting seafood.

Tomatillo-Avocado Vinaigrette:

¼ pound fresh tomatillos, husks removed, rinsed well

1 garlic clove

½ teaspoon stemmed, seeded, deveined, and chopped jalapeño

2 tablespoons fresh lemon juice or lime juice

2 tablespoons extra-virgin olive oil

1 small ripe Hass avocado, pitted, peeled, and cut into ½-inch dice

2 tablespoons chopped fresh cilantro leaves

Kosher salt

Freshly ground black pepper

Cherry Tomato Salsa:

1 cup cherry tomatoes, halved

¼ red onion, minced

½ jalapeño, stemmed, seeded, deveined, and minced

2 tablespoons fresh lime juice

1 tablespoon minced fresh cilantro leaves

Kosher salt

Freshly ground black pepper

Grilled Loup de Mer:

4 (4-ounce) fresh loup de mer fillets, each about 1 inch thick

1 tablespoon extra-virgin olive oil

1 tablespoon finely julienned fresh basil

Juice of 1 lemon

Kosher salt

Freshly ground black pepper

To Assemble:

Fresh basil sprigs

Prepare the Tomatillo-Avocado Vinaigrette: Preheat the oven to 400°F.

Arrange the tomatillos, garlic, and chopped jalapeño in a small baking dish. Bake until the tomatillos are tender, 10 to 15 minutes. Scrape into a food processor fitted with the stainless-steel blade and puree. Strain through a medium-fine strainer into a bowl. Whisk in the lemon or lime juice. Then, whisking continuously, slowly drizzle in the olive oil. Stir in the avocado and cilantro. Season to taste with salt and pepper and set aside.

Prepare the Cherry Tomato Salsa: In a bowl, stir together the tomatoes, onion, minced jalapeño, lime juice, and cilantro. Season to taste with salt and pepper. Set aside.

Preheat an outdoor or indoor grill or the broiler.

Prepare the Grilled Loup de Mer: When the grill or broiler is hot, put the loup de mer fillets on a plate. In a small bowl, stir together the olive oil, basil, and lemon juice. Season the fish lightly on both sides with salt and pepper, and then brush all over with the oil-basil-lemon mixture.

Grill or broil the fish just until nicely seared with grill marks or golden brown, about 4 minutes per side. Then transfer the fillets to a heatproof dish, cover with foil, and leave to rest near the grill or broiler for 10 to 15 minutes more; the residual heat in the fillets will continue to cook them through while leaving them still moist in the center.

Assemble the dish: Spoon some of the Tomatillo-Avocado Vinaigrette into the centers of four dinner plates. Place a loup de mer fillet on top of the vinaigrette. Spoon the Cherry Tomato Salsa on top of and alongside the fish. Garnish with basil sprigs and serve immediately.

Nutrition Facts Per Serving: Calories: 273; Calories from Fat: 147; Total Fat: 16.49g; Saturated Fat: 1.88g; Monounsaturated Fat: 10.39g; Polyunsaturated Fat: 4.42g; Cholesterol: 0mg; Sodium: 30mg; Total Carbohydrate: 10.15g; Dietary Fiber: 3.23g; Sugars: 4.81g; Protein: 24.80g

Grilled Salmon with Cucumber-Yogurt Sauce and Warm Potato-Vegetable Salad

SERVES 4

When you have three different yet compatible preparations coming together on a single dinner plate, it can feel as if you're feasting, even if the entire dish is low in fat and calories. This recipe, with its crispy-moist fish, warm vegetables, and cool yogurt sauce, is a perfect example.

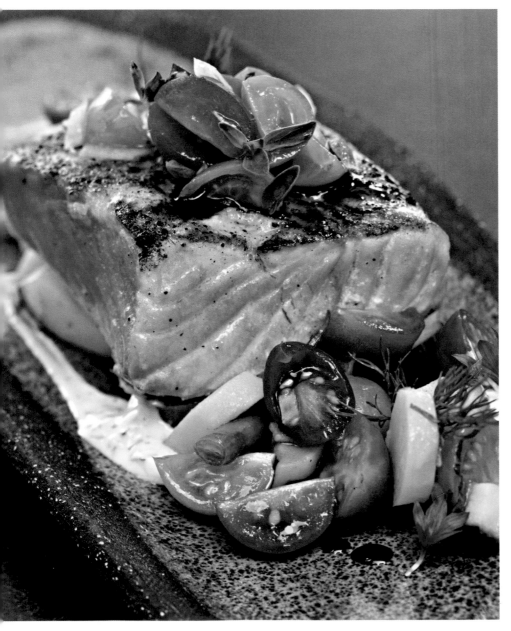

Warm Potato-Vegetable Salad:

1 pound fingerling potatoes or other small boiling potatoes

Kosher salt

1 cup fresh green beans, cut into 1-inch pieces

1 cup Champagne vinegar

1 tablespoon sugar

Freshly ground black pepper

½ medium red onion, cut into ¼-inch dice

¼ cup homemade Vegetable Stock (page 274) or good-quality canned low-sodium broth

1 cup cherry tomatoes, halved

1 tablespoon chopped fresh flat-leaf parsley leaves

Cucumber-Yogurt Sauce:

1 cup nonfat plain Greek yogurt

Grated zest of 2 lemons

Juice of 2 lemons

½ cup chopped fresh dill

½ medium red onion, cut into ¼-inch dice

2 English (hothouse) cucumbers, halved, seeded, and cut into ¼-inch dice

Kosher salt

Freshly ground black pepper

Grilled Salmon:

4 (6-ounce) fresh wild salmon fillets

Extra-virgin olive oil, for brushing

Kosher salt

Freshly ground black pepper

To Assemble:

2 tablespoons balsamic vinegar

Fresh baby basil sprigs

Dill sprigs

Several hours before serving, start the Warm Potato-Vegetable Salad: Rinse the potatoes, leaving their skins on. Put them in a saucepan with enough cold water to cover well and add a sprinkling of salt. Bring to a boil over high heat; then, adjust the heat to maintain a steady boil and cook until the potatoes are just tender enough to be pierced easily with a long metal skewer, about 15 minutes.

While the potatoes are cooking, bring a saucepan of water to a boil. Blanch the green beans in the boiling water until tender-crisp, 2 to 3 minutes, then transfer them to a large bowl filled with ice and water and shock them to stop the cooking process. Drain well and set aside. Refill the bowl with ice and water.

When the potatoes are done, drain them well, transfer to the prepared ice bath, and leave until thoroughly cooled, about 30 minutes.

Meanwhile, in a large bowl, stir together the vinegar, sugar, and salt and pepper to taste. Set aside.

Drain and peel the potatoes, using your fingertips and, if necessary, a small, sharp knife to slip off their skins. Cut each potato crosswise into discs about ¼ inch thick and add them to the vinegar mixture. Add the red onion, toss gently, cover with plastic wrap, and marinate in the refrigerator for 3 to 4 hours. Set aside the blanched green beans along

with the Vegetable Stock, halved tomatoes, and chopped parsley.

About 1 hour before serving, prepare the Cucumber-Yogurt Sauce: In a bowl, stir together the yogurt, lemon zest, lemon juice, dill, and red onion. Fold in the cucumber and season to taste with salt and pepper. Cover with plastic wrap and refrigerate.

Prepare the Grilled Salmon: Preheat an outdoor or indoor charcoal or gas grill, or a broiler.

Lightly brush the salmon fillets on both sides with olive oil and season lightly with salt and pepper. Grill to the desired degree of doneness, about 4 minutes per side per 1 inch of thickness for medium, 5 minutes per side for medium-well.

While the salmon is cooking, complete the Warm Potato-Vegetable Salad: In a sauté pan, stir together the Vegetable Stock and the potato mixture and warm over medium heat. Stir in the blanched green beans, tomatoes (reserving several pieces for garnish), and parsley. Taste and adjust the seasonings with salt and pepper.

Assemble the dish: Spread some of the Cucumber-Yogurt Sauce on each of four serving plates. Spoon the Warm Potato-Vegetable Salad on top to form even beds. Place a salmon fillet on top of each bed of salad. Spoon more cucumber sauce around each fillet, transferring the rest to a serving bowl to pass at the table. Place the reserved cherry tomatoes on top of the salmon. Drizzle the salmon, tomatoes, and plates with the balsamic vinegar. Garnish with baby basil and dill sprigs. Serve immediately.

WOLFGANG'S HEALTHY TIPS

→ Notice how a variety of contrasts— warm and cool, crispy and soft, tangy and sweet—and different shapes and colors enhance the pleasures this dish offers, encouraging you to slow down and savor every bite.

→ Try the recipe with other kinds of grilled fish fillets, or with chicken breasts or lean red meat.

→ The potato-vegetable salad works well as a side dish for any other grilled seafood, poultry, or meat. You can also add other vegetables to the mixture, such as baby peas, diced roasted bell pepper, or broccoli florets.

→ The Cucumber-Yogurt Sauce also works as a salad dressing or as a dip for crudités or baked chips.

Nutrition Facts Per Serving: Calories: 366; Calories from Fat: 104; Total Fat: 11.65g; Saturated Fat: 2.03g; Monounsaturated Fat: 7.41g; Polyunsaturated Fat: 2.21g; Cholesterol: 25mg; Sodium: 82mg; Total Carbohydrate: 41.08g; Dietary Fiber: 4.81g; Sugars: 14.84g; Protein: 23.03g

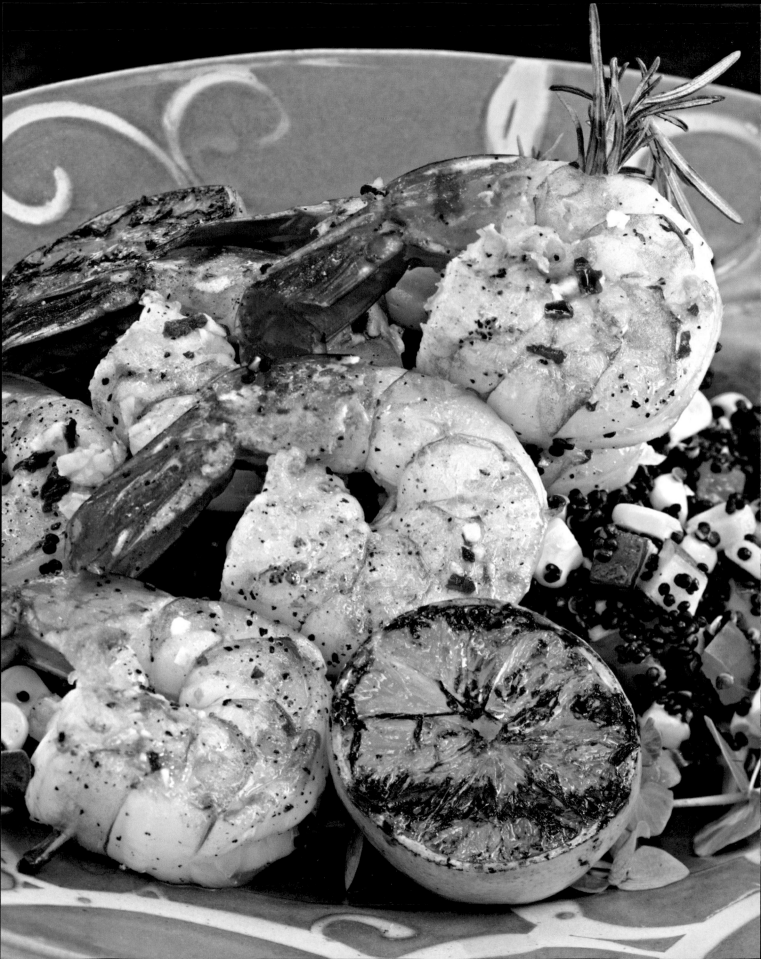

Grilled Shrimp on Rosemary Skewers with Grilled Limes and Quinoa and Grilled Vegetable Pilaf

SERVES 4

Before there were ever such things as skewers, rustic cooks sharpened small branches of fragrant herbs to scent food while holding it together over the fire. Grilling the limes that will be squeezed over the shrimp at the table makes their juices taste even sweeter and richer.

1 teaspoon grated lime zest

3 tablespoons fresh lime juice

1 tablespoon extra-virgin olive oil

½ tablespoon red pepper flakes

2 or 3 fresh basil leaves, cut into fine julienne strips

2 garlic cloves, minced

1½ pounds extra-large shrimp (16 to 20 per pound), peeled and deveined, tails left on if desired

2 limes, halved

8 sturdy fresh rosemary sprigs, each 6 to 8 inches long

1 recipe Quinoa and Grilled Vegetable Pilaf (page 204)

Kosher salt

Freshly ground black pepper

In a large nonreactive bowl, whisk together the lime zest, lime juice, olive oil, red pepper flakes, basil, and garlic. Add the shrimp, stir to coat them evenly, cover with plastic wrap, and refrigerate for at least 1 hour and up to 3 hours.

Preheat an outdoor grill, an indoor countertop grill, a ridged grill pan, or the broiler. With the tip of a small, sharp knife, carefully remove any visible seeds from the lime halves. Set the limes aside.

Strip the leaves from each rosemary sprig, leaving just a tuft at one end. With a knife or kitchen shears, carefully trim the bare end of each branch to a point.

Remove the shrimp from the marinade and skewer them on the rosemary sprigs, passing the point of each branch through both the head and tail end of each shrimp.

Start preparing the Quinoa and Grilled Vegetable Pilaf.

As soon as the pilaf is ready, season the shrimp on both sides with salt and pepper to taste. Grill the shrimp until they turn bright pink all over, 1 to 2 minutes per side, turning the skewers once with long-handled tongs. At the same time, grill the lime halves with their cut sides facing the heat.

Serve immediately, arranging beds of quinoa pilaf on a platter or individual serving plates and placing the skewers on top and the grilled lime halves on the side. Encourage guests to use a fork to slide the shrimp carefully off their skewers, then squeeze the warm lime halves over the shrimp.

WOLFGANG'S HEALTHY TIPS

→ Here's another good example of a complete healthy meal on a plate—lean protein, fresh vegetables, and a whole grain all together in a colorful presentation that tastes as good as it looks.

→ Feel free to serve the shrimp skewers on their own. Without the pilaf, they're just 165 calories per serving, 34 of those from fat.

Nutrition Facts Per Serving (including Quinoa and Grilled Vegetable Pilaf): Calories: 368; Calories from Fat: 97; Total Fat: 10.94g; Saturated Fat: 1.75g; Monounsaturated Fat: 2.61g; Polyunsaturated Fat: 0.60g; Cholesterol: 214mg; Sodium: 1,393mg; Total Carbohydrate: 31.25g; Dietary Fiber: 5.71g; Sugars: 6.25g; Protein: 31.20g

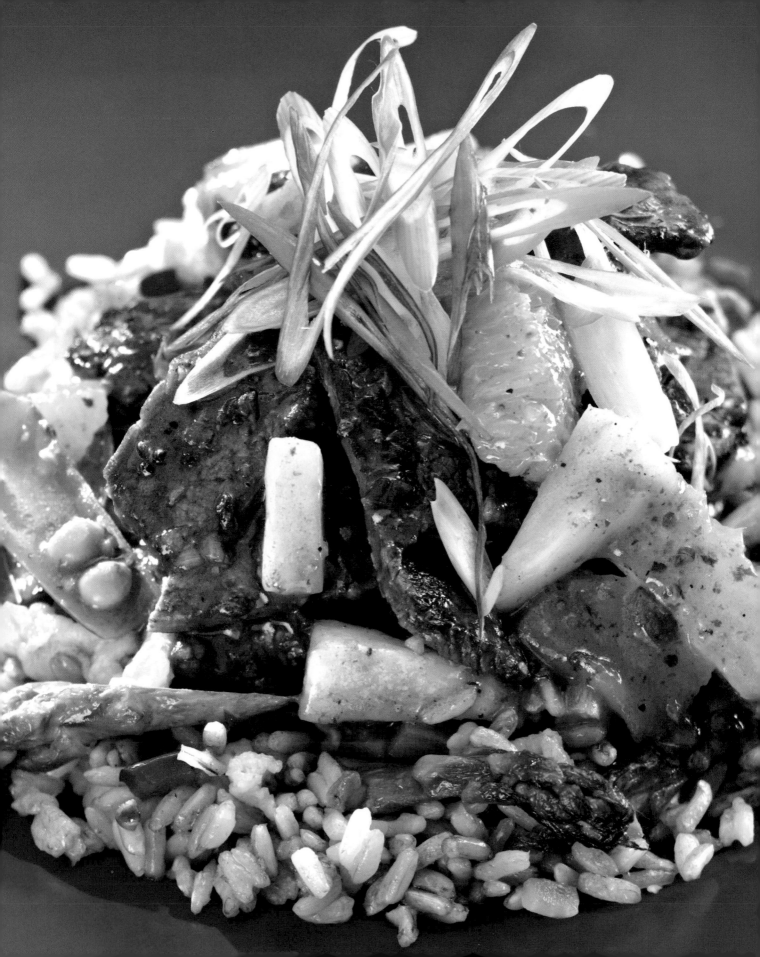

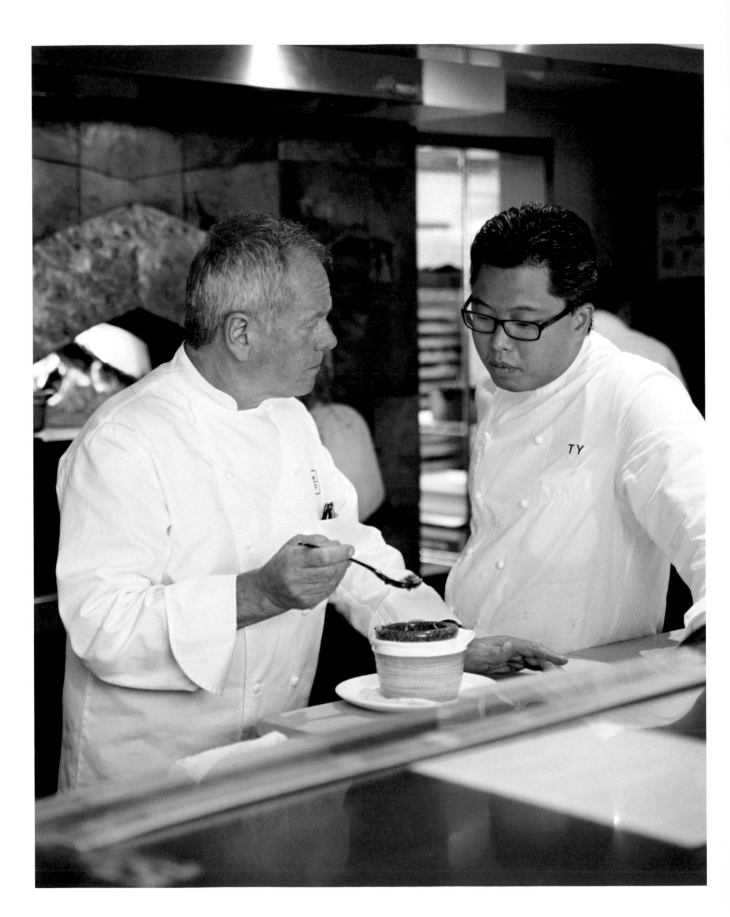

POULTRY AND MEAT MAIN DISHES

"What's for dinner?"

That's one of the questions you hear most often in homes everywhere when evening approaches, and more often than not the answer involves some sort of poultry or red meat. So many of us associate robust chicken, turkey, beef, pork, and lamb dishes with comforting, satisfying meals at the end of our busy days. And what we don't want to hear so much, especially after a long and tiring day, is an answer involving the word "healthy."

I've created all of the recipes in this chapter to change how people look at healthy main courses. Whether they feature poultry or meat, they are all as big in flavor as they are low in calories and fat. Many have also been developed as one-plate recipes—that is, they combine a protein along with grain and vegetable sides to form a balanced meal that will help you leave the table feeling completely happy without overindulging.

And the options don't end with the recipes that follow. You'll also find main-dish salads on pages 73–97 that feature more red meats along with poultry, as well as main-course pastas on pages 101–117. And many of the salads, soups, and side dishes throughout this book can be served as vegetarian or vegan dishes that work wonderfully as the centerpieces of a meal.

Have a great dinner!

→ Sautéed Chicken Breasts with Tomatoes and Sherry Vinegar Sauce

→ Butterflied Garlic-Parsley Chicken with Brown Rice Mushroom Risotto

→ Spice-Rubbed Chicken Breasts and Fried Rice Bowls

→ Northern Indian Chicken Curry with Sweet Potatoes and Brown Basmati Rice

→ Tandoori-Style Chicken Kabobs with Mango Ginger Chutney

→ Barbecued Chicken with Sweet-and-Spicy Barbecue Sauce and Mashed Grilled Vegetables

→ Turkey-Mushroom Burgers with Wolfgang's "Secret Sauce"

→ Turkey Piccata with Winter Squash Puree

→ Stir-Fried Orange-Pineapple Beef with Fried Rice

→ Beef Stew with Winter Vegetables

→ Stir-Fried Orange-Flavored Ground Pork in Radicchio Cups

→ Pan-Seared Pork Chops with Sautéed Cabbage

→ Sautéed Lamb with Zucchini, Eggplant, and Moroccan Harissa-Yogurt Sauce

→ Healthy Reisfleisch with Beef and Turkey Kielbasa

★ Paella-Style Shrimp Reisfleisch

★ Vegetarian Reisfleisch

Sautéed Chicken Breasts with Tomatoes and Sherry Vinegar Sauce

SERVES 4

One of the heartiest, healthiest chicken dishes I know, this recipe simmers boneless, skinless chicken breasts in a tangy-sweet vinegar-and-tomato sauce and then presents them on a bed of pasta tossed with the sauce.

4 boneless skinless chicken breast halves

½ teaspoon kosher salt

¼ teaspoon freshly ground black pepper

All-purpose flour, for dusting

1½ tablespoons extra-virgin olive oil

2 medium shallots, minced

2 garlic cloves, minced

2 teaspoons chopped fresh thyme leaves

½ cup sherry vinegar or red wine vinegar

½ pound whole wheat or whole-grain pasta such as bow ties or large macaroni

3 cups canned diced tomatoes

¾ cup homemade Chicken Stock (page 271) or good-quality canned low-sodium broth

1 tablespoon tomato paste

1 tablespoon honey

2 teaspoons minced fresh chervil

2 teaspoons minced fresh dill

2 teaspoons minced fresh flat-leaf parsley

Season the chicken breasts all over with salt and pepper, then dust them lightly with flour.

In a large, heavy nonstick sauté pan, heat the olive oil over medium-high heat. As soon as it is hot enough to shimmer slightly and swirl easily around the pan, add the chicken breasts, starting skinned side down, and sauté just until golden brown, 4 to 5 minutes per side. Remove the chicken to a platter and cover with aluminum foil to keep warm.

Bring a large pot of lightly salted water to a boil.

Meanwhile, drain all but a thin coating of fat from the pan in which you cooked the chicken. Add the shallots, garlic, and thyme and sauté for 1 minute. Add the vinegar and stir and scrape with a wooden spoon to deglaze the pan. Raise the heat to high, bring the liquid to a boil, and cook until it has reduced by half.

While the liquid is reducing, add the pasta to the boiling water and cook until al dente—tender but still slightly chewy—following the manufacturer's suggested cooking time.

Stir the tomatoes, chicken stock, tomato paste, and honey into the reduced vinegar mixture. Simmer briskly, stirring occasionally, until the sauce has thickened slightly but is still loose and juicy.

Carefully return the chicken breasts to the pan, nestling them into the sauce.

Reduce the heat to maintain a gentle simmer and continue cooking until the chicken is done, about 6 minutes more.

Remove the chicken from the sauce and set aside. Drain the pasta and add it to the sauce, tossing thoroughly to coat.

To serve, spoon the pasta and sauce into a large, shallow pasta serving bowl or individual pasta bowls. Arrange the chicken on top. Garnish with the chervil, dill, and parsley.

WOLFGANG'S HEALTHY TIPS

→ If you would prefer another kind of starchy side dish, by all means leave out the pasta, and serve the chicken with something else to soak up the delicious juices, such as couscous, plain steamed brown rice, Brown Rice Mushroom Risotto (page 198), or one of the mashed potato recipes on pages 194–195.

→ This recipe would also work very well with turkey breast cutlets or with lean slices of pork tenderloin.

Nutrition Facts Per Serving: Calories: 509; Calories from Fat: 91; Total Fat: 10.19g; Saturated Fat: 2.35g; Monounsaturated Fat: 5.95g; Polyunsaturated Fat: 1.89g; Cholesterol: 152mg; Sodium: 661mg; Total Carbohydrate: 40.50g; Dietary Fiber: 4.63g; Sugars: 10.06g; Protein: 58.11g

Butterflied Garlic-Parsley Chicken with Brown Rice Mushroom Risotto

SERVES 4

One of my favorite ways to roast a chicken involves butterflying it, a step that ensures it cooks quickly and evenly, yielding breast meat as juicy as the dark meat. For healthy results, resist the crispy brown skin if you can! The Brown Rice Mushroom Risotto makes a satisfying accompaniment and is surprisingly easy, since it's prepared in a pressure cooker.

Brown Rice Mushroom Risotto (page 198)

1 whole frying chicken (about 4 pounds), butterflied by your butcher (or by following instructions below)

½ cup coarsely chopped fresh flat-leaf parsley leaves

8 garlic cloves, minced

Kosher salt

Freshly ground black pepper

2 tablespoons extra-virgin olive oil

Preheat the oven to 450°F.

Start preparing the Brown Rice Mushroom Risotto (page 198).

While the oven is heating and the risotto is cooking, prepare the chicken. If the butcher hasn't butterflied it for you, do it yourself: Using poultry shears, working slowly and deliberately, cut along each side of the backbone from neck to tail, and remove the backbone. Turn the bird breast side up, spread it open, and flatten it with a firm blow from the heel of your hand.

From the neck opening, gently ease your fingertips between the skin and the meat to loosen the skin all over the breast, taking care not to tear the skin. From underneath the breast skin, work your fingertips gently underneath the skin of the thighs to loosen that as well.

In a small bowl, stir together the parsley and garlic. Carefully spoon the mixture underneath the loosened skin of the chicken and, massaging the skin from the outside, spread the mixture as evenly as possible over the breast and thighs.

Season the chicken generously all over with salt and pepper.

Heat an ovenproof skillet large enough to hold the chicken over high heat. Add the olive oil and swirl it in the skillet. As soon as you begin to see slight wisps of smoke from the oil, carefully place the chicken skin side down in the skillet. Sear the chicken, undisturbed, gradually reducing the heat to medium, until the skin has turned golden brown and crisp, 5 to 7 minutes. With tongs, carefully turn the chicken skin side up.

Put the skillet with the chicken into the preheated oven and cook until the chicken is deep golden brown and the juices run clear when the thickest part of the thigh is pierced with a thin skewer, 10 to 15 minutes.

Remove the chicken from the skillet with tongs and transfer it to a cutting board. Cover with aluminum foil and let rest for about 10 minutes.

With a large, sharp knife, cut the chicken into four equal pieces.

Spoon the Brown Rice Mushroom Risotto onto individual heated serving plates and arrange the chicken on top. (Advise guests to remove the skin from the chicken if they desire a lower-fat dish.)

WOLFGANG'S HEALTHY TIPS

→ In case you think that the risotto is what makes the overall dish low fat, the chicken on its own—eaten with the skin removed—comes in at around 305 calories per serving, with 103 calories (33.8 percent) from fat. Eat the skin with it, though, and you more than double the calories, with most of the extra calories coming from fat.

→ If you like, serve the chicken with another whole-grain side such as couscous or Farro and Root Vegetable Pilaf (page 201).

Nutrition Facts Per Serving (without chicken skin, including Brown Rice Mushroom Risotto): Calories: 546; Calories from Fat: 158; Total Fat: 17.64g; Saturated Fat: 3.49g; Monounsaturated Fat: 10.88g; Polyunsaturated Fat: 3.26g; Cholesterol: 137mg; Sodium: 369mg; Total Carbohydrate: 42.04g; Dietary Fiber: 2.52g; Sugars: 1.35g; Protein: 46.90g

Spice-Rubbed Chicken Breasts and Fried Rice Bowls

SERVES 4

Steamed, fragrantly seasoned chicken breasts quickly become a complete, casual meal when they are served on top of bowls filled with my equally fast recipe for Vegetable Fried Rice (page 196).

4 (4-ounce) boneless skinless chicken breast halves

1 tablespoon minced fresh ginger

1 tablespoon minced garlic

1 tablespoon minced scallion

½ teaspoon red pepper flakes

½ teaspoon kosher salt

1 tablespoon cornstarch

½ recipe Vegetable Fried Rice (page 196)

Trim any visible fat and connective tissue from the edges of the chicken breasts and put them on a plate. In a blender, combine the ginger, garlic, scallion, red pepper flakes, and salt. Add the cornstarch and 1 tablespoon cold water and pulse until the mixture forms a fine, smooth paste. Spread the mixture evenly on top of the chicken breasts. Set aside.

Bring a saucepan of water to a boil, or prepare a countertop steamer following the manufacturer's instructions. Arrange the chicken breasts side by side in a steamer basket that fits snugly on top of the saucepan, or in the countertop steamer's tray. Steam the chicken until it is cooked through and the internal temperature of a breast registers 165°F on an instant-read thermometer inserted into its thickest part, 8 to 10 minutes.

Meanwhile, prepare the Vegetable Fried Rice, reserving that recipe's cilantro and scallion garnishes. As soon as it is ready, divide it among four heated large individual serving bowls, or mound it on heated serving plates.

When the chicken breasts are done, transfer them to a cutting board. With a sharp knife, cut each breast crosswise at a 45-degree angle into slices about ¼ inch thick. Fan out each sliced breast across the rice in each bowl or on each plate. Garnish with the cilantro and scallions. Serve immediately.

WOLFGANG'S HEALTHY TIPS

→ As this recipe demonstrates, steaming is one of the easiest, quickest ways to prepare lean, juicy chicken breasts. (You can also broil the chicken breasts, without changing the recipe in any other way.) The great flavor comes from an easy spice paste that coats each boneless, skinless piece. Feel free to vary the seasonings to your taste once you've tried this version.

→ Note that the chicken breasts on their own are very low in calories: just 280 per serving, with only 36 calories per serving from fat.

→ The spice rub will also work well on your favorite fish fillets, which would also be delicious over the rice.

→ If you prefer, serve the chicken even more simply on top of steamed brown rice or more seasoned Brown Sushi Rice (page 200).

Nutrition Facts Per Serving (including Vegetable Fried Rice): Calories: 499; Calories from Fat: 79; Total Fat: 48.91g; Saturated Fat: 2.37g; Monounsaturated Fat: 3.94g; Polyunsaturated Fat: 2.59g; Cholesterol: 174mg; Sodium: 387mg; Total Carbohydrate: 40.27g; Dietary Fiber: 6.40g; Sugars: 5.98g; Protein: 58.05g

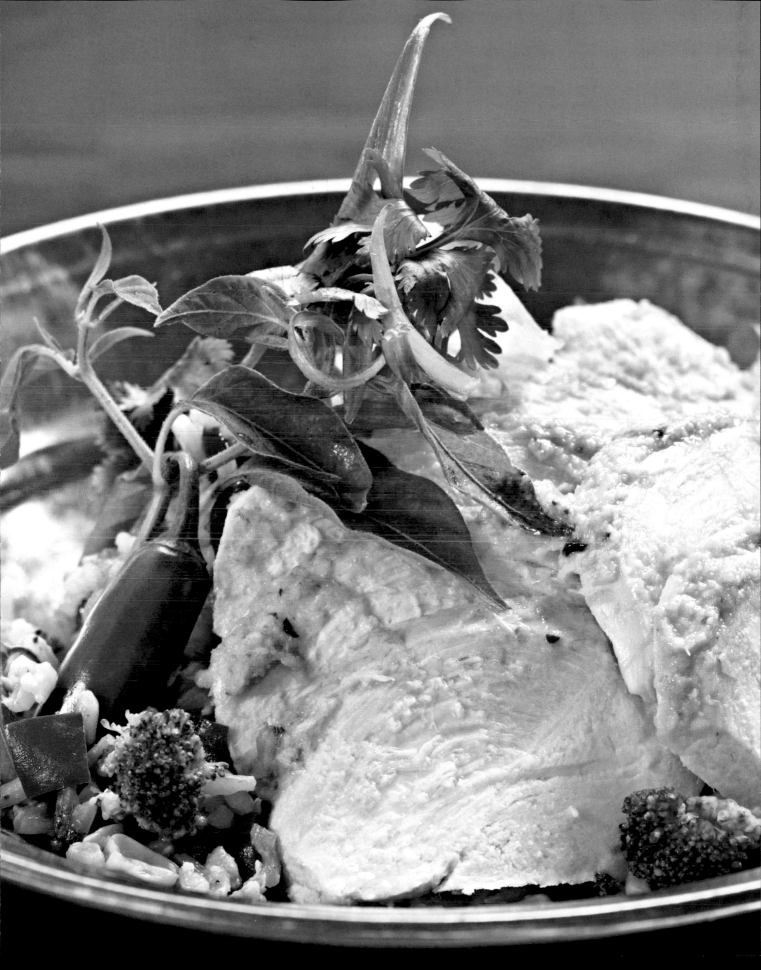

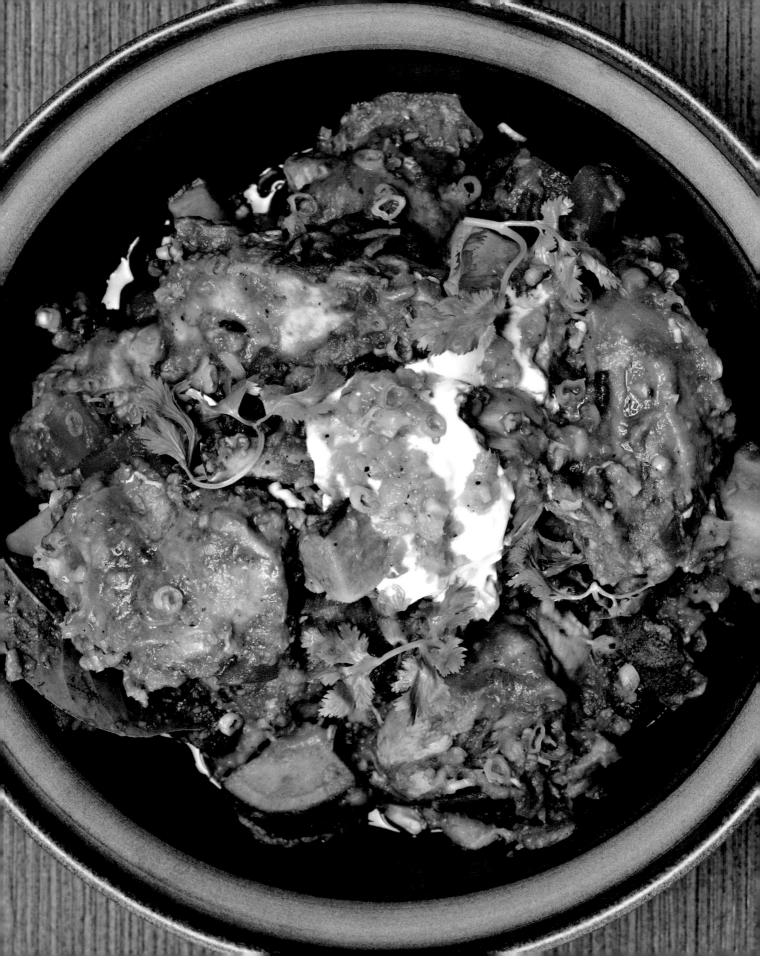

Northern Indian Chicken Curry with Sweet Potatoes and Brown Basmati Rice

SERVES 4 TO 6

You'll find this flavorful curry very easy to make, since the chicken pieces go right into the stew without browning—which also cuts down on the fat in the recipe.

3 pounds bone-in chicken pieces, skin and visible fat removed

1½ teaspoons kosher salt, plus more as needed

3 teaspoons freshly ground black pepper, plus more as needed

2 tablespoons unsalted butter

2 medium yellow onions, sliced

1½ tablespoons dark brown sugar

1½ tablespoons minced garlic

1½ tablespoons minced fresh ginger

1 tablespoon minced green jalapeño

1 bay leaf

1 tablespoon Curry Powder (page 285) or packaged store-bought curry powder

2 cups diced tomatoes

1 tablespoon tomato paste

2 tablespoons seedless raisins

¾ pound orange-fleshed sweet potatoes or ruby yams, scrubbed and cut into 1-inch cubes

3 cups homemade Chicken Stock (page 271) or good-quality canned low-sodium broth

2 cups steamed brown basmati or regular brown rice

1 tablespoon finely chopped fresh cilantro leaves, for garnish

1 tablespoon thinly sliced scallions, for garnish

¾ cup nonfat plain yogurt, for garnish (optional)

Mango-Ginger Chutney (pages 156–157), for garnish (optional)

Season the chicken pieces all over with ½ teaspoon of the salt and ½ teaspoon of the black pepper. Set aside at room temperature.

In a large saucepan, melt the butter over medium heat. Add the onions and sauté, stirring constantly, just until they turn glossy, 1 to 2 minutes. Season with the remaining 1 teaspoon salt and 2½ teaspoons black pepper, and the sugar. Continue to sauté, stirring, until the onions have turned soft but have not yet browned, about 5 minutes.

Add the garlic, ginger, jalapeño, bay leaf, and Curry Powder. Sauté, stirring, until the spices turn aromatic, 1 to 2 minutes. Add the seasoned chicken pieces, tomatoes, tomato paste, raisins, sweet potatoes, and 2 cups of the chicken stock. Slowly bring to a boil, stirring occasionally.

As soon as the mixture boils, reduce the heat to maintain a gentle simmer and cook, stirring occasionally, until the chicken is cooked through and the sweet potatoes are tender, about 45 minutes, adding more stock as necessary to keep the curry moist. Taste and adjust the seasonings with salt and pepper. Discard the bay leaf.

To serve, spoon the rice onto individual serving plates, spoon the chicken, sweet potatoes, and sauce over it, and garnish with cilantro and scallions. Spoon the yogurt and Mango-Ginger Chutney (if using) on top or pass them as condiments at the table.

WOLFGANG'S HEALTHY TIPS

→ The sweet potatoes in this recipe help modest portions of chicken go a long way, providing a filling, satisfying main course. Used here in place of the regular white potatoes you might find in a traditional curry, they are also richer in vitamins and minerals.

→ Including brown rice as part of the recipe enhances the fiber content and soaks up every drop of delicious sauce. For extra convenience, look in your market's grain section for sealed plastic containers of precooked brown rice, ready to heat up quickly in your microwave oven just before serving.

→ If you like, prepare a double batch of the curry. Let the additional portions cool, remove the chicken meat from the bones, and pack the meat, sauce, and sweet potatoes into individual-serving sealable containers to store in the freezer for healthy, convenient future meals.

Nutrition Facts Per Serving (based on 4 servings): Calories: 549; Calories from Fat: 104; Total Fat: 11.65g; Saturated Fat: 4.97g; Monounsaturated Fat: 4.21g; Polyunsaturated Fat: 2.47g; Cholesterol: 190mg; Sodium: 614mg; Total Carbohydrate: 45.19g; Dietary Fiber: 5.88g; Sugars: 12.84g; Protein: 58.72g

Tandoori-Style Chicken Kabobs with Mango-Ginger Chutney

SERVES 4

This recipe delivers big flavors with its spicy but not-too-hot marinade and its sweet-and-tangy tropical chutney. It works equally well for a warm-weather cookout or indoors at other times of year. For a fun presentation after cooking, insert the pointed end of each skewer into a halved cabbage placed cut side down on a serving platter.

Chicken Kabobs:

1½ pounds boneless skinless chicken pieces, half white meat, half dark meat

¾ teaspoon whole cumin seeds

¾ teaspoon whole coriander seeds

1 cup nonfat plain yogurt

1 tablespoon honey

1 tablespoon finely chopped scallion

1½ teaspoons finely chopped fresh ginger

1½ teaspoons finely chopped garlic

¾ teaspoon freshly ground black pepper

¾ teaspoon kosher salt, plus more as needed

½ teaspoon red pepper flakes

¼ cup coarsely chopped fresh cilantro leaves

Mango-Ginger Chutney:

¾ teaspoon peanut oil

½ medium red onion, diced

¼ teaspoon kosher salt

⅛ teaspoon freshly ground black pepper

¼ jalapeño, finely chopped

1 tablespoon minced fresh ginger

½ stalk fresh lemongrass, tough outer leaves removed, heart cut into 1-inch pieces, or 1 (3-by-¼-inch) strip lemon zest

¾ teaspoon dark brown sugar

3 tablespoons rice wine vinegar

1 large mango, peeled, pitted, and cut into ¼-inch dice

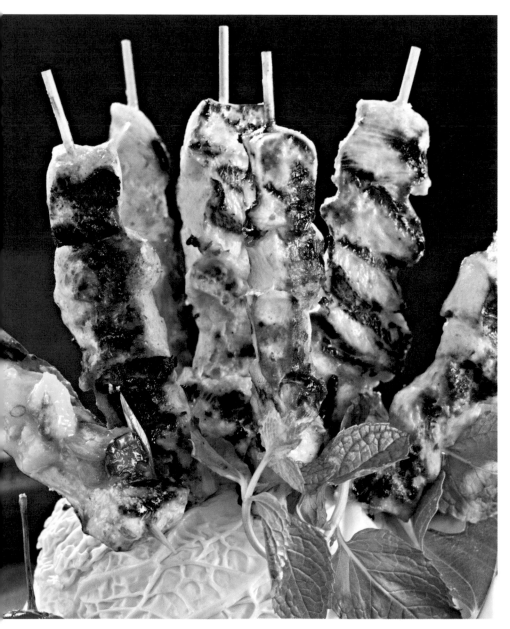

Zest of ½ orange

Juice of ½ orange

Prepare the Chicken Kabobs: If using bamboo or wooden skewers, place eight in a shallow dish, add cold water to cover, and leave them to soak for about an hour.

Cut the chicken into 1-inch chunks and thread them on the skewers. Arrange the skewers in a shallow, nonreactive dish.

In a small dry skillet, toast the whole cumin seeds and coriander seeds over medium-low heat, stirring frequently, just until they are fragrant and slightly darkened in color, 1 to 2 minutes. Transfer to a dish to cool.

Place the toasted seeds in a blender with the yogurt, honey, scallion, ginger, garlic, black pepper, salt, and red pepper flakes. Blend thoroughly. Add the cilantro leaves and process until they are pureed and thoroughly blended.

Pour the marinade over the skewers, turning them to coat the chicken evenly. Cover with plastic wrap and marinate in the refrigerator for 2 hours.

Prepare the Mango-Ginger Chutney: In a medium sauté pan, heat the peanut oil over medium heat. Add the onion and sauté until tender, about 4 minutes. Add the salt, pepper, jalapeño, ginger, lemongrass or lemon zest, and brown sugar. Continue to cook, stirring frequently, until the sugar has melted completely and begun to turn syrupy, 1 to 2 minutes more. Carefully stir in the vinegar and cook, stirring, for about 3 minutes more. Stir in the mango, orange zest, and orange juice and cook, stirring frequently, until the chutney is

thick, 5 to 7 minutes more. Transfer to a stainless-steel or glass bowl and let cool to room temperature. Transfer the cooled chutney to a food processor fitted with the stainless-steel blade and pulse until coarsely pureed. Transfer to a bowl, cover with plastic wrap, and refrigerate.

Grill the Chicken Kabobs: Preheat an outdoor grill, an indoor countertop grill, a ridged stovetop grill pan, or a broiler.

Remove the chicken kabobs from the marinade, shaking off excess marinade. Season the kabobs to taste with salt. Grill until the chicken is golden brown on all sides and cooked through, about 10 minutes total.

Serve the kabobs on a platter or individual plates, passing the chutney alongside at the table. Reserve any extra chutney for another use.

WOLFGANG'S HEALTHY TIPS

→ With its combination of light and dark meat, this offers something for every preference, but feel free to make it with all breast meat or all thigh meat if you like.

→ Serve as a light yet satisfying appetizer, allowing 1 skewer per person.

→ The recipe works equally well with turkey or lean pork.

→ If you like, try turning it into a salad, pushing the chunks of chicken off the skewers onto a bed of mixed greens or baby spinach leaves.

Nutrition Facts Per Serving: Calories: 434; Calories from Fat: 64; Total Fat: 7.16g; Saturated Fat: 2.19g; Monounsaturated Fat: 3.06g; Polyunsaturated Fat: 1.91g; Cholesterol: 185mg; Sodium: 502mg; Total Carbohydrate: 26.53g; Dietary Fiber: 2.21g; Sugars: 22.96g; Protein: 59.34g

Barbecued Chicken with Sweet-and-Spicy Barbecue Sauce and Mashed Grilled Vegetables

SERVES 6 TO 8

If you're looking for a perfect summertime cookout feast, look no further. This combination of smoky-tasting mashed vegetables and spicy-sweet chicken packs a lot of flavor for its lean calorie count. Leftovers are great cold.

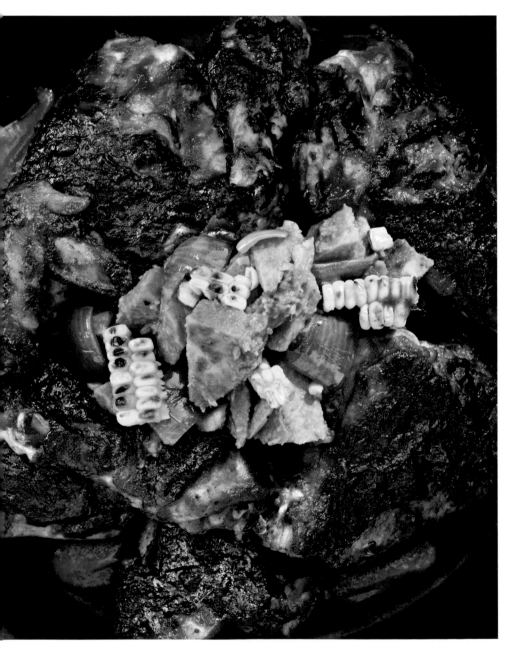

Sweet-and-Spicy Barbecue Sauce:

3 tablespoons peanut oil or vegetable oil

1 red onion, coarsely chopped

1 red bell pepper, stemmed, seeded, deveined, and coarsely chopped

1 cup fresh pineapple chunks

3 small fresh hot red or green chiles, stemmed, seeded, deveined, and minced

1 cup plus 3 tablespoons tomato ketchup

⅔ cup red wine vinegar

⅓ cup tomato paste

½ cup packed dark brown sugar

¼ cup low-sodium soy sauce

½ tablespoon kosher salt

1 teaspoon ground coriander

1 teaspoon ground cinnamon

Barbecued Chicken:

1 whole chicken, cut into 8 pieces, breasts and thighs boned, drumsticks and wings left bone-in, skin removed from all pieces

Extra-virgin olive oil, for brushing

Kosher salt

Freshly ground black pepper

Mashed Grilled Vegetables:

2 orange-fleshed sweet potatoes, trimmed, cut diagonally into ½-inch-thick slices, and parboiled in boiling water to cover until barely tender, drained thoroughly

4 ears corn, parboiled in boiling water until barely tender, drained thoroughly

2 large sweet yellow or red onions, cut into ½-inch-thick slices

Extra-virgin olive oil, for brushing

½ cup fresh orange juice

Kosher salt

Freshly ground black pepper

Prepare the Sweet-and-Spicy Barbecue Sauce: In a large saucepan, heat the peanut oil or vegetable oil over medium-high heat. Add the onion, red bell pepper, pineapple, and chiles and sauté, stirring occasionally, until tender and golden brown, about 15 minutes. Stir in the ketchup, vinegar, tomato paste, sugar, soy sauce, salt, coriander, and cinnamon. Bring to a boil, reduce the heat to low and simmer, stirring occasionally, for 20 minutes.

In a food processor or a blender, taking care to follow the manufacturer's instructions to avoid spattering, puree the sauce, working in batches if necessary and transferring the pureed batches to a nonreactive bowl. Set aside. If you make the sauce ahead, let it cool to room temperature before covering and refrigerating.

Prepare the Barbecued Chicken: Preheat a charcoal or gas grill, arranging one part of the fire for direct-heat cooking, the other part for indirect-heat cooking.

Very lightly brush the chicken pieces all over with oil and season with salt and pepper. Put the pieces directly over the hottest part of the fire and cook until evenly seared a deep golden color, about 3 minutes per side. Then, with long grilling tongs, move the pieces to the cooler part of the grill not directly over the heat. With a grill basting brush, baste the pieces generously on both sides with some of the sauce. Cover the grill and

cook until the chicken registers 165°F on a grilling thermometer inserted into the thickest part of the meat, 7 to 10 minutes per side. (Dark meat will take a few minutes longer than white meat.) As the chicken pieces are done, transfer them to a heated platter and cover with aluminum foil.

Meanwhile, prepare the Mashed Grilled Vegetables: During the last 6 minutes or so of cooking the chicken, very lightly brush the sweet potato, corn, and onion with oil. Arrange the vegetables over the hotter part of the cooking surface and grill until evenly browned, turning occasionally, about 6 minutes total.

While the chicken and vegetables are cooking, gently warm the remaining barbecue sauce. (Discard any sauce that has touched the basting brush to avoid cross-contamination.)

Remove the vegetables from the grill, transferring the corn and onions to a cutting board and the sweet potatoes to a bowl. Cover the bowl to keep the sweet potatoes warm. Using a paper towel to protect your hand, steady one end of an ear of corn on the cutting board and use a sharp knife to cut off the kernels several rows at a time, carefully cutting downward from one end to the other parallel to the cob. Transfer the kernels to another bowl. Coarsely chop the onion slices and add them to the corn. Add the orange juice to the sweet potatoes, along with ½ cup of the warmed barbecue sauce. Use a fork to mash the sweet potatoes into very coarse chunks. Stir in the corn kernels and chopped onions and season to taste with salt and pepper.

Mound the mashed vegetables on a serving platter or individual plates. Arrange the chicken pieces around the vegetable mixture. Transfer the remaining warmed sauce to a sauceboat to pass at the table.

WOLFGANG'S HEALTHY TIPS

→ People sometimes worry about grilled chicken drying out, especially when it's grilled without skin. The barbecue sauce helps keep it moist, though, and removing the chicken pieces to a foil-covered platter the moment an instant-read thermometer tells you they're done helps keep them juicy.

→ Grilling a generous amount of sweet potatoes, corn, and onions along with the poultry, and then turning them into a rustic mash, transforms this dish into a vegetable main course garnished with meat—a healthier balance of foods.

→ Of course, you can also make the mash on its own to go with other grilled foods, although it benefits from the extra moisture and flavor contributed by a little of the sauce you've made for the chicken.

Nutrition Facts Per Serving (based on 6 servings): Calories: 565; Calories from Fat: 126; Total Fat: 14.09g; Saturated Fat: 3.51g; Mono unsaturated Fat: 6.38g; Polyunsaturated Fat: 4.20g; Cholesterol: 97mg; Sodium: 832mg; Total Carbohydrate: 74.95g; Dietary Fiber: 6.59g; Sugars: 45.92g; Protein: 33.50g

Turkey-Mushroom Burgers with Wolfgang's "Secret Sauce"

SERVES 4

Sometimes, you just crave a big, juicy burger that's bursting with flavor. This recipe fully satisfies that craving, sacrificing none of the qualities of a great burger while keeping the fat and calories surprisingly low.

Wolfgang's "Secret Sauce":

¼ cup good-quality low-fat mayonnaise

2 tablespoons tomato ketchup

1 tablespoon bottled tomato-based barbecue sauce

1 tablespoon finely chopped red onion

½ tablespoon chopped cornichons or sweet pickles

1 teaspoon chopped fresh flat-leaf parsley

2 teaspoons lemon juice

Turkey-Mushroom Burgers and Onions:

3 slices multigrain bread

6 tablespoons nonfat milk

¾ pound white mushrooms, wiped clean, stem ends trimmed

1½ tablespoons extra-virgin olive oil

3 tablespoons chopped shallot

2 teaspoons chopped garlic

Kosher salt

Freshly ground black pepper

2 tablespoons Dijon mustard

1 teaspoon chopped fresh thyme

1¼ pounds extra-lean ground turkey

2 teaspoons chopped fresh flat-leaf parsley

Nonstick cooking spray

1 large yellow or red onion, cut into ½-inch-thick slices

To Assemble:

4 good-quality whole wheat or multigrain hamburger buns, split

1 beefsteak tomato, cut crosswise into 4 slices, each ¼ inch thick

4 butter lettuce leaves, rinsed and patted dry

Prepare Wolfgang's "Secret Sauce": In a small bowl, stir together the mayonnaise, ketchup, barbecue sauce, onion, cornichons, parsley, and lemon juice. Cover with plastic wrap and refrigerate until ready to use.

Prepare the Turkey-Mushroom Burgers: Trim and discard the crusts from the bread slices and crumble the trimmed slices into a bowl. Pour the milk over the crumbled bread and set aside to soak.

With a chef's knife or in a food processor fitted with the stainless-steel blade, finely chop the mushrooms.

In a large nonstick sauté pan, heat the olive oil over medium-high heat. Add the chopped mushrooms, shallot, and garlic and season with pinches of salt and pepper. Sauté, stirring frequently with a wooden spoon, until the mushrooms are tender and the liquid they release has evaporated, about 10 minutes.

Stir in the mustard and thyme. Transfer to a rimmed baking sheet and spread out the mushrooms evenly with a spoon. Let cool.

When the mushrooms are completely cool, transfer them to a large bowl and add the turkey, parsley, and soaked crumbled bread. With clean hands, mix the ingredients together thoroughly. Form four individual patties about ¾ inch thick. Season on both sides with salt and pepper.

Heat a countertop electric griddle or grill, a stovetop griddle or grill pan, or a large nonstick skillet to medium-high heat (or, if the weather is nice, prepare a fire in an outdoor grill). Spray with nonstick cooking spray (or, away from the grill fire, spray the cooking grid with nonstick cooking spray before placing it on the grill). Cook the burgers until they are nicely browned and still look juicy, 4 to 5 minutes per side. At the same time, lightly spray the onion slices on both sides with nonstick cooking spray, season to taste with salt and pepper, and cook them alongside the burgers until nicely browned, 2 to 3 minutes per side. When the turkey burgers are done, transfer them to a heatproof platter and cover loosely with aluminum foil; the residual heat will continue to cook them to perfect doneness without drying them out.

Assemble the dish: Lightly toast the cut sides of the buns on the griddle or grill or in the pan. Coarsely chop the onions.

Spread some of the sauce on the bottom half of each bun. Place a turkey burger on top. Garnish with onions, tomato, and lettuce. Serve immediately, passing additional sauce on the side.

→ For the healthiest results, start with the leanest ground turkey you can find. If your butcher doesn't offer it, buy boneless turkey pieces, trim away all skin and visible fat, cut into 1-inch chunks, and spread on a tray. Firm them up in the freezer for 30 minutes, and then pulse in a food processor with the stainless-steel blade until evenly chopped with a slightly coarse texture.

→ Lean ground turkey can be dry when cooked. That's why I enhance the burger mixture with sautéed mushrooms and some soaked multigrain bread, which adds both moisture and flavor. Try doing this with ground chicken or any lean ground meat.

→ If you're craving a cheeseburger, look for reduced-fat sliced cheeses, and place a slice on top of each burger while they cook on their second sides.

Nutrition Facts Per Serving: Calories: 540; Calories from Fat: 148; Total Fat: 16.51g; Saturated Fat: 3.07g; Monounsaturated Fat: 7.41g; Polyunsaturated Fat: 6.02g; Cholesterol: 78mg; Sodium: 738mg; Total Carbohydrate: 53.70g; Dietary Fiber: 6.26g; Sugars: 13.27g; Protein: 45.76g

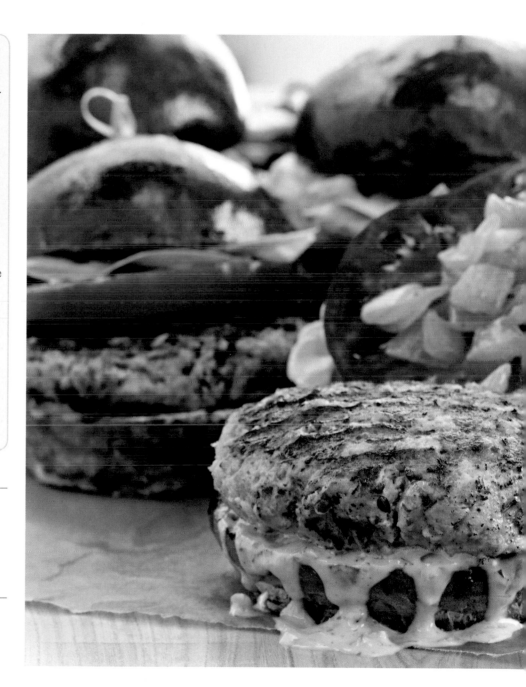

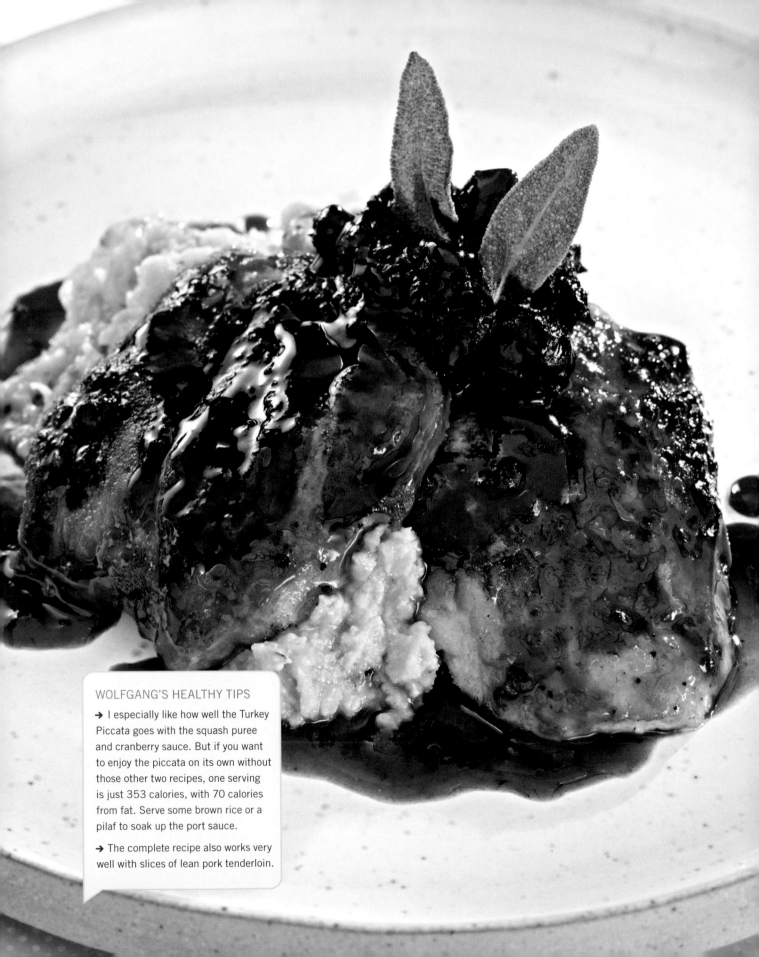

WOLFGANG'S HEALTHY TIPS

→ I especially like how well the Turkey Piccata goes with the squash puree and cranberry sauce. But if you want to enjoy the piccata on its own without those other two recipes, one serving is just 353 calories, with 70 calories from fat. Serve some brown rice or a pilaf to soak up the port sauce.

→ The complete recipe also works very well with slices of lean pork tenderloin.

Turkey Piccata with Winter Squash Puree

SERVES 4

If you want something for Thanksgiving that's different and very healthy but still tastes traditional, try this festive and beautiful recipe. Or make it any time and feel like it's the holidays.

½ cup Cranberry Sauce with Zinfandel (page 206) or good-quality store-bought cranberry chutney or chunky cranberry sauce

Juice of ½ lemon

1 tablespoon unsalted butter, cut into 2 or 3 pieces

Winter Squash Puree:

1 pound fresh butternut squash, unpeeled, seeds and strings removed, cut into large chunks

1 pound fresh acorn squash, unpeeled, seeds and strings removed, cut into large chunks

3 tablespoons honey

¼ teaspoon ground allspice

¼ teaspoon ground cinnamon

¼ teaspoon ground ginger

Turkey Piccata:

1½ pounds boneless skinless turkey breast, cut into 8 equal slices

Kosher salt

Freshly ground black pepper

8 whole fresh sage leaves, plus more for optional garnish

2 ounces thinly sliced prosciutto (about 4 long, thin slices), slices halved

All-purpose flour, for dusting

½ tablespoon vegetable oil

½ cup port

1 cup homemade Chicken Stock (page 271) or good-quality canned low-sodium broth

If using the Cranberry Sauce with Zinfandel (page 206), prepare it a day in advance.

About 1¾ hours before serving time, start preparing the Winter Squash Puree: Preheat the oven to 375°F.

In a single layer in a baking pan, put the squash pieces, peel side down, and add 1 cup water. Cover the pan securely with aluminum foil and bake until the squash pieces are tender, about 1 hour. Set aside at room temperature until cool enough to handle.

Carefully remove the foil and, with a metal spoon, scoop the flesh away from the squash shells, transferring it to a heatproof bowl. Mash the squash with a potato masher until smooth. Add the honey and evenly sprinkle in the allspice, cinnamon, and ginger. Stir until thoroughly blended. Cover the bowl with foil and place it over a pan of gently simmering water to keep it warm until serving time. Leave the oven on, resetting it to its lowest temperature.

Prepare the Turkey Piccata: Season one side of each turkey slice with salt and pepper, then turn them seasoned side down. Place a sage leaf on top of the center of each slice and season with pepper. Top with a slice of prosciutto

and press down firmly with your palm to seal the prosciutto and turkey together. Evenly but lightly dust both sides of each slice with flour.

Heat a large, heavy nonstick sauté pan over medium-high heat. Add the oil. Working in batches if necessary to avoid overcrowding, carefully add the slices, prosciutto side down, and sauté until golden, 2 to 3 minutes. With a spatula, carefully turn them over and sear the other side until golden, 2 to 3 minutes more. Remove from the pan and keep warm in the oven on a heatproof platter covered with foil.

Return the pan to the heat. Pour in the port and stir and scrape with a wooden spoon to deglaze the pan. Stir in the stock and lemon juice and simmer briskly until reduced by half, 5 to 7 minutes. Stirring briskly with a whisk, add the butter a piece at a time until it melts to form a thick, rich sauce. Cover and keep warm.

Stir the Winter Squash Puree and mound it in the centers of 4 heated dinner plates. Rest two turkey scaloppini, prosciutto side up, on top. Spoon some pan sauce over and around the turkey. Spoon some cranberry sauce on top of the turkey and garnish with extra sage. Pass the remaining pan sauce and cranberry sauce at the table.

Nutrition Facts Per Serving (including Winter Squash Puree and Cranberry Sauce with Zinfandel): Calories: 539; Calories from Fat: 71; Total Fat: 7.97g; Saturated Fat: 3.39g; Monounsaturated Fat: 3.12g; Polyunsaturated Fat: 1.45g; Cholesterol: 127mg; Sodium: 450mg; Total Carbohydrate: 54.65g; Dietary Fiber: 5.38g; Sugars: 25.91g; Protein: 50.11g

Stir-Fried Orange-Pineapple Beef with Fried Rice

SERVES 4

In this classic example of an Asian-style one-plate meal, quickly stir-fried slices of lean steak in a citrus-scented sauce are complemented by heaping servings of wholesome brown rice and vegetables.

½ recipe Vegetable Fried Rice (page 196)

1 tablespoon cornstarch

2 tablespoons orange juice

Nonstick cooking spray

1 pound well-trimmed flank steak, all visible fat removed, meat cut across the grain into slices about ⅛ inch thick

Kosher salt

Freshly ground black pepper

1 tablespoon peanut oil

2 teaspoons finely chopped garlic

2 teaspoons finely chopped fresh ginger

2 teaspoons finely chopped scallion

2 teaspoons grated orange zest

¼ teaspoon red pepper flakes (optional)

¾ cup homemade Chicken Stock (page 271) or good-quality canned low-sodium broth

1 tablespoon low-sodium soy sauce

1 tablespoon packed dark brown sugar

1 medium seedless orange, segmented (see page 289)

1 cup bite-size fresh pineapple wedges

Begin preparing the Vegetable Fried Rice (page 196), reserving the recipe's scallion garnish.

When the rice is almost ready, start the stir-fry. In a small bowl, combine the cornstarch and the orange juice and stir well to form a slurry. Set aside.

Preheat a nonstick stovetop or electric wok. When it is hot, spray its cooking surface evenly with nonstick cooking spray. Scatter in the steak slices, season quickly with salt and pepper, and stir-fry, using a nonstick spatula to keep the slices moving all over the wok's surface, just until the meat is evenly browned, about 3 minutes. Transfer the meat to a bowl and set aside.

Place the peanut oil in the wok. As soon as it is hot, add the garlic, ginger, scallion, orange zest, and, if you like, red pepper flakes, and stir-fry just until aromatic, about 30 seconds. Add the stock, soy sauce, sugar, and cornstarch slurry and stir until the mixture starts bubbling and thickens, about 1 minute.

Return the steak slices to the wok, add the orange segments and pineapple wedges, and stir briefly to coat them evenly with the sauce. Taste and adjust the seasonings as needed with a little more salt and pepper.

Divide the fried rice among four heated large individual serving plates or bowls.

Spoon the steak, fruit, and sauce on top of each serving of fried rice. Garnish with the reserved scallions. Serve immediately.

WOLFGANG'S HEALTHY TIPS

→ The stir-fried steak mixture on its own, which comes in at about 302 calories per serving, derives only about 35 percent of those calories from fat (107 calories), thanks to the fresh fruit. Adding the fried brown rice brings the dish's total fat calorie percentage down to a very healthy 29 percent.

→ Flank steak is one of the leaner beef cuts you can choose, but make sure to trim away any visible fat beforehand. The meat is flavorful but on the tougher side, which makes stir-frying an excellent way to cook it, because the steak is thinly sliced across the grain to maximize its tenderness during the quick cooking process.

Nutrition Facts Per Serving (including Vegetable Fried Rice): Calories: 521; Calories from Fat: 150; Total Fat: 16.70g; Saturated Fat: 5.67g; Monounsaturated Fat: 7.82g; Polyunsaturated Fat: 3.22g; Cholesterol: 101mg; Sodium: 337mg; Total Carbohydrate: 56.83g; Dietary Fiber: 7.99g; Sugars: 18.28g; Protein: 33.95g

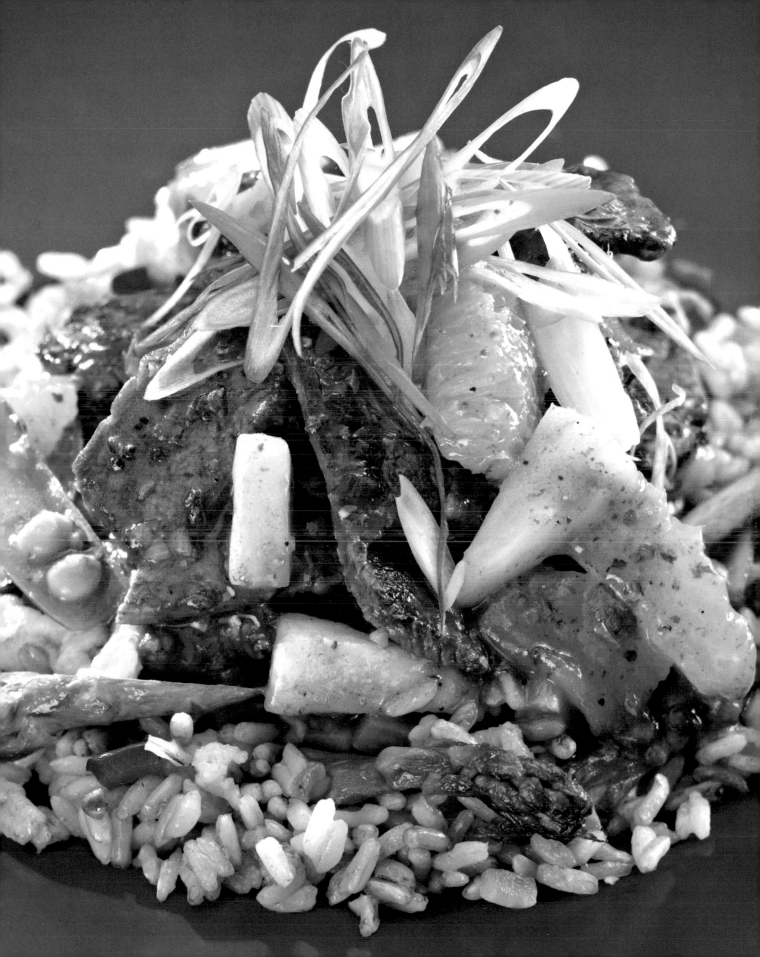

Beef Stew with Winter Vegetables

SERVES 4 TO 6

It may sound like a contradiction to say that a beef stew is low in fat. But it's all a matter of proportion. This recipe, which provides virtually a whole meal in a bowl, contains far more vegetables than meat, but leaves you feeling as if you have feasted.

1½ pounds beef shoulder

¼ cup whole wheat flour

1 teaspoon kosher salt, plus more as needed

¼ teaspoon freshly ground black pepper, plus more as needed

Nonstick cooking spray

1 tablespoon extra-virgin olive oil

1 large onion, coarsely chopped

2 large garlic cloves, minced

1 celery stalk, coarsely chopped

¼ cup tomato paste

1 cup dry red wine

4 cups homemade Beef Stock (page 272) or good-quality canned low-sodium broth

¼ cup balsamic vinegar

1 bay leaf

2 teaspoons minced fresh thyme leaves, or 1 teaspoon dried thyme

½ pound sweet potato, peeled and cut into 1-inch pieces

¼ pound parsnips, cut into 1-inch pieces

1 medium carrot, cut into 1-inch chunks

2 cups button mushrooms, trimmed and wiped clean with a damp cloth

4 cups steamed brown rice, or Brown Rice Mushroom Risotto (page 198), for serving

2 tablespoons minced fresh flat-leaf parsley leaves, for garnish

Cut the beef into 1-inch cubes, trimming away excess fat and any gristle.

In a plastic food storage bag large enough to hold all the meat with room to spare, combine the flour, salt, and pepper. Add the meat to the bag and shake until all the beef cubes are coated with the flour mixture.

Heat a large, heavy saucepan over medium-high heat. Spray with nonstick cooking spray and add the oil. Working in batches to prevent overcrowding, brown the beef cubes on all sides, removing them from the pan as they are browned.

Pour off any excess fat from the pan and spray with more nonstick cooking spray. Add the onion, garlic, and celery and sauté, stirring frequently, until translucent, 5 to 7 minutes. Add the tomato paste and cook, stirring, until it darkens slightly, about 1 minute more.

Add the wine to the pan and bring it to a boil, stirring and scraping with a wooden spoon to deglaze the pan. Return the meat to the pan. Add the stock, balsamic vinegar, bay leaf, and thyme. Cover, reduce the heat to maintain a bare simmer, and cook until tender, about 1 hour.

Stir in the sweet potato, parsnips, and carrot. Cover and continue simmering until the vegetables are tender, about 20 minutes more.

About 10 minutes before serving time, heat a large nonstick sauté pan over medium-high heat. Spray with nonstick cooking spray, add the mushrooms and sauté until lightly browned, about 5 minutes.

Remove the bay leaf from the stew. Stir in the mushrooms. Taste the sauce and add more salt and pepper, if necessary.

Mound 1 cup of the brown rice into each of four shallow soup bowls and ladle the stew around it. Garnish with the parsley.

WOLFGANG'S HEALTHY TIPS

→ The first step in making a healthy beef stew is to choose a lean cut of meat, such as widely available shoulder, and to ask the butcher to trim away all visible fat before cutting it into cubes. At home, before cooking, it's a good idea to go through the meat again and quickly (but carefully) trim away any more fat you see.

→ Browning the meat adds flavor to the stew. But you don't need too much oil to do that, and the dusting of seasoned whole wheat flour adds color and helps to thicken the sauce.

→ Feel free to vary the root vegetables depending on what is available and what you like.

Nutrition Facts Per Serving (based on 4 servings, including steamed brown rice): Calories: 734; Calories from Fat: 134; Total Fat: 14.89g; Saturated Fat: 4.83g; Monounsaturated Fat: 7.68g; Polyunsaturated Fat: 2.39g; Cholesterol: 129mg; Sodium: 1,193mg; Total Carbohydrate: 86.95g; Dietary Fiber: 10.96g; Sugars: 13.10g; Protein: 55.65g

Stir-Fried Orange-Flavored Ground Pork in Radicchio Cups

SERVES 4 AS A MAIN COURSE, 8 AS AN APPETIZER

Eating the well-seasoned, juicy pork-and-vegetable mixture in radicchio cups (you can substitute iceberg lettuce cups) turns a stir-fry into a sort of fun, filling main-course salad that can also be enjoyed in half portions as an appetizer.

2 tablespoons low-sodium soy sauce

1 tablespoon brown sugar

2 teaspoons minced fresh ginger

1 teaspoon minced garlic

1 teaspoon freshly ground black pepper

Grated zest of 1 orange

1 pound lean ground pork

8 large cup-shaped radicchio leaves, free of tears

Juice of 2 oranges

1 tablespoon cornstarch

2 tablespoons peanut oil

2 tablespoons rice vinegar

2 tablespoons bottled hoisin sauce

4 medium fresh shiitake mushrooms, stemmed, caps cut into thin strips (about 1 cup)

1 cup julienned carrot

1 cup bean sprouts

2 cups cooked brown rice

2 cups packed baby spinach leaves, cut into thin julienne strips

½ cup finely julienned scallions

Nutrition Facts Per Serving (based on 4 servings): Calories: 450; Calories from Fat: 128; Total Fat: 14.32g; Saturated Fat: 3.95g; Monounsaturated Fat: 6.85g; Polyunsaturated Fat: 3.51g; Cholesterol: 62mg; Sodium: 532mg; Total Carbohydrate: 47.21g; Dietary Fiber: 5.05g; Sugars: 13.69g; Protein: 30.26g

In a large nonreactive bowl, stir together the soy sauce, brown sugar, ginger, garlic, pepper, and orange zest. Add the ground pork and stir thoroughly with a fork to combine the meat and seasonings. Cover with plastic wrap and marinate in the refrigerator for at least 2 hours.

About 15 minutes before cooking begins, remove the pork from the refrigerator.

Prepare the radicchio cups. Fill a bowl with ice and water and immerse the leaves in the ice water to make them extra-crisp.

In a small nonreactive bowl, stir together the orange juice and cornstarch until the cornstarch has dissolved completely. Set aside. Measure the peanut oil, rice vinegar, and hoisin sauce into small individual bowls and have them ready on the counter close to the stove, along with the pork mixture, shiitake mushrooms, carrots, and bean sprouts.

Heat a large nonstick wok or sauté pan over medium-high heat. When the wok or pan is hot, add the peanut oil. When the oil is hot enough to swirl easily and just beginning to give off the slightest wisps of smoke, carefully add the pork mixture. Stir-fry the pork, moving it around the wok or pan in a constant motion with a wok spatula or large metal spoon, breaking up the meat into small pieces as you stir. Continue stir-frying until the pork is cooked through and lightly browned, about 4 minutes. Add the mushrooms, carrots, and bean sprouts

and stir-fry until they are combined with the pork and softened slightly.

Pour in the rice vinegar and quickly stir and scrape to deglaze the pan and mix the vinegar with the meat. Add the brown rice. Quickly stir the cornstarch mixture and add it, along with the hoisin sauce, to the pan. Continue stir-frying until a glossy, thickly sauced mixture forms, 3 to 5 minutes more.

Drain the radicchio cups and quickly pat them dry with paper towels. Divide the julienned spinach evenly among the cups. Spoon the ground pork mixture on top of the spinach. Garnish with julienned scallions. Transfer the cups to a serving platter or individual plates and serve immediately.

WOLFGANG'S HEALTHY TIPS

→ This recipe is a perfect example of how finely cut-up vegetables can "disappear" into a dish, making it a great way to get children—or grown-ups—to eat more vegetables.

→ For the leanest ground pork, grind it yourself: Buy a lean cut, such as pork loin. Trim away all visible fat and cut the meat into even 1-inch cubes. Chill them in the freezer for about 30 minutes, until firm. Then pulse in a food processor fitted with the stainless-steel blade until evenly, coarsely chopped.

→ The preparation works very well with lean ground lamb or ground chicken, too.

Pan-Seared Pork Chops with Sautéed Cabbage

SERVES 4

My recipe for Sautéed Cabbage with Canadian Bacon and Wine Vinegar (page 188) turns simple lean pork chops—first pan-seared and then finished cooking in the oven—into a complete, filling main-course plate.

4 (8-ounce) bone-in center loin pork chops, trimmed of fat

Kosher salt

Freshly ground pepper

1 tablespoon finely chopped fresh thyme

2 tablespoons extra-virgin olive oil

1 recipe Sautéed Cabbage with Canadian Bacon and Wine Vinegar (page 188)

½ cup homemade Chicken Stock (page 271) or good-quality canned low-sodium broth

2 tablespoons whole-grain mustard

2 tablespoons bottled hoisin sauce

1 tablespoon finely chopped fresh fines herbes (a mix of flat-leaf parsley, chives, tarragon, and chervil, or any combination of these)

Fresh flat-leaf parsley leaves, for garnish

Preheat the oven to 400°F.

Heat a large, heavy-bottomed, oven-proof skillet or sauté pan over medium-high heat. Meanwhile, pat the pork chops dry with paper towels and sprinkle them on both sides with salt and pepper to taste and the thyme.

Add the oil to the hot skillet. As soon as the oil is hot enough to swirl around easily, add the pork chops, spacing them about 1 inch apart in the pan. Cook, undisturbed, until their undersides are golden brown, 2 to 3 minutes. Use tongs to turn them over and sear about 1 minute longer.

Transfer the skillet to the oven and roast until the chops are cooked through but still slightly pink at the center, 12 to 15 minutes.

Meanwhile, make the Sautéed Cabbage. Cover and keep warm.

When the pork chops are done, transfer them to a platter and cover with aluminum foil to keep warm.

Pour off all of the fat from the skillet in which the pork chops were cooked. Return the skillet to the stovetop over medium-high heat and pour in the stock. With a wooden spoon, stir and scrape to deglaze the pan. Boil it briefly, stirring, until it has reduced slightly. Stir in the mustard, hoisin sauce, and fines herbes. Taste and adjust the seasonings with salt and pepper.

To serve, distribute the Sautéed Cabbage among individual heated serving plates. If you like, carve the meat from each chop's bone in thick slices and fan them around the cabbage, placing the bone on top of the cabbage; or simply rest a pork chop on the side of the cabbage on each plate. Spoon the pan sauce lightly over and around each chop. Garnish with parsley and serve immediately.

WOLFGANG'S HEALTHY TIPS

→ This same recipe would work equally well with lean lamb cutlets, small steaks, or chicken breasts. The most important thing is to trim fat from the protein before cooking—or before eating.

→ Chinese hoisin sauce, a traditional condiment usually made from fermented soybeans, has an intense savory-sweet flavor and thick consistency that I like to use to give body to quick sauces in place of the traditional *fond de veau*, or veal reduction, used in classic French cooking. Though hoisin is high in sodium, a little goes a long way. Bottled hoisin is widely available in the Asian foods section of supermarkets.

→ If you like, serve this with a grain dish such as Brown Rice Mushroom Risotto (page 198).

Nutrition Facts Per Serving (including Sautéed Cabbage): Calories: 422; Calories from Fat: 127; Total Fat: 14.13g; Saturated Fat: 3.59g; Monounsaturated Fat: 8.57g; Polyunsaturated Fat: 1.97g; Cholesterol: 131mg; Sodium: 655mg; Total Carbohydrate: 20.92g; Dietary Fiber: 5.51g; Sugars: 10.69g; Protein: 47.24g

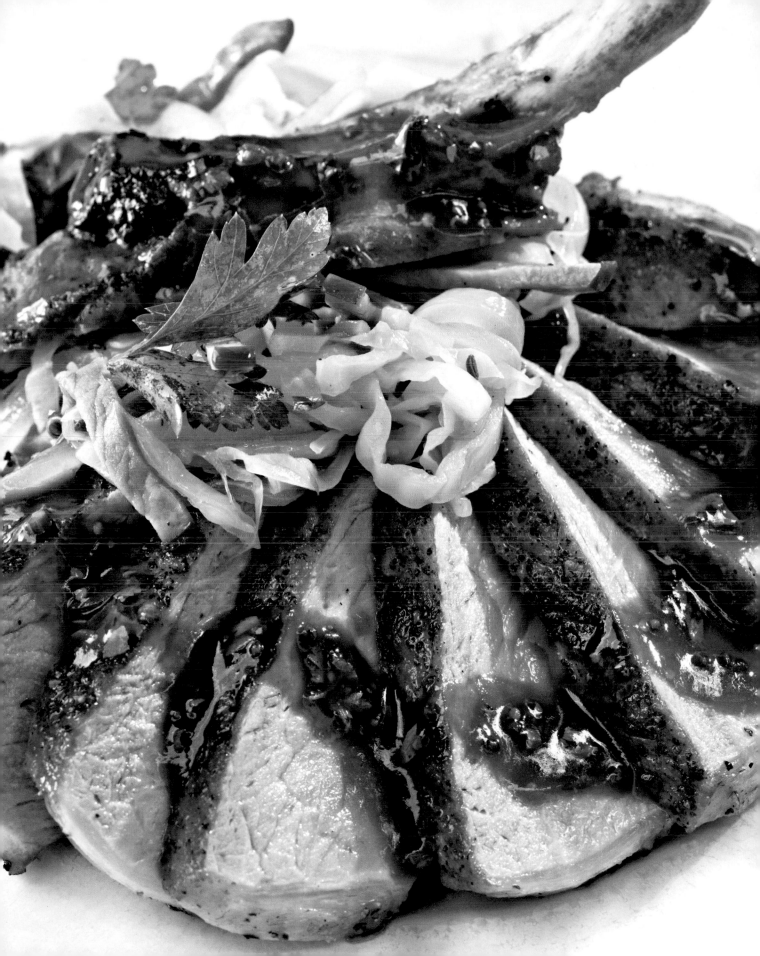

Sautéed Lamb with Zucchini, Eggplant, and Moroccan Harissa-Yogurt Sauce

SERVES 4

Here's a perfect recipe for when you crave something exotic yet still familiar tasting and comforting. Look for the Moroccan seasoning paste called harissa in ethnic markets or well-stocked supermarkets, or online. If you like, serve the lamb, vegetables, and sauce on top of grilled pita bread, Indian naan, or another favorite flatbread.

2 tablespoons extra-virgin olive oil

1 pound small eggplant, cut into ½-inch cubes

1 pound zucchini, cut into ½-inch cubes

Kosher salt

Freshly ground black pepper

2 garlic cloves, finely chopped

2 sprigs fresh thyme

½ pound fresh tomatoes, peeled, seeded (see page 288), and cut into ½-inch cubes

4 (4-ounce) lamb tenderloin medallions, well trimmed

¾ cup dry white wine

¾ cup homemade Beef Stock (page 272), Chicken Stock (page 271), or good-quality canned low-sodium broth

½ tablespoon chopped fresh oregano

1 teaspoon harissa paste

1 teaspoon honey

¼ cup nonfat plain Greek yogurt

Coarse sea salt, for sprinkling (optional)

In a large, heavy, nonstick saucepan, heat 1 tablespoon of the olive oil over medium-high heat. Add the eggplant and zucchini cubes, season with salt and pepper to taste, and add the garlic and thyme sprigs. Sauté, stirring frequently, until tender, about 10 minutes.

Add the tomatoes and stir thoroughly, just until the tomatoes are heated through, about 2 minutes. Taste and, if necessary, add a little more salt and pepper. Remove and discard the thyme sprigs. Cover the vegetables and keep warm.

In a nonstick sauté pan large enough to hold all the lamb without crowding, heat the remaining 1 tablespoon olive oil over medium-high heat. Season the lamb medallions on both sides with salt and pepper and add them to the pan. Cook to the desired degree of doneness (3 to 4 minutes per side for medium-rare), turning once. Transfer to a warmed plate and cover with aluminum foil to keep warm.

Carefully pour off the fat from the pan. Return the pan to the heat, add the white wine, and stir and scrape with a wooden spoon to deglaze the pan. Bring the wine to a boil and cook until it has reduced slightly, 3 to 4 minutes. Stir in the stock and oregano and continue boiling until the liquid has reduced to a syrupy consistency, 7 to 10 minutes more.

Reduce the heat to low and stir in the harissa paste and honey until blended. Add the yogurt and stir just until blended and heated through. Remove from the heat, taste, and adjust the seasonings with a little salt and pepper, if necessary.

Before serving, carve each lamb medallion across the grain into thick slices. Arrange the sliced meat and the vegetables on a serving platter or individual plates, drizzling them with the harissa-yogurt mixture. Sprinkle the lamb with a little sea salt, if you like, and serve.

WOLFGANG'S HEALTHY TIPS

→ The lively, but not too hot, spices in this dish make you stop and savor every bite, so you'll feel fully satisfied by the end of the meal.

→ Each serving contains a lot more vegetables than it does meat, yet you'll come away from the table feeling as if you've had a robust red-meat meal.

→ The nonfat Greek yogurt cools down the spiciness of the harissa a bit and adds a wonderful rich flavor without fat.

Nutrition Facts Per Serving: Calories: 340; Calories from Fat: 104; Total Fat: 11.61g; Saturated Fat: 3.31g; Monounsaturated Fat: 6.97g; Polyunsaturated Fat: 1.32g; Cholesterol: 83mg; Sodium: 247mg; Total Carbohydrate: 21.43g; Dietary Fiber: 7.51g; Sugars: 13.07g; Protein: 29.97g

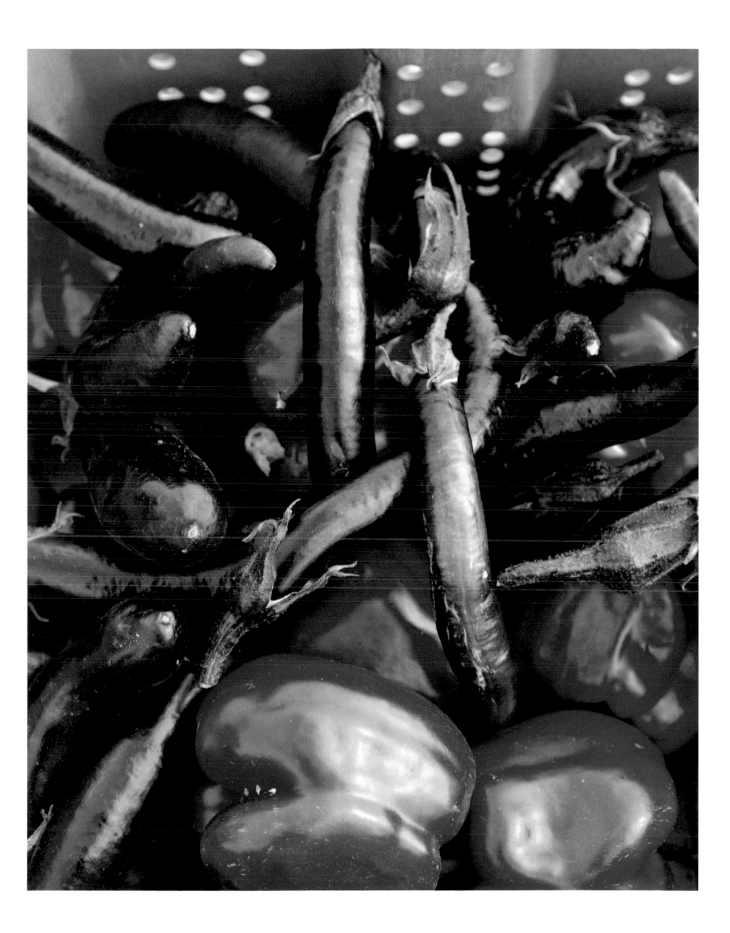

Healthy Reisfleisch with Beef and Turkey Kielbasa

SERVES 8

When I was growing up in Austria, this slowly simmered casserole of rice and meat (*reisfleisch* literally means "rice-meat") was one of our favorite suppers, a delicious, economical way to feed a family. Here, I've found a way not only to cook it much more quickly using an electric pressure cooker, but also to make it healthier with brown rice, lower-fat meats, and extra vegetables.

1 tablespoon unsalted butter

1½ cups diced red bell pepper

1½ cups diced yellow onion

1½ cups diced celery

1½ cups diced carrot

2 garlic cloves, minced

2 cups long-grain brown rice

2¼ cups Chicken Stock (page 271) or good-quality canned low-sodium broth

2 teaspoons fresh lemon juice

1 pound smoked turkey kielbasa sausage, cut into ¼-inch slices

1 pound lean beef steak, such as top sirloin, well trimmed of excess fat and cut into bite-size pieces

1 tablespoon sweet paprika

1 to 2 teaspoons red pepper flakes (optional)

Kosher salt

Freshly ground black pepper

1½ cups frozen peas

2 tablespoons chopped fresh flat-leaf parsley leaves, for serving

Set the pressure cooker timer to 10 minutes and preheat for 5 minutes.

In the pressure cooker pot, melt the butter and cook until it starts to turn a light nut-brown color. Immediately add the bell pepper, onion, celery, carrot, and garlic. Sauté, stirring frequently, until the vegetables turn glossy and begin to soften slightly, about 3 minutes.

Add the rice, broth, lemon juice, sausage, beef, paprika, red pepper flakes (if using), and salt and pepper to taste. Stir well.

Secure the lid on the pressure cooker and seal the steam vent. Reset the timer to 15 minutes.

When the time is up, allow the pressure to release naturally for 10 minutes. Then, open the steam vent to release any remaining pressure. Uncover the pressure cooker, add the frozen peas, and fluff the rice lightly with a fork to distribute the peas through the rice.

Resecure the lid and leave for 5 minutes to allow the peas to heat through.

Scoop the reisfleisch into bowls or onto serving plates and garnish with the parsley.

> WOLFGANG'S HEALTHY TIPS
>
> • This is one of the best examples I know of how a small amount of red meat can be made to stretch a long way. In my childhood, we did that for economic reasons, but today it's an excellent approach for good health, too.
>
> • The chewiness of the brown rice and the robust but not overwhelming spiciness of this dish helps you slow down and savor every mouthful, making this especially satisfying.
>
> • Though the dish's Austrian name suggests it contains meat, you can use the recipe as a basis for similar— and similarly named—preparations containing other forms of animal protein, or none at all, like the two variations that follow.

Nutrition Facts Per Serving: Calories: 426; Calories from Fat: 49; Total Fat: 5.50g; Saturated Fat: 2.27g; Monounsaturated Fat: 2.27g; Polyunsaturated Fat: 0.96g; Cholesterol: 66mg; Sodium: 715mg; Total Carbohydrate: 51.95g; Dietary Fiber: 5.56g; Sugars: 8.07g; Protein: 29.24g

Variation: Paella-Style Shrimp Reisfleisch

For a version reminiscent of Spain's popular rice dish, start by shelling 2 pounds of large fresh shrimp, reserving the shells and cutting the shrimp lengthwise in half. Briskly simmer the shells in 3 cups vegetable stock until the liquid has reduced to 1 cup; strain out and discard the shells. In the pressure cooker, heat 1 tablespoon olive oil and sauté the same aromatic vegetables as in the Healthy Reisfleisch; add the brown rice, 3 cups canned diced tomatoes in their liquid, the lemon juice, the strained broth, red pepper flakes, if desired, and ½ teaspoon saffron threads. Stir well. Cook under pressure for 12 minutes, then let the pressure release naturally for 10 minutes. Vent off any remaining pressure and remove the lid. Arrange the shrimp halves on top of the rice, resecure the lid, and cook under pressure for 1 minute more, release the pressure. With a fork, gently fold in the shrimp while fluffing the rice. Serve garnished with parsley.

Variation: Vegetarian Reisfleisch

For a meat-free "rice-meat," follow the main Healthy Reisfleisch recipe, sautéing the aromatic vegetables in olive oil in the pressure cooker. Cook the rice in 2¼ cups vegetable stock along with the lemon juice and other seasonings under pressure for 12 minutes before letting the pressure release naturally for 10 minutes and then venting off any remaining pressure. Uncover the cooker and stir in 1½ cups each of small broccoli florets, fresh green beans cut into 1-inch pieces, and fresh asparagus cut into 1-inch pieces. Resecure the lid and cook under pressure for 3 minutes more; release the pressure valve, uncover the cooker, and serve, garnished with parsley.

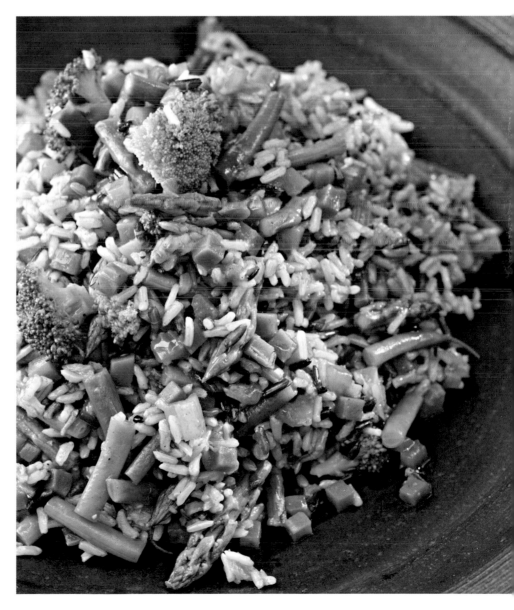

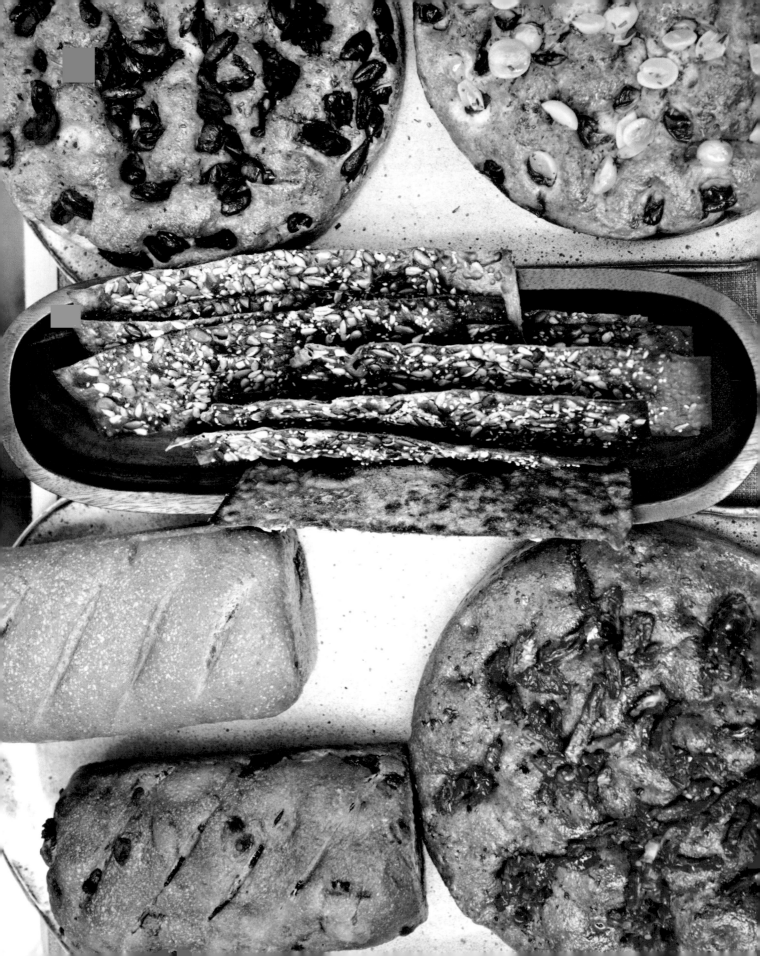

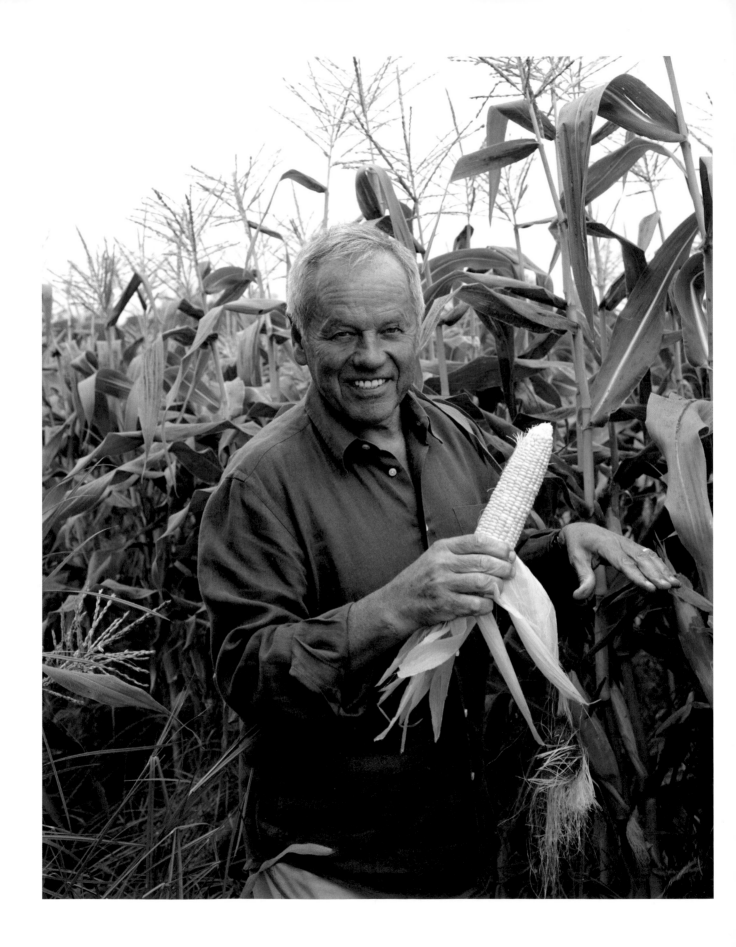

SIDE DISHES

You might be surprised to find that this chapter is one of the largest in the book. But that reflects the way almost all the experts say we should eat today for maximum health—filling most of our plates with fresh vegetable and whole-grain dishes and then adding animal proteins almost like garnishes, or leaving them off the plate completely.

That's certainly the way I now try to eat, and more and more, my chefs and I see it's the way guests in our restaurants prefer to eat, too. People today love all kinds of sides they wouldn't have thought to order a generation ago. In fact, many of these recipes reflect the ever-more-popular small-plates approach to composing a meal with several different shared portions of delicious dishes that often feature whatever was freshest and best at the farmers' market.

You'll find that these recipes are some of the most versatile in this book. You can eat them alongside a main course, to be sure. But most would also work well as appetizers, or as featured attractions in a vegetarian or vegan meal. However you enjoy them, you'll also find examples in each recipe of a fresh approach to cooking that maximizes flavor and nutrients while minimizing fat.

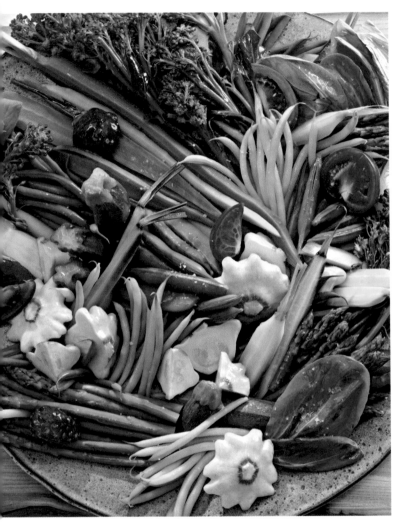

A platter of perfectly cooked, hot, fresh, tender-crisp vegetables in all kinds of colors and shapes is a centerpiece on my family's dinner table. And it's so easy to put together that you don't really need a recipe—just some simple instructions. Besides, the way I like to prepare it, the platter is different every time.

I'll explain.

Every Sunday, I take my young sons to our nearby farmers' market. That's one of the best, most fun ways I know to educate them about all the wonderful vegetables and fruits there are, and to get them excited about eating them. We walk together up and down the aisles, looking to see what's new and in season at all the different stalls, and talking with the farmers themselves. Often, we'll be offered samples to taste. And I'll always let the boys pick out the vegetables (and fruits, too) they're most excited about, for us to take home and cook. Each visit, depending on the season and what we like the most, yields a different harvest. Before we leave the market, of course, we also stop by a flower stand to bring home a big bouquet for their mother.

Before we sit down to eat, and while I'm trimming and peeling those vegetables that need it, and cutting up the larger ones into bite-size chunks that are evenly sized for even cooking, I'll bring water to a boil in a large pan that has a steamer insert. Then, I'll cook each vegetable individually, starting with those thicker and denser ones that need to be cooked longer and finishing with those that cook more quickly; that way, they'll all still be fairly warm when served.

Here's how a typical platter might go:

→ **Asparagus,** pencil-thin spears, tough stem ends simply snapped off where they naturally break, stalks then steamed for about 2 minutes.

→ **Bok choy,** baby-size heads, trimmed and halved lengthwise, steamed for about 3 minutes.

→ **Broccoli,** crowns cut into small florets and stems peeled and cut into pieces about the same size as the florets, or long, thin stalks of broccoli rabe, steamed for about 3 minutes.

→ **Carrots,** in a variety of colors, medium-size, trimmed with an inch or two of stalk remaining, peeled, and halved lengthwise, steamed for about 8 minutes.

→ **Haricots verts,** slender green or yellow French-style fresh beans, trimmed, steamed for about 2 minutes.

→ **Kohlrabi,** the big root trimmed and thickly peeled, then cut into thick slices that I stack and cut again into big sticks like steak fries, steamed for 4 to 5 minutes.

→ **Snow peas** or **sugar snap peas,** trimmed or stringed if necessary, steamed for 2 to 3 minutes.

→ **Summer squashes,** including baby zucchini and pattypan squashes, left whole, halved, or quartered depending on size, steamed for 3 to 4 minutes.

→ **Tomatoes,** larger ones cut into wedges, small cherry, pear, or grape tomatoes left whole or halved depending on size, left raw.

The cooking times are all approximate, because they'll vary with the size and freshness of the individual vegetable. So, how do you know how long to cook them? It's simple: Around the time you think a vegetable is ready, carefully remove a piece and try it: If it's brightly colored and tender-crisp, easy to bite into but still with a little crunch, it's ready.

As each vegetable is done, I transfer it straight from the steamer basket to a heated platter, lightly sprinkle it with sea salt, and lightly drizzle it with extra-virgin olive oil. And I immediately start the next vegetable steaming. I might also add to the platter some vegetables I've cooked simply in other ways, such as Roasted Tomatoes Provençal (page 180), Caramelized Brussels Sprouts (page 186), or Grilled Cauliflower Steaks (page 191).

Once the entire platter is filled with a variety of vegetables, we might start eating it as an appetizer. Or we'll serve it as a side dish to go with a main course that's been cooking as the vegetables are steamed.

My sons love vegetables this way. We all do. I'd like to encourage you to make this a healthy tradition in your family, too.

Roasted Tomatoes Provençal

SERVES 4 TO 8

While reducing the oil in the pesto to only a single tablespoon, I've based this easy recipe on a classic southern French way to cook tomatoes. For the best flavor, I recommend making it only in summer, when you can get good, delicious, sun-ripened tomatoes.

4 ripe but firm medium sun-ripened tomatoes

Kosher salt

Freshly ground black pepper

¼ cup fresh whole wheat or multigrain bread crumbs

¼ cup Light Pesto (page 281), plus more as needed for serving

Preheat the oven to 400°F.

Halve the tomatoes horizontally. With the tip of a small, sharp knife, cut out the core at the stem end of each tomato. Place the tomatoes cut side up in a baking dish. Season their cut surfaces well with salt and pepper.

In a small bowl, stir together the bread crumbs and Light Pesto. Place a spoonful of the mixture on top of each tomato half, distributing it evenly. With the back of a spoon, gently spread the mixture over the cut surface of each half.

Roast until the tomatoes are hot and the bread crumb topping is golden brown, about 15 minutes.

Serve hot, lukewarm, or at room temperature. If you like, drizzle a little extra Light Pesto over the tomato halves before serving.

WOLFGANG'S HEALTHY TIPS

→ Yes, more than a third of the calories per serving—43.2 percent, to be exact—come from fat. But virtually all of that comes from the Light Pesto's olive oil, a healthy fat.

→ In addition to serving these tomatoes as a side for grilled seafood or lean poultry or meat, offer them as an appetizer or as part of an antipasto buffet.

Nutrition Facts Per Serving (based on 4 servings): Calories: 74; Calories from Fat: 32; Total Fat: 3.68g; Saturated Fat: 0.55g; Monounsaturated Fat: 3.17g; Polyunsaturated Fat: 0.69g; Cholesterol: 0mg; Sodium: 28mg; Total Carbohydrate: 9.28g; Dietary Fiber: 2.61g; Sugars: 5.03g; Protein: 2.36g

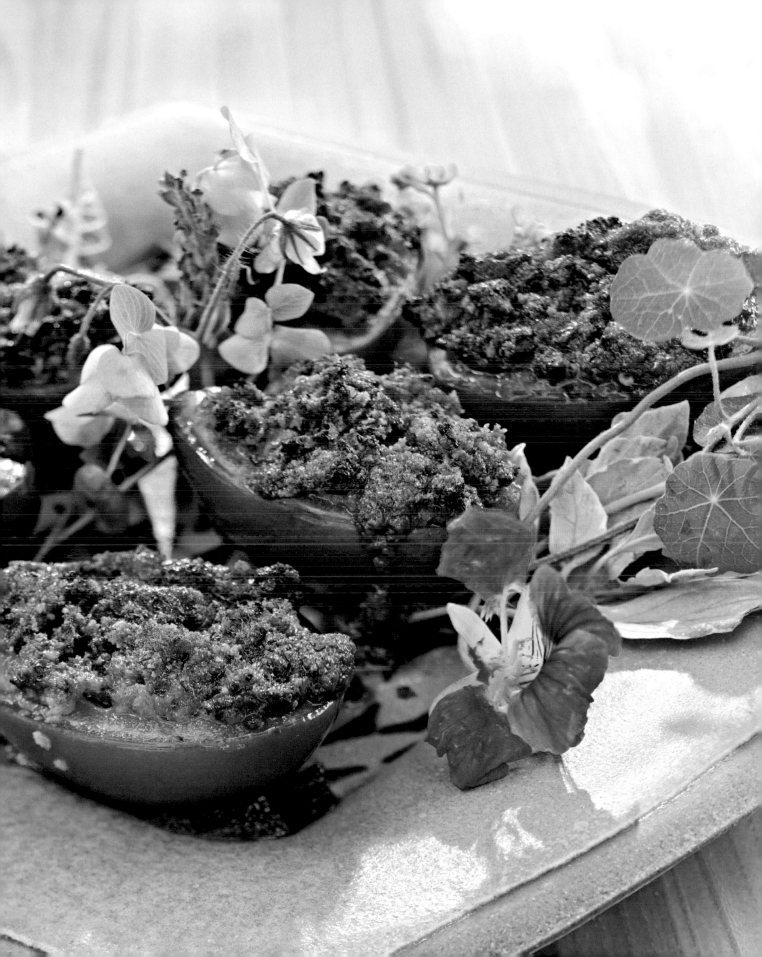

Sautéed Baby Spinach with Garlic and Chile Flakes

SERVES 4

It's no wonder that health-conscious eaters order steamed or lightly sautéed spinach so often in restaurants. The vegetable is very low in calories, rich in nutrients, flavorful, and a beautiful green color. Here's one of my favorite ways to cook it.

½ tablespoon extra-virgin olive oil

1 large garlic clove, minced

1 pound baby spinach leaves, rinsed and patted thoroughly dry

¼ teaspoon red pepper flakes

Pinch of sugar

Kosher salt

Freshly ground black pepper

In a large nonstick skillet, heat the olive oil over medium-high heat. As soon as it is hot enough to swirl easily, add the garlic. Sauté just until fragrant, about 30 seconds.

Add the spinach and red pepper flakes and cook, stirring continuously, just until the leaves have wilted and turned bright green, about 1 minute. Season with the sugar and salt and pepper to taste. Serve immediately.

WOLFGANG'S HEALTHY TIPS

→ The fat in this low-calorie side comes almost entirely from the healthful olive oil used in sautéing, which helps to develop the garlic's flavor before the spinach is added.

→ Although spinach has a distinctive astringent taste, it is still fairly bland. That's why touches of bold seasonings like balsamic vinegar and red pepper flakes have such a big impact on the dish.

Nutrition Facts Per Serving: Calories: 42; Calories from Fat: 17; Total Fat: 1.92g; Saturated Fat: 0.31g; Monounsaturated Fat: 1.24g; Polyunsaturated Fat: 0.37g; Cholesterol: 0mg; Sodium: 89mg; Total Carbohydrate: 4.53g; Dietary Fiber: 2.52g; Sugars: 0.63g; Protein: 3.30g

Eggplant, Zucchini, and Tomato Gratin

SERVES 4

Some of my favorite summer vegetables, widely available year-round, join together in this simple French-style baked side dish, perfect with any kind of meat, poultry, or seafood. Traditionally, the eggplant and zucchini are first fried. But you get leaner, cleaner-tasting results by spraying them with a little nonstick cooking spray and broiling or grilling them.

Olive oil–flavored nonstick cooking spray

1 tablespoon minced garlic

½ teaspoon red pepper flakes (optional)

4 cups canned diced tomatoes

2 teaspoons sugar

2 teaspoons minced fresh thyme, fresh oregano, or fresh basil leaves

Kosher salt

Freshly ground black pepper

¾ pound slender Asian eggplants, cut lengthwise into slices ¼ inch thick

¾ pound zucchini, cut lengthwise into slices ¼ inch thick

2 ounces shredded reduced-fat mozzarella (about ½ cup)

1 tablespoon freshly grated Parmesan

Heat a nonstick skillet over medium heat. Spray with the nonstick cooking spray. Add the garlic and red pepper flakes (if using) and sauté, stirring, until fragrant, about 30 seconds. Add the diced tomatoes, sugar, herbs, and salt and pepper to taste. Cook, stirring occasionally, until most of the liquid has evaporated and a thick but still fluid sauce forms, 10 to 15 minutes. Remove from the heat.

Preheat the oven to 450°F.

Heat a ridged stovetop grill pan, a countertop electric grill, or the broiler. Place the eggplant and zucchini slices on a clean work surface, season lightly with salt and pepper, and spray on both sides with nonstick cooking spray.

Working in batches to avoid over-crowding, cook the eggplant and zucchini slices on the grill pan, grill, or under the broiler until golden brown, 2 to 3 minutes per side. Transfer to a plate and set aside.

Spray a shallow baking dish with nonstick cooking spray. Spread about a third of the tomato sauce on the bottom. Layer the eggplant and zucchini slices over the sauce, overlapping them slightly. Spread another third of the tomato sauce on top. Sprinkle evenly with the cheeses.

Bake in the oven until heated through, bubbling, and golden brown, about 25 minutes. When the gratin is almost done, gently reheat the remaining sauce. Serve the gratin hot or at room temperature, spooning it from the gratin dish onto individual heated plates. Pass the warmed sauce on the side.

WOLFGANG'S HEALTHY TIPS

→ Serve double-size portions as a light summer main dish accompanied by your favorite whole-grain pilaf or brown rice.

→ Try this as an appetizer, too, or as part of a buffet.

→ If you have really sweet, firm, sun-ripened tomatoes available, substitute 1½ to 2 pounds of them for the canned tomatoes. Cut them into slices, remove the watery seed sacs, spray the slices with nonstick cooking spray, lightly season with salt, and broil or grill briefly before layering them with the eggplant and zucchini.

Nutrition Facts Per Serving: Calories: 127; Calories from Fat: 26; Total Fat: 2.97g; Saturated Fat: 1.80g, Monounsaturated Fat: 0.82g; Polyunsaturated Fat: 0.36g; Cholesterol: 10mg; Sodium: 458mg; Total Carbohydrate: 20.50g; Dietary Fiber: 6.27g; Sugars: 12.16g; Protein: 7.85g

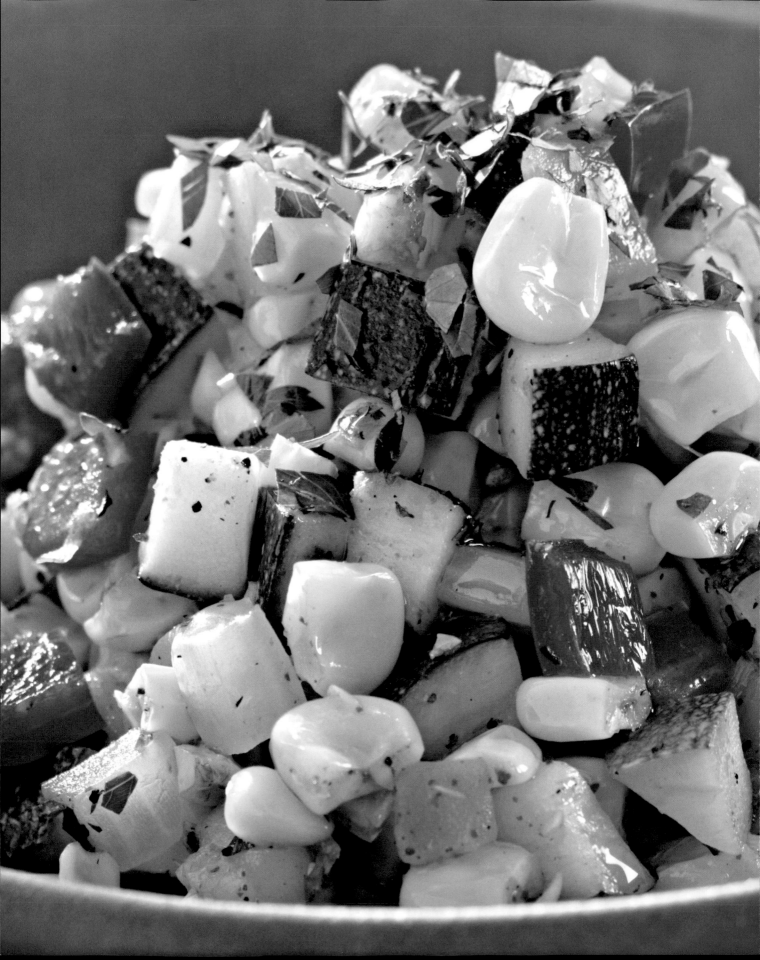

Summer Vegetable Succotash

SERVES 4

Succotash, which gets its name from a Narragansett tribal word meaning "boiled corn kernels," is one of the most flavorful side dishes of summer and autumn. Traditional versions include lima beans, but I've substituted zucchini for an even easier preparation.

3 large ears white or yellow sweet corn

1½ tablespoons extra-virgin olive oil

2 medium zucchini, cut into ¼-inch dice

2 celery stalks, darker green leafy ends trimmed, cut into ¼-inch dice

1 red bell pepper, stemmed, seeded, and cut into ¼-inch dice

1 medium white onion, cut into ¼-inch dice

1 tablespoon minced garlic

½ tablespoon minced fresh thyme leaves

1 bay leaf

Juice of ½ lime

Pinch of cayenne

Kosher salt

Freshly ground black pepper

1 tablespoon chopped fresh flat-leaf parsley, for serving

Steadying one end of an ear of corn on a slip-resistant cutting board, use a sharp knife to cut off the kernels several rows at a time, cutting downward from one end to the other, parallel to the cob. Transfer the kernels to a bowl. Repeat with the remaining corn.

In a heavy cast-iron skillet, heat 1 tablespoon of the olive oil over medium-high heat. When it is hot enough to flow easily, add the corn kernels and sauté, stirring frequently, until they barely begin turning golden brown, 7 to 10 minutes. Transfer the corn to a bowl and set aside. Carefully wipe out the skillet with paper towels.

Return the skillet to the heat. Heat the remaining ½ tablespoon olive oil and, when it is hot, add the zucchini, celery, bell pepper, onion, and garlic. Sauté until the vegetables are tender but not yet browned, about 10 minutes. Stir in the thyme, bay leaf, lime juice, cayenne, and salt and black pepper to taste and continue to cook for 3 minutes more. Stir in the reserved sautéed corn kernels and cook for about 3 minutes more. Remove the bay leaf. Serve immediately, garnished with the parsley.

WOLFGANG'S HEALTHY TIPS

→ Instead of boiling the corn here, I sauté it in a heavy skillet with a little healthy olive oil (traditional recipes use bacon fat or butter), which caramelizes the corn's natural sugars for a rich flavor.

→ The lively seasonings in this recipe—garlic, fresh lime juice, and cayenne—also contribute to giving a low-fat dish big flavor.

Nutrition Facts Per Serving: Calories: 189; Calories from Fat: 59; Total Fat: 6.58g; Saturated Fat. 1.18g, Monounsaturated Fat. 4.19g; Polyunsaturated Fat: 1.21g; Cholesterol: 0mg; Sodium: 43mg; Total Carbohydrate: 31.29g; Dietary Fiber: 5.15g; Sugars: 13.00g; Protein: 5.88g

Caramelized Brussels Sprouts

SERVES 4

The growing popularity of Brussels sprouts has a lot to do with the fact that people are discovering how good they can be when they aren't boiled too long and are even slightly browned during cooking. Serve with your favorite roast or grilled meat, poultry, or seafood.

Kosher salt

1½ pounds Brussels sprouts, trimmed and halved lengthwise

Nonstick cooking spray

½ tablespoon dark brown sugar

Freshly ground black pepper

¼ cup homemade Chicken Stock (page 271), Vegetable Stock (page 274), or good-quality canned low-sodium broth

1 tablespoon chopped fresh flat-leaf parsley, for serving

Bring several inches of water to a boil in a large saucepan. Fill a large bowl with ice cubes and water.

When the water is boiling, salt the water, if you like. Add the Brussels sprouts and cook just until the water returns to a boil and the sprouts turn bright green, 1 to 2 minutes. Drain and immediately immerse the Brussels sprouts in the ice water. Let cool for several minutes. Drain thoroughly, and pat the sprouts completely dry with a clean kitchen towel or paper towels.

Heat a cast-iron skillet or a sauté pan large enough to hold all the Brussels sprouts in a single layer, or if necessary, 2 smaller pans. Spray them evenly with nonstick cooking spray. Sprinkle the bottoms evenly with the sugar and place the Brussels sprouts cut sides down in the pan. Sprinkle lightly with salt and pepper.

Cook until the undersides of the Brussels sprouts are caramelized and a deep brown color, 5 to 7 minutes. Drizzle with the stock and continue to cook, stirring, to glaze the sprouts, 1 to 2 minutes more.

Serve from the skillet, or transfer to a serving bowl or plates. Garnish with the parsley. Serve immediately.

> WOLFGANG'S HEALTHY TIPS
>
> → Nonstick cooking spray makes this recipe almost fat free. But even a splurge of 1 tablespoon unsalted butter, melted and swirled in the pan before you sprinkle in the sugar, adds just 25 calories per serving, 24 of which come from fat, for a side that still gets only 29 percent of its calories from fat.
>
> → Blanching the Brussels sprouts—briefly boiling them and then plunging them into ice water—preserves their bright green color, making this dish as appealing to the eye as it is delicious.

Nutrition Facts Per Serving: Calories: 64; Calories from Fat: 2; Total Fat: 0.33g; Saturated Fat: 0.08g; Monounsaturated Fat: 0.04g; Polyunsaturated Fat: 0.21g; Cholesterol: 0mg; Sodium: 68mg; Total Carbohydrate: 13.62g; Dietary Fiber: 5.05g; Sugars: 4.62g; Protein: 4.71g

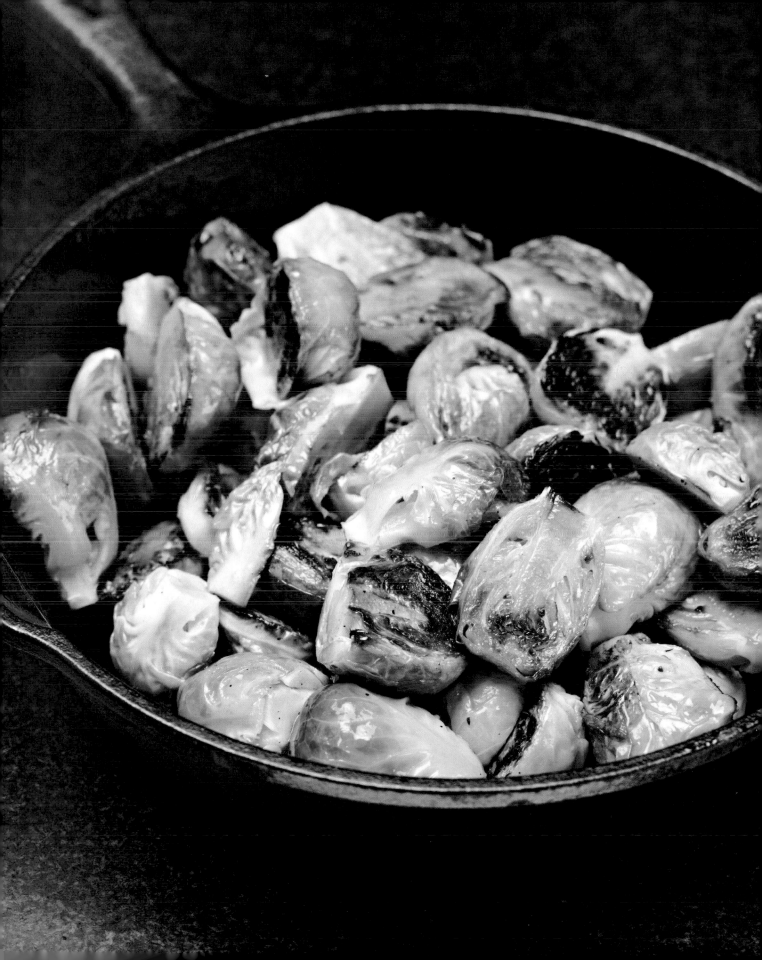

Sautéed Cabbage with Canadian Bacon and Wine Vinegar

SERVES 4

The late great movie writer-director Billy Wilder, an Austrian-born American like me, always loved a less lean version of this tangy central European–style side dish when I made it for him at Spago. Serve it with roast, broiled, or grilled pork chops (see page 168) or other meats or poultry.

½ tablespoon extra-virgin olive oil

1 teaspoon whole caraway seeds

1 small white onion, thinly sliced

2 slices Canadian bacon (about 2 ounces total), cut into thin julienne strips

½ cup white wine vinegar

½ medium head green or white cabbage, cored and cut crosswise into thin strips

1 tablespoon minced fresh flat-leaf parsley

1 tablespoon minced fresh chives, for serving

In a large nonstick skillet, heat the olive oil over medium-high heat. Add the caraway seeds and onion and sauté, stirring continuously, until the onion is glossy and starting to turn tender, about 2 minutes.

Add the Canadian bacon and continue sautéing, stirring frequently, until the onion just begins to turn golden, 3 to 5 minutes more. Add the vinegar, raise the heat to high, and stir and scrape with a wooden spoon to deglaze the pan. Immediately add the cabbage and stir until it is just heated through and slightly wilted, 3 to 4 minutes. Stir in the parsley.

Serve immediately, garnished with the chives.

WOLFGANG'S HEALTHY TIPS

→ Lean Canadian bacon replaces the much fattier bacon used in the traditional version of this Austrian recipe. If you like, you could also try lean turkey bacon. Or leave out the meat completely for a vegan version.

→ Thin slices of a tart-sweet, crisp green apple such as a Granny Smith or a Fuji variety make an excellent addition, stirred in with the cabbage.

→ You can also make the recipe with cider vinegar in place of the white wine vinegar, if you like, to add a slightly fruity tang.

Nutrition Facts Per Serving: Calories: 97; Calories from Fat: 24; Total Fat: 2.60g; Saturated Fat: 0.62g; Monounsaturated Fat: 1.75g; Polyunsaturated Fat: 0.32g; Cholesterol: 7mg; Sodium: 229mg; Total Carbohydrate: 13.15g; Dietary Fiber: 4.79g; Sugars: 6.62g; Protein: 5.49g

Roasted Root Vegetable Medley

SERVES 12 TO 16

For a holiday or other special-occasion meal, you want to go all out with your side dishes. Yet this colorful and flavorful one, featuring eight different kinds of root vegetables and a whole head of garlic, is surprisingly simple to prepare. Leftovers are also good served cold the next day with your leftover roast.

8 slender carrots, peeled and trimmed

8 baby turnips, peeled and trimmed

8 fingerling potatoes, scrubbed clean under cold running water, peels left on

2 large parsnips, peeled and trimmed

1 medium orange-flesh or ruby sweet potato, scrubbed clean under cold running water, peel left on

1 medium yellow onion, peeled

1 kohlrabi bulb, peeled

1 small celery root (celeriac) bulb, peeled

1 small head garlic, cloves separated, left unpeeled

2 sprigs fresh rosemary, sage, or thyme

Olive oil–flavored nonstick cooking spray

Kosher salt

Freshly ground black pepper

Chopped fresh flat-leaf parsley or chives, for serving

Preheat the oven to 400°F.

Prepare the vegetables, making sure that all the pieces are roughly the same 1-inch size or thickness for even cooking, and cutting off and discarding any green tops. Leave the carrots and baby turnips whole. Halve the cleaned potatoes lengthwise. Cut the parsnips diagonally into 1-inch chunks. Cut the sweet potato into 1-inch chunks. Halve the onion, then cut each half into quarters. Cut the kohlrabi into thick wedges. Halve the celery root and cut each half crosswise into slices 1 inch thick. Separate the head of garlic into individual cloves, leaving them unpeeled.

Put all the vegetable pieces, garlic cloves, and herb sprigs in a large baking dish. Spray with nonstick cooking spray and toss until lightly and evenly coated. Season well with salt and black pepper, and toss to coat evenly.

Roast, stirring occasionally to ensure even roasting, until the vegetables are golden brown and tender enough to be pierced easily with the tip of a metal skewer or small, sharp knife, about 45 minutes. Present the vegetables in their baking dish or transfer them to a heated platter. Garnish with parsley or chives just before serving.

WOLFGANG'S HEALTHY TIPS

→ With the only fat coming from traces in the vegetables themselves and the nonstick cooking spray, this dish is amazingly lean, especially when you consider how rich it tastes—partly the result of the natural sugars present in the roots caramelizing during roasting.

→ Feel free to vary the kinds and amounts of root vegetables you include, guided by your tastes and what looks best at the market.

→ The whole garlic cloves not only help to scent the other vegetables, but they also provide a delicious bonus. Once roasted, they'll be as soft as butter and have a full, almost sweet flavor. Squeeze them from their skins and use as a condiment with your main dish, or spread on whole-grain bread to enjoy with your meal.

Nutrition Facts Per Serving (based on 12 servings): Calories: 161; Calories from Fat: 2; Total Fat: 0.31g; Saturated Fat: 0.09g; Monounsaturated Fat: 0.05g; Polyunsaturated Fat: 0.17g; Cholesterol: 0mg; Sodium: 85mg; Total Carbohydrate: 37.29g; Dietary Fiber: 5.71g; Sugars: 6.75g; Protein: 4.33g

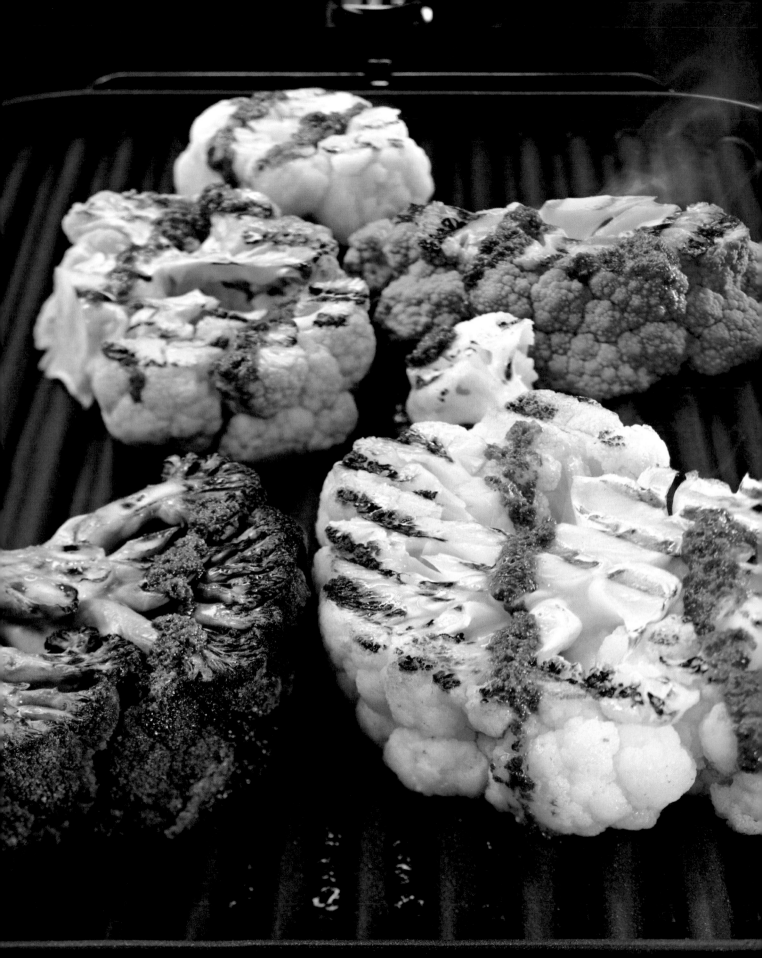

Grilled Cauliflower Steaks

SERVES 4

When cut vertically into whole steaks and then grilled, ordinary cauliflower becomes extraordinarily delicious, making a good side dish for grilled meat, poultry, or seafood—or a very lean vegetarian main dish or appetizer on its own. When multiplying the recipe for a party, look for heads of beautiful purple, green, and orange cauliflower at the farmers' market or a good greengrocer to make a beautiful kaleidoscopic presentation.

1 large head cauliflower

Kosher salt

Olive oil–flavored nonstick cooking spray

Freshly ground black pepper

¼ cup Light Pesto (page 281)

Remove the leaves from the cauliflower head and trim the base even with the bottom of the head. Set aside.

Bring a large pot of water, deep enough to immerse the whole cauliflower head, to a boil. Fill a bowl large enough to hold the cauliflower with ice cubes and water.

When the water reaches a full boil, lightly salt the water, if desired. Immerse the head of cauliflower in the boiling water. As soon as the water returns to a boil, use a large, sturdy slotted spoon or wire skimmer to remove the cauliflower from the pot and transfer it to the ice water to cool for at least 2 to 3 minutes.

Drain the cooled cauliflower head thoroughly and pat it dry with paper towels. Transfer to a cutting board.

With a large, sharp knife, and starting toward the center, carefully cut the head of cauliflower vertically into slices about ¾ inch thick. You should get at least 4 large "steaks" and several other good-size slices; reserve any smaller pieces for another use.

Heat a large nonstick ridged stovetop grill pan or electric countertop grill to medium-high heat. Spray the cauliflower slices on both sides with nonstick cooking spray and season to taste on both sides with salt and pepper.

Place the cauliflower steaks on the grill pan or grill. Cook until deep golden brown, about 5 minutes per side. If you like, drizzle some of the Light Pesto over the steaks after turning them, to help release the sauce's fragrance; or transfer the grilled cauliflower steaks to a heated platter or individual serving plates and pass the pesto separately for each person to drizzle over their portion.

WOLFGANG'S HEALTHY TIPS

→ The drizzle of pesto sauce in the recipe adds bright green color and an extra punch of flavor. But if you're being very strict about fat, eat the cauliflower steak alone without the pesto. Each serving will be 52 calories, with only 1 calorie from fat. But the fat in the sauce comes from healthful olive oil.

→ If you serve this as a main dish, accompany it with steamed brown rice or another whole-grain side such as Farro and Root Vegetable Pilaf (page 201).

Nutrition Facts Per Serving (with Light Pesto): Calories: 86; Calories from Fat: 31; Total Fat: 3.68g; Saturated Fat: 0.60g; Monounsaturated Fat: 3.10g; Polyunsaturated Fat: 0.55g; Cholesterol: 0mg; Sodium: 29mg; Total Carbohydrate: 12.06g; Dietary Fiber: 2.79g; Sugars: 6.89g; Protein: 2.71g

Sautéed Wild Mushrooms with Garlic, Shallots, and Balsamic Vinegar

SERVES 4

With their earthy, deep flavor and chewy textures, mushrooms are often compared to meat in the way they can satisfy even dedicated carnivores. And the many different kinds you can find in markets of so-called "wild" mushrooms, most now commercially cultivated, makes them an even more varied pleasure. I love to serve them sautéed as a side dish for any kind of protein.

1 pound mixed fresh wild mushrooms, such as maitake, porcini, chanterelles, shiitakes, oysters, or morels

2 teaspoons extra-virgin olive oil

1 shallot, minced

1 garlic clove, minced

Kosher salt

Freshly ground black pepper

3 cups packed baby arugula leaves

2 tablespoons aged balsamic vinegar

1 tablespoon finely chopped fresh chives or flat-leaf parsley

With a clean, damp cloth or paper towels, wipe the mushrooms clean. Trim any tough stems. Cut any mushroom clusters or slender mushrooms lengthwise, or wide mushroom caps crosswise, into slices ¼ inch thick.

In a large nonstick skillet, heat the olive oil over high heat. As soon as it swirls easily, add the sliced mushrooms. Sauté, stirring continuously, just until the juices released by the mushrooms have evaporated and the mushrooms have begun to brown, 7 to 10 minutes. Stir in the shallot and garlic and sauté until aromatic, about 1 minute more. Season to taste with salt and pepper.

Arrange a bed of arugula on individual serving plates or on a serving platter or bowl. Spoon the mushrooms on top. Drizzle with the balsamic vinegar and garnish with the chives or parsley.

WOLFGANG'S HEALTHY TIPS

→ Rapid sautéing with a little oil over high heat intensifies the flavor of the mushrooms by evaporating much of their moisture.

→ The touch of balsamic vinegar, with its concentrated sweet-and-sour syrupiness, further highlights the flavor of the mushrooms, making the dish taste extra rich without extra fat.

→ You can also serve the mushrooms on top of even larger beds of arugula or mixed greens as a salad—garnished, if you like, with a light sprinkle of crumbled goat cheese or shaved Parmesan.

Nutrition Facts Per Serving: Calories: 76; Calories from Fat: 20; Total Fat: 2.27g; Saturated Fat: 0.33g; Monounsaturated Fat: 1.65g; Polyunsaturated Fat: 0.29g; Cholesterol: 0mg; Sodium: 16mg; Total Carbohydrate: 10.39g; Dietary Fiber: 4.58g; Sugars: 2.84g; Protein: 2.25g

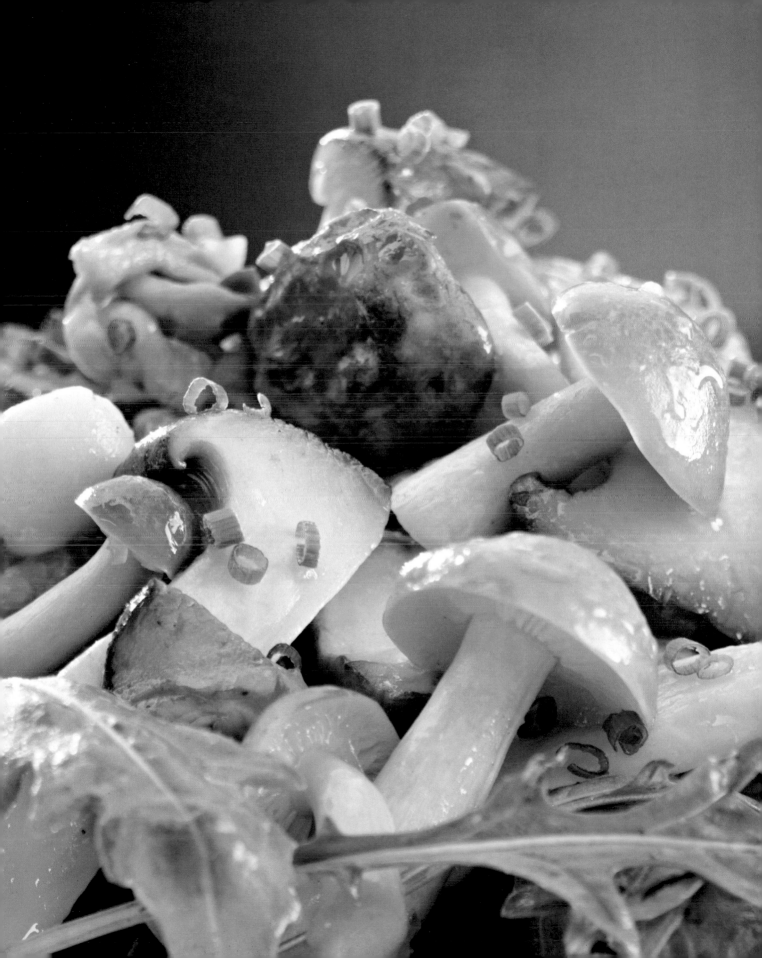

It isn't surprising that potatoes are among the most popular side dishes. Earthy and filling, they satisfy admirably. And, being relatively bland, they provide cooks with a canvas for adding all sorts of enhancements.

Too often, those additions—butter, cream, or cheese—can be high in fat. But that doesn't have to be the case. As the following three recipes show, mashed potatoes can taste luxurious and indulgent while staying lean. Use these as inspiration for your own mashed potato creations.

Here's a hint: Try enhancing the mixture with some other light but flavor-packed sauce or condiment such as Light Pesto (page 281), Onion Soubise (page 283), or Roasted Garlic (page 284).

Mashed Yukon Gold Potatoes with Brown Butter

SERVES 4

With its bright yellow color and rich flavor, the now widely available Yukon gold potato variety has become what you might genuinely call the "gold standard" for mashed potatoes. This healthy version works equally well as an everyday or special-occasion side.

1½ pounds Yukon gold potatoes, peeled, cut in uniform chunks

Kosher salt

3 tablespoons unsalted butter

½ cup buttermilk

Freshly ground white pepper

Freshly grated nutmeg

1 tablespoon minced fresh flat-leaf parsley leaves or chives

Put the potatoes in a pot and add cold water to cover by several inches. Salt the water generously. Bring to a boil over high heat; reduce the heat to maintain a simmer. Simmer the potatoes until just fork-tender, about 30 minutes.

About 5 minutes before the potatoes are done, melt the butter in a small skillet over medium heat. Continue cooking until the butter turns a light nut-brown color, 2 to 3 minutes; watch carefully to avoid burning, and remove the skillet from the heat as soon as the butter starts to brown.

At the same time, bring the buttermilk to a boil in a small saucepan over medium heat. Reduce the heat to very low and keep warm.

As soon as the potatoes are done, drain them thoroughly. Pass the potatoes through a ricer or a food mill into a heatproof bowl.

Vigorously stir the brown butter and the hot buttermilk into the potatoes until thoroughly combined. Season to taste with salt and white pepper and a dash of freshly grated nutmeg.

Cover the bowl; if not serving immediately, set the bowl over a pan of simmering water to keep the potatoes warm. Transfer to a serving dish. Garnish with the parsley or chives.

WOLFGANG'S HEALTHY TIPS

→ This is a good example of how a little richness can go a long way. Just a little butter supplies most of the fat in this recipe, and browning it intensifies its flavor, adding a deep, nutty taste to the puree.

→ The hint of nutmeg also enriches the flavor of the mashed potatoes. For the best taste, buy whole nutmeg and grate it fresh with a special fine-toothed nutmeg grater, which usually has a hatch in which you can store the whole acorn-size spice.

Nutrition Facts Per Serving: Calories: 234; Calories from Fat: 75; Total Fat: 8.43g; Saturated Fat: 5.69g; Monounsaturated Fat: 2.32g; Polyunsaturated Fat: 0.41g; Cholesterol: 23mg; Sodium: 42mg; Total Carbohydrate: 34.89g; Dietary Fiber: 2.44g; Sugars: 2.64g; Protein: 5.08g

Variation: Horseradish Mashed Potatoes

Prepared horseradish, usually found in the refrigerated case of supermarkets and sometimes in the Jewish foods section, adds a pleasant bite to a side that goes especially well with beef and other meat dishes. Follow the recipe for Mashed Yukon Gold Potatoes, but simply melt the butter without letting it brown. During mashing, add 1 tablespoon plain prepared horseradish.

Variation: Wasabi Mashed Potatoes

A touch of the Japanese horseradish known as wasabi, available dried in the Asian foods section of the supermarket or as a paste at the sushi counters found in many markets, adds a lively kick of flavor and beautiful green color to this puree. Follow the recipe for Mashed Yukon Gold Potatoes, omitting the butter, and mash into the potatoes 2 teaspoons wasabi powder, stirred to a paste in 2 teaspoons water, or about 1 tablespoon prepared wasabi paste, adding more or less to taste.

Vegetable Fried Rice

SERVES 8 AS A SIDE DISH, 4 AS A MAIN COURSE

Fried rice can be so full of colors, shapes, and flavors that it feeds the eye as well as the body. Although it's a perfect side dish to Asian or non-Asian main dishes alike, I sometimes like it as a light main dish on its own. Because the stir-frying goes so quickly here, be sure to have all the ingredients prepped and arranged in easy reach and order of use before you start cooking.

4 cups cooked and cooled brown rice, preferably made a day ahead

2 tablespoons peanut oil or vegetable oil

2 garlic cloves, minced

1 small yellow onion, minced

1 teaspoon minced fresh ginger

¼ to ½ teaspoon red pepper flakes

½ pound sugar snap peas, strings removed

½ pound bite-size broccoli florets

½ cup fresh corn kernels (from about 1 small ear)

½ small red bell pepper, stemmed, seeded, and cut into ¼-inch dice

8 asparagus spears, trimmed and cut diagonally into ¼-inch slices

1 large egg, lightly beaten

2 tablespoons low-sodium soy sauce

Kosher salt

Freshly ground black pepper

2 tablespoons coarsely chopped fresh cilantro leaves, for garnish

2 scallions, thinly sliced, for garnish

In a mixing bowl, gently rub the cold rice between your fingers to separate it into individual grains.

Heat a nonstick wok or a large, heavy nonstick skillet over medium-high heat. Add the oil. When it is hot enough that it is barely beginning to show slight wisps of smoke, add the garlic, onion, ginger, and red pepper flakes. With a stir-fry spatula or a long-handled wooden spatula or spoon, stir constantly until fragrant, about 1 minute.

Add the sugar snap peas and broccoli and stir-fry just until their color brightens, about 30 seconds. Add the corn, bell pepper, and asparagus and continue stir-frying. Then add the rice and stir-fry for 2 minutes more.

Drizzle the beaten egg around the rim of the wok or skillet so that it cooks before it touches the rice. Quickly stir the egg, breaking it up into small curds and folding it into the rice. Sprinkle in the soy sauce and stir well. Season the fried rice to taste with salt and pepper.

Heap the rice into individual large heated bowls or a large serving bowl, or onto a platter, or serve from the wok or skillet. Garnish with the cilantro and scallions. Serve immediately.

WOLFGANG'S HEALTHY TIPS

→ Spoon the fried rice into large individual serving bowls and top it with your favorite protein, such as Spice-Rubbed Chicken Breasts (page 152) or other simple grilled, broiled, or steamed poultry, meat, seafood, or tofu, to make a complete main course.

→ Alternatively, stir sliced or chopped leftovers into the rice mixture, just long enough before the end of cooking to heat them up.

→ For an even lower-fat version, feel free to substitute 3 egg whites for the egg, or use some of the fat-free egg product sold in cartons in your supermarket's refrigerated section. Leave out the egg for a vegan version.

Nutrition Facts Per Serving (based on 8 servings): Calories: 219; Calories from Fat: 43; Total Fat: 4.81g; Saturated Fat: 1.03g; Monounsaturated Fat: 2.14g; Polyunsaturated Fat: 1.64g; Cholesterol: 23mg; Sodium: 78mg; Total Carbohydrate: 37.43g; Dietary Fiber: 6.26g; Sugars: 5.88g; Protein: 7.75g

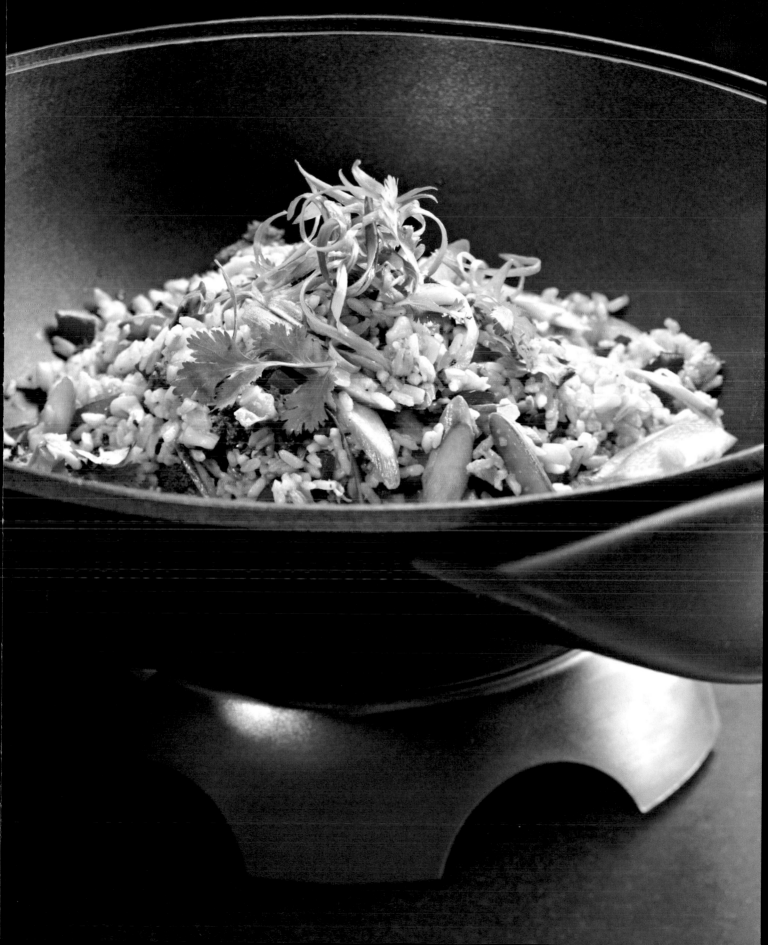

Brown Rice Mushroom Risotto

SERVES 4

I've discovered that cooking brown rice in a pressure cooker with stock, sautéed mushrooms, and seasonings produces a creamy, chewy consistency surprisingly similar to that of classic Italian risotto—and so much healthier.

1½ tablespoons extra-virgin olive oil

1 tablespoon minced garlic

1 tablespoon minced shallot

2 cups coarsely chopped fresh mushrooms of any kind

1 cup brown rice

1½ cups homemade Chicken Stock (page 271) or Vegetable Stock (page 274), or good-quality canned low-sodium broth

1 tablespoon port

Kosher salt

Freshly ground black pepper

2 recipes Onion Soubise (page 283)

1 cup fresh peas or frozen baby peas

2 tablespoons finely chopped fresh flat-leaf parsley or chives

¼ cup freshly grated Parmesan (optional)

In an electric pressure cooker pot with the lid off, heat the olive oil. Add the garlic and shallot and sauté, stirring, until tender, about 3 minutes. Add the mushrooms and cook, stirring regularly, until most of the moisture they give up has evaporated, 10 to 15 minutes.

Add the rice and stir well to combine with the mushroom mixture. Stir in the stock and port and salt and pepper to taste. Secure the lid on the pressure cooker, bring to full pressure, and set the timer for 15 minutes.

Meanwhile, prepare the Onion Soubise.

When the rice is done, release the pressure and carefully remove the lid. Taste the rice. If it seems not quite tender enough, secure the lid, bring back to pressure, and cook about 2 minutes more before releasing the pressure and removing the lid again.

Once the rice is completely cooked, add the peas to the pressure cooker without stirring them into the rice. Secure the lid back on the pressure cooker and leave for 5 minutes to allow the peas to steam under residual heat. Then, uncover and stir the peas into the rice mixture.

Stir in the hot Onion Soubise. Taste and adjust the seasonings.

Serve immediately, garnished with the parsley or chives and Parmesan, if desired.

WOLFGANG'S HEALTHY TIPS

→ I love this as a healthy side with a meat or poultry main dish such as Sautéed Lamb with Zucchini and Eggplant (page 170) or Butterflied Garlic-Parsley Chicken (page 151). You could also serve this as an appetizer.

→ For a vegetarian or vegan main course, sauté additional mushrooms of your choosing and spoon them on top of each portion of the risotto, as shown in the photo.

→ I enjoy a little Parmesan on my risotto, though it is optional. Just 1 tablespoon of Parmesan adds 21 calories per serving, 12 of them from fat, and also ups the sodium count by 76mg if you're watching your salt intake.

Nutrition Facts Per Serving: Calories: 345; Calories from Fat: 86; Total Fat: 9.62g; Saturated Fat: 1.48g; Monounsaturated Fat: 5.89g; Polyunsaturated Fat: 1.38g; Cholesterol: 0mg; Sodium: 250mg; Total Carbohydrate: 57.83g; Dietary Fiber: 4.66g; Sugars: 12.60g; Protein: 8.68g

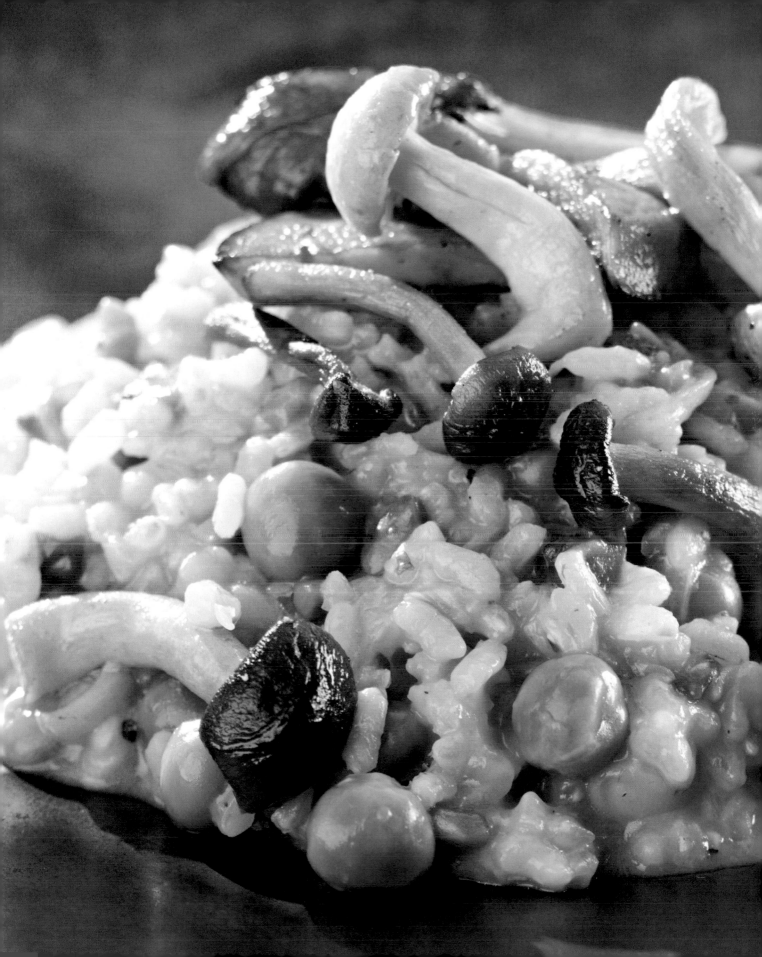

Brown Sushi Rice

MAKES ABOUT 2 CUPS; FOUR ½-CUP SERVINGS

The rice traditionally used as a base for sushi has a wonderful flavor thanks to a few very simple seasonings. I think they work especially well with the nutty flavor of brown rice, to make an easy, delicious side for all sorts of Asian-style foods.

1 cup medium-grain brown rice

1 tablespoon low-sodium soy sauce

3 tablespoons rice wine vinegar

1½ tablespoons honey

Rinse the rice under cold running water. Drain well.

Put the rice in a rice cooker or a heavy saucepan. Add 2 cups water and ½ tablespoon of the soy sauce. Set the rice cooker for 45 minutes; or bring the water to a boil in the pan, reduce the heat to maintain a bare simmer, cover, and cook until all the liquid has been absorbed, about 45 minutes. Turn off the rice cooker or remove the pan from the heat and set aside, covered, to rest for 10 minutes.

In a small bowl, stir together the remaining ½ tablespoon soy sauce, the rice wine vinegar, and the honey until the honey has dissolved completely.

Transfer the rice to a bowl. Sprinkle the soy sauce mixture over the rice and, with a large spoon, stir and toss the rice to combine. Let cool at room temperature for about 15 minutes, stirring every few minutes.

Serve the rice lukewarm, as a base for rice bowls, molded as a base for Tuna Tataki (page 135) or other seared or raw Asian-style seafood, or as a side dish.

WOLFGANG'S HEALTHY TIPS

→ If you like, make a quick, simple stir-fry of vegetables and some scrambled egg (or egg whites or fat-free egg product) or firm tofu cubes and stir it into the warm rice to make an easy vegetarian or vegan (without the egg) main course.

→ Make an extra batch of the recipe and refrigerate in a covered container to enjoy at lunch the next day, either as the basis for an Asian-flavored rice salad or simply rolled up inside slices of lean cold cuts for a casual meal.

→ Feel free to substitute other whole grains such as barley, farro, or quinoa for up to half of the brown rice to vary the dish.

Nutrition Facts Per Serving: Calories: 199; Calories from Fat: 10; Total Fat: 1.17g; Saturated Fat: 0.25g; Monounsaturated Fat: 0.46g; Polyunsaturated Fat: 0.46g; Cholesterol: 0mg; Sodium: 140mg; Total Carbohydrate: 43.11g; Dietary Fiber: 1.66g; Sugars: 6.58g; Protein: 3.79g

Farro and Root Vegetable Pilaf

SERVES 4

Farro, an ancient ancestor of wheat, forms the foundation here for an earthy, nutty, flavorful side dish rich in fiber and other nutrients.

2 tablespoons extra-virgin olive oil

1 large carrot, cut into ¼-inch dice

1 large celery stalk, cut into ¼-inch dice

1 medium yellow onion, cut into ¼-inch dice

1 small fennel bulb, trimmed and cut into ¼-inch dice

½ pound uncooked farro (about 1¼ cups)

Kosher salt

Freshly ground black pepper

In a saucepan, heat the olive oil over medium-high heat. When it is hot enough to swirl easily, add the carrot, celery, onion, and fennel. Sauté, stirring frequently, until the vegetables are tender and lightly browned, 5 to 7 minutes.

Add the farro to the pan and stir until lightly toasted and fragrant, about 1 minute. Add 2 quarts water, season to taste with salt and pepper, and bring to a boil. Reduce the heat to very low, cover the pot, and cook until the farro is tender, about 25 minutes.

Pour the farro into a fine-mesh strainer to drain. Return to the pot, cover, and keep warm until serving time.

WOLFGANG'S HEALTHY TIPS

→ Although the root vegetables and touch of olive oil enhance the flavor of the grain, you could also partially or fully replace the water with vegetable stock or chicken stock to give the farro even more flavor.

→ Leftovers (or an extra batch) are also good served cold as a salad, drizzled with a light dressing.

→ Some people sensitive to gluten find the gluten in farro more easily digestible. Check with your doctor.

Nutrition Facts Per Serving: Calories: 275; Calories from Fat: 65; Total Fat: 7.23g; Saturated Fat: 1.11g; Monounsaturated Fat: 5.03g; Polyunsaturated Fat: 1.09g; Cholesterol: 0mg; Sodium: 53mg; Total Carbohydrate: 48.76g; Dietary Fiber: 9.68g; Sugars: 2.84g; Protein: 6.81g

Farro Risotto with Wild Mushrooms

SERVES 4

Although risotto is traditionally made with plump short-grain Italian rice varieties like Arborio, you can also produce a creamy-tasting low-fat side with other grains, like the farro in this earthy-tasting recipe.

Wild Mushroom Puree:

½ tablespoon extra-virgin olive oil

1 tablespoon minced shallot

½ pound assorted wild mushrooms, such as chanterelles, morels, porcini, shiitakes, creminis, and portobellos, trimmed, wiped clean, and cut into ¼-inch dice

2 tablespoons dry sherry or Madeira

1 cup homemade Chicken Stock (page 271), Vegetable Stock (page 274), or good-quality canned low-sodium broth

Kosher salt

Freshly ground black pepper

Farro Risotto:

2 tablespoons extra-virgin olive oil

¼ cup minced shallot

1 cup uncooked farro

4 cups homemade Vegetable Stock (page 274) or good-quality canned low-sodium broth, plus a little extra as needed, heated to a bare simmer in a saucepan

Kosher salt

Freshly ground black pepper

½ tablespoon sherry vinegar

2 tablespoons minced fresh fines herbes (a mix of chives, chervil, dill, or flat-leaf parsley or any combination of these)

Prepare the Wild Mushroom Puree: In a sauté pan, heat the olive oil over medium-high heat. Add the shallot and sauté, stirring frequently, until it begins to turn glossy and tender, 2 to 3 minutes. Raise the heat slightly, add the mushrooms and sauté, stirring frequently, until the mushrooms are tender and most of their liquid has evaporated. Add the sherry or Madeira and stir and scrape with a wooden spoon to deglaze the pan. Stir in the stock. When it is hot, carefully puree the mixture with an immersion blender; or transfer it to a blender, in batches if necessary, and puree, following manufacturer's instructions to avoid spattering. Season to taste with salt and pepper. Set aside.

Prepare the Farro Risotto: In a large saucepan, heat the olive oil over medium-high heat. Add the shallot and sauté until glossy and tender, 2 to 3 minutes. Add the farro and stir until the grains are completely coated with the oil and smell slightly toasty, about 1 minute. Add ½ cup of the hot stock, reduce the heat slightly to maintain a light simmer, and cook, stirring continuously, until most of the liquid has been absorbed, about 3 minutes. Continue adding stock in this way, ½ cup at a time, while stirring constantly, until the farro grains are tender but still slightly firm and chewy, 20 to 25 minutes.

Stir in the reserved Wild Mushroom Puree and cook until the mixture is heated through. Season to taste with salt and pepper. Stir in the sherry vinegar.

Spoon the risotto into heated shallow serving bowls or plates. Garnish with the fines herbes and serve immediately.

WOLFGANG'S HEALTHY TIPS

→ Try this as a base for simple grilled proteins such as chicken breasts, shrimp, or scallops. Combined with a small portion of a higher-fat cut, this low-fat side can also bring your meal within an overall 30 percent calories from fat.

→ Made with vegetable stock, this becomes a filling vegan main dish.

→ Feel free to prepare the risotto with regular cultivated mushrooms if wild varieties are not available.

Nutrition Facts Per Serving: Calories: 270; Calories from Fat: 78; Total Fat: 8.69g; Saturated Fat: 1.29g; Monounsaturated Fat: 6.23g; Polyunsaturated Fat: 1.17g; Cholesterol: 0mg; Sodium: 699mg; Total Carbohydrate: 38.47g; Dietary Fiber: 7.40g; Sugars: 1.49g; Protein: 9.49g

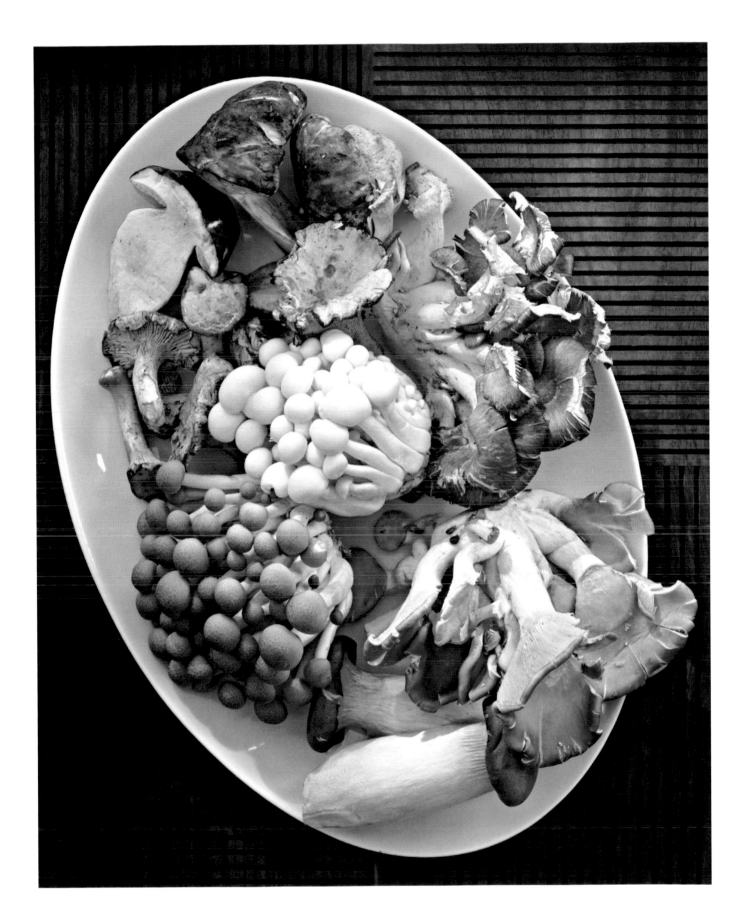

Quinoa and Grilled Vegetable Pilaf

SERVES 4

The ancient Latin American grain called quinoa (pronounced *keen-wah*) has a nutty flavor and light yet chewy texture that make it a very exciting base for a pilaf to serve with all kinds of main courses. You'll find it in a spectrum of colors ranging from black and purple to red and pink to deep orange to bright yellow and pale tan. I especially like this recipe with grilled foods like my Grilled Shrimp on Rosemary Skewers with Grilled Limes (page 145).

1½ cups quinoa

3 cups homemade Chicken Stock (page 271), Vegetable Stock (page 274), or good-quality canned low-sodium broth

1 large Japanese eggplant, cut lengthwise into slices ⅓ inch thick

1 large zucchini, trimmed and cut lengthwise into slices ⅓ inch thick

1 large red bell pepper, quartered, stemmed, seeded, and deveined

1 ear sweet corn

2 tablespoons extra-virgin olive oil

Kosher salt

Freshly ground black pepper

1 tablespoon chopped fresh flat-leaf parsley leaves

1 tablespoon chopped fresh chervil leaves

1 tablespoon chopped fresh chives

1 tablespoon chopped fresh mint leaves

Preheat an outdoor grill, an indoor countertop grill or ridged grill pan, or a broiler.

Put the quinoa in a fine-mesh strainer and rinse under cold running water. Transfer to a medium saucepan and add the stock. Bring to a boil over medium-high heat; then reduce the heat to low, cover the pan, and cook until the quinoa is tender and all the liquid has been absorbed, about 15 minutes. Set aside and keep warm.

Meanwhile, when the grill or broiler is hot, lightly brush the eggplant and zucchini slices, bell pepper quarters, and corn with the oil and season lightly with salt and pepper. Place on the grill or under the broiler and cook until the eggplant, zucchini, and pepper are nicely browned on both sides and tender, 3 to 5 minutes per side, and the corn is golden brown or very slightly charred all over, 5 to 7 minutes total.

As the vegetables are done, transfer them to a clean cutting board. As soon as they are cool enough to handle, cut the eggplant, zucchini, and peppers into ⅓-inch dice. Carefully steadying one end of the corn ear on the board and cutting downward with the knife parallel to the cob, cut the corn kernels from the cob.

Transfer the warm cooked quinoa to a heated serving bowl. Run the tines of a fork through it to separate the grains. Add all the vegetable pieces and the herbs, toss well, and season to taste with salt and pepper. Serve immediately.

WOLFGANG'S HEALTHY TIPS

→ Try other grilled and diced vegetables in the pilaf, such as sweet onions, shiitake mushroom caps, asparagus, and even carrots.

→ Look for other kinds of quinoa besides the standard pale brownish-yellow "white" quinoa. You'll find that red and black each have a slightly different, more pronounced flavor and chewier texture.

Nutrition Facts Per Serving: Calories: 203; Calories from Fat: 63; Total Fat: 7.06g; Saturated Fat: 1.08g; Monounsaturated Fat: 5.05g; Polyunsaturated Fat: 0.93g; Cholesterol: 0mg; Sodium: 430mg; Total Carbohydrate: 25.61g; Dietary Fiber: 4.63g; Sugars: 5.45g; Protein: 7.64g

Dal

SERVES 8 AS A SIDE DISH, 4 AS A MAIN DISH

Although most people in the West think of this popular Indian lentil recipe as a side dish, perhaps alongside Northern Indian Chicken Curry (page 155) or Tandoori-Style Chicken Kabobs (page 156), it also makes an excellent vegetarian main course accompanied by steamed brown rice, basmati rice, or another grain you like.

WOLFGANG'S HEALTHY TIPS

→ I call for orange lentils, also some-times labeled pink lentils, because they have a beautiful coral color and a lovely, mild flavor. But try other varieties, including Indian yellow, brown, or black lentils, or even French green or Puy lentils.

→ Being fairly bland and earthy, lentils take a lot of salt to bring out their flavor. If you are on a sodium-restricted diet, feel free to cut back on the salt you add.

→ If you are not vegetarian or vegan, try making the dal with chicken stock and replacing the oil with ghee, the Indian clarified butter that is sold commercially in ethnic markets, for an even richer flavor.

¼ cup canola oil or vegetable oil

1½ cups diced onion

2 cups orange lentils

2 tablespoons minced garlic

2 jalapeños, stemmed, seeded, deveined, and minced

2 tablespoons finely minced fresh ginger

2 tablespoons homemade Curry Powder (page 285) or good-quality store-bought curry powder

1 tablespoon whole cumin seeds, toasted in a dry sauté pan just until fragrant, then crushed with a mortar and pestle, plus more as needed

1 tablespoon dark brown sugar, plus more as needed

1 tablespoon kosher salt, plus more as needed

1 teaspoon freshly ground black pepper, plus more as needed

1 bay leaf

¾ cup canned diced tomatoes

½ tablespoon rice vinegar

8 cups homemade Vegetable Stock (page 274) or good-quality canned low-sodium broth

In a large saucepan, heat the oil over medium heat. Add the onion and sauté, stirring frequently, just until softened but without browning, 3 to 5 minutes.

Add the lentils, garlic, jalapeños, ginger, Curry Powder, cumin, sugar, salt, pepper, and bay leaf. Sauté until the herbs and spices are fragrant, 1 to 2 minutes. Add the tomatoes and rice vinegar and stir and scrape to deglaze the pan.

Add the stock, raise the heat to high, and bring to a boil, stirring occasionally; then reduce the heat to maintain a simmer and cook, uncovered, stirring occasionally, until the lentils are tender, 15 to 20 minutes. Remove the bay leaf. Before serving, taste and adjust the seasonings, if necessary, with a little more cumin, sugar, salt, and pepper.

Nutrition Facts Per Serving (based on 8 servings): Calories: 282; Calories from Fat: 67; Total Fat: 7.52g; Saturated Fat: 0.65g; Monounsaturated Fat: 4.61g; Polyunsaturated Fat: 2.26g; Cholesterol: 0mg; Sodium: 1,465mg; Total Carbohydrate: 37.78g; Dietary Fiber: 16.22g; Sugars: 5.24g; Protein: 16.71g

Cranberry Sauce with Zinfandel

MAKES ABOUT 2 CUPS; SIXTEEN 2-TABLESPOON SERVINGS

I have always enjoyed making my own cranberry sauce for special holiday meals. It has a more complex, less processed-tasting flavor and texture than the store-bought kind.

3 cups whole unsweetened fresh
or frozen cranberries

1 cup Zinfandel or other dry red wine

½ cup packed dark brown sugar

2 tablespoons grated orange zest

½ tablespoon ground ginger

½ teaspoon freshly ground
black pepper

1 cinnamon stick

In a nonreactive saucepan, combine all the ingredients. Bring to a boil over medium-high heat, stirring occasionally; then reduce the heat to maintain a simmer. Continue to cook, stirring occasionally, until the mixture is thick and the berries are glazed in thick syrup, 20 to 30 minutes.

Remove the pan from the heat and set aside until cool. Remove the cinnamon stick. Transfer to a covered nonreactive container and refrigerate until serving. Serve chilled or at room temperature.

WOLFGANG'S HEALTHY TIPS

→ For very few calories, this traditional accompaniment adds great distinction not only to turkey but also ham or any other kind of roast, broiled, or grilled meat, poultry, or game.

→ Store any leftover cranberry sauce in a covered nonreactive dish in the refrigerator. The day after a big meal, try spreading some on sliced whole-grain bread to make sandwiches with your leftover roast.

→ Once you've tried the recipe, feel free to vary the seasonings to taste. You could try star anise, a piece of vanilla bean, or even ½ teaspoon red pepper flakes for a spicier version.

Nutrition Facts Per Serving: Calories: 49; Calories from Fat: 0; Total Fat: 0.04g; Saturated Fat: 0.01g; Monounsaturated Fat: 0.01g; Polyunsaturated Fat: 0.01g; Cholesterol: 0mg; Sodium: 2mg; Total Carbohydrate: 9.93g; Dietary Fiber: 1.07g; Sugars: 7.44g; Protein: 0.13g

Cinnamon-Swirl Bread

MAKES TWO 9-INCH LOAVES

I like this healthy version of the classic bread sliced and toasted with my morning coffee. It's a great recipe to prepare for Sunday brunch, and is also excellent for sandwiches.

1 recipe Whole Wheat Yeast Dough
(page 287)

Nonstick cooking spray

⅓ cup sugar

1 tablespoon ground cinnamon

Prepare the Whole Wheat Yeast Dough. After the dough has rested, covered, for 10 minutes, divide it into two equal pieces. On a lightly floured work surface and with clean hands, gently roll and shape each piece to make an even ball shape. Cover the balls with a damp kitchen towel and let rest at room temperature for 20 minutes.

Using a lightly floured rolling pin, roll out each ball to form a 9-by-12-inch rectangle.

Evenly spray the insides of two 9-inch loaf pans with nonstick cooking spray. In a small bowl, stir together the sugar and cinnamon.

Lightly brush the surface of each rectangle with cold water. Starting at the nearest 9-inch edge of each rectangle, evenly sprinkle each piece of dough with the cinnamon-sugar mixture up to 1 inch from the opposite edge.

Starting at the nearest 9-inch edge, tightly roll up each rectangle of dough. Place one roll, seam down, in each prepared loaf pan. Cover the pans with a damp towel and let rise at warm room temperature until doubled in volume, about 45 minutes.

Preheat the oven to 375°F.

With a sharp knife, lightly score three or four evenly spaced diagonal slashes across the top of each loaf. Bake the loaves until golden brown, about 45 minutes. Carefully turn them out of the pans onto a wire rack to cool before slicing with a bread knife.

WOLFGANG'S HEALTHY TIPS

→ Seedless raisins make a great addition to the loaf, dotted on top of the cinnamon sugar before you roll up each rectangle of dough.

→ After the loaves have cooled completely, you can seal one in a freezer bag and store it in the freezer for several weeks, thawing it in the refrigerator before use.

Nutrition Facts Per Serving (2 slices, each ½ inch thick): Calories: 137; Calories from Fat: 35; Total Fat: 3.99g; Saturated Fat: 0.59g; Monounsaturated Fat: 2.81g; Polyunsaturated Fat: 0.58g; Cholesterol: 0mg; Sodium: 70mg; Total Carbohydrate: 22.95g; Dietary Fiber: 1.99g; Sugars: 4.74g; Protein: 3.09g

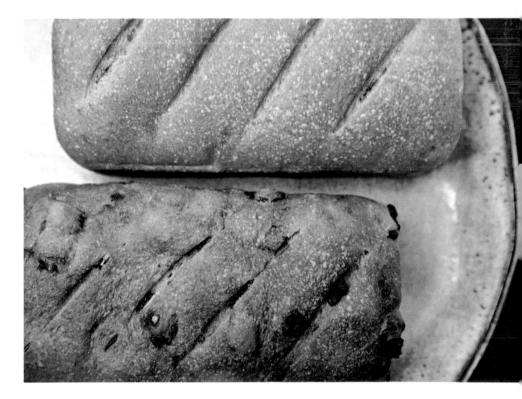

Grape and Rosemary Focaccia

MAKES ONE 10-INCH ROUND LOAF; 12 SINGLE-SLICE SERVINGS

In this version of the popular Italian flatbread, made with my Whole Wheat Yeast Dough (page 287), I love the combination of sweet grapes and savory fresh herbs. Use red or green seedless grapes depending on availability and what you prefer.

1 recipe Whole Wheat Yeast Dough (page 287)

Nonstick cooking spray

1 cup seedless grapes, halved

2 teaspoons extra-virgin olive oil

1 tablespoon chopped fresh rosemary leaves

Pinch of kosher salt

Prepare the Whole Wheat Yeast Dough.

Line a 10-inch cake pan with a circle of parchment paper. Spray the paper with nonstick cooking spray.

After the dough has rested, covered, for 10 minutes, remove it from the bowl and press it into the prepared pan. Cover it with a damp kitchen towel and let rest at room temperature for 20 minutes.

With clean fingertips, press down firmly all over the dough to create regularly spaced dimples in which to place the grape halves. Place the grapes in the dimples. Cover with the towel and leave to rise at room temperature until the dough has doubled in size and almost enclosed the grapes, 45 minutes to 1 hour.

Preheat the oven to 375°F.

Remove the towel. Brush the dough with the olive oil and sprinkle evenly with the rosemary and the salt.

Bake for 10 minutes, then reduce the temperature to 350°F and continue baking until the bread is deep golden brown, about 30 minutes more.

Serve hot, warm, or at room temperature, cut into 12 wedges or squares.

WOLFGANG'S HEALTHY TIPS

→ Serve this as an accompaniment to a light lunchtime salad or as part of a brunch buffet.

→ While the calories from fat in this recipe come in at exactly 30 percent, if you can spare some extra calories from a heart-healthy fat, add some walnut pieces along with the grapes.

Nutrition Facts Per Serving: Calories: 200; Calories from Fat: 60; Total Fat: 6.75g; Saturated Fat: 1.02g; Monounsaturated Fat: 4.77g; Polyunsaturated Fat: 0.96g; Cholesterol: 0mg; Sodium: 108mg; Total Carbohydrate: 30.81g; Dietary Fiber: 2.87g; Sugars: 3.51g; Protein: 4.71g

Variation: Olive Focaccia, Sun-Dried Tomato Focaccia, or Cherry Tomato Focaccia

For a more savory version, replace the grapes with your choice of 1 cup of your favorite black or green marinated or cured pitted and halved olives; 1 cup of thoroughly drained oil-packed sun-dried tomatoes, halved; or 1 cup of halved and seeded red or yellow cherry tomatoes.

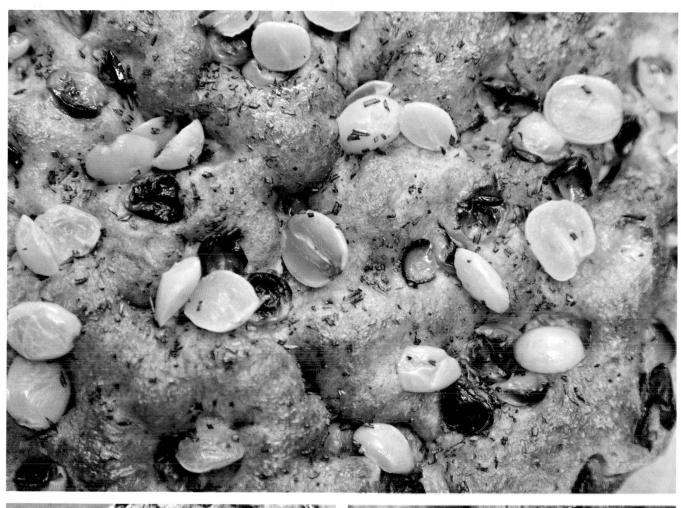

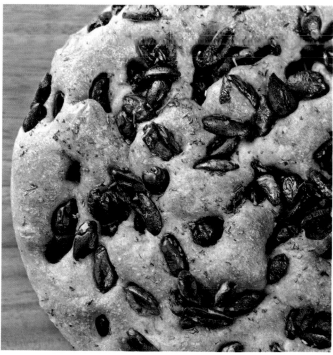

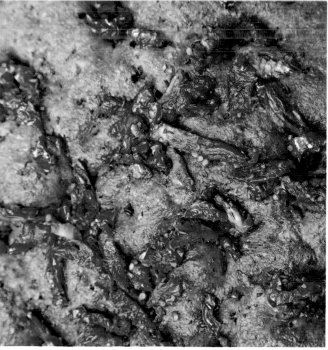

Chocolate-Cherry Bread

MAKES TWO 9-INCH LOAVES

Make this variation on my whole wheat bread dough as a treat for a special brunch. I also like a slice or two toasted with my morning coffee. But, to me, it can also be an enjoyable dessert!

1 recipe Whole Wheat Yeast Dough (page 287)

1 cup dried cherries, rehydrated in warm water for 15 minutes, thoroughly drained

1 cup semisweet chocolate chips

Nonstick cooking spray

Prepare the Whole Wheat Yeast Dough up to the point at which it has been kneaded in the stand mixer at medium speed for 8 to 10 minutes. Add the rehydrated drained cherries and the chocolate chips to the mixer bowl and continue mixing at medium speed until thoroughly combined, about 2 minutes more.

Remove the bowl from the mixer, cover with a damp kitchen towel, and let rest at room temperature for 10 minutes.

Divide the dough into two equal pieces. On a lightly floured work surface and with clean hands, gently roll and shape each piece to make an even ball shape. Cover the balls with a damp kitchen towel and let rest at room temperature for 20 minutes.

Evenly spray two 9-inch loaf pans with nonstick cooking spray.

With your hands, shape each ball of dough into a 9-inch loaf shape and transfer it to a prepared loaf pan. Cover the pans with a damp towel and let rise at warm room temperature until doubled in volume, about 45 minutes.

Preheat the oven to 375°F.

With a sharp knife, lightly score three or four evenly spaced diagonal slashes across the top of each loaf. Bake the loaves in the preheated oven until golden brown, about 45 minutes.

Carefully turn the loaves out of the pans onto a wire rack to cool before slicing with a bread knife.

WOLFGANG'S HEALTHY TIPS

→ Yes, the chocolate pushes the fat calories above 30 percent. But this could certainly fit into a day of healthy eating.

→ For an extra-lean loaf, you could also cut down on how much chocolate you use. Or you could even leave out the chocolate completely and add more of the dried cherries or another dried fruit for a delicious low-fat fruit bread.

Nutrition Facts Per Serving (2 slices, each ½ inch thick): Calories: 188; Calories from Fat: 60; Total Fat: 6.72g; Saturated Fat: 2.26g; Monounsaturated Fat: 3.75g; Polyunsaturated Fat: 0.72g; Cholesterol: 0mg; Sodium: 72mg; Total Carbohydrate: 30.42g; Dietary Fiber: 2.69g; Sugars: 10.50g; Protein: 3.47g

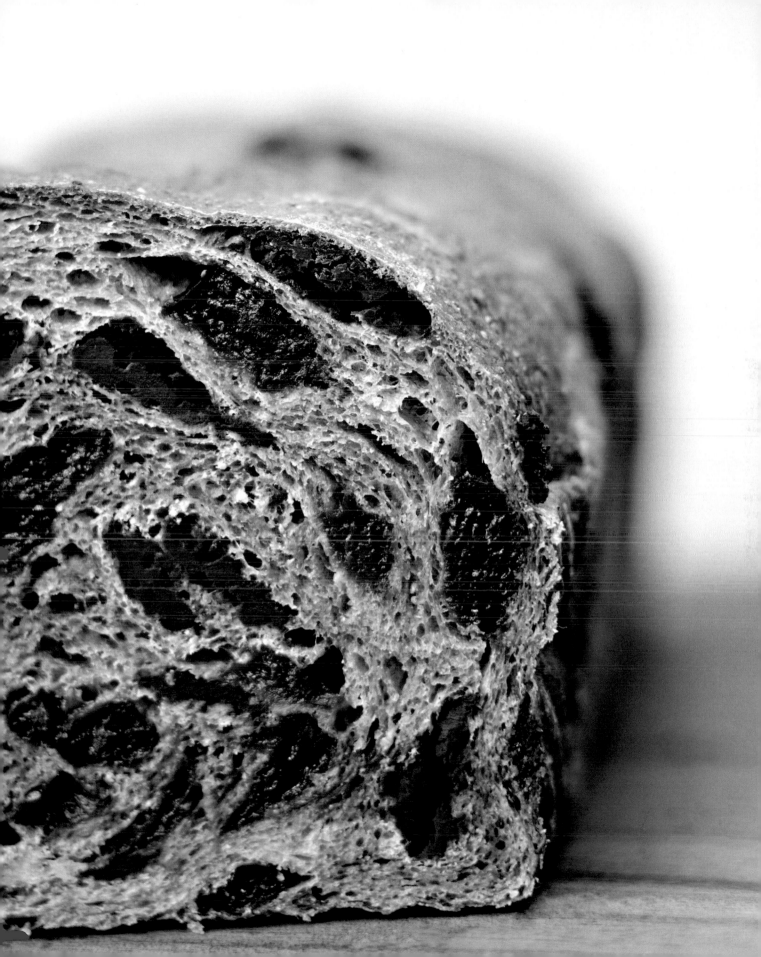

Spago Seeded Multigrain Flatbread

MAKES ABOUT 16 TRIANGULAR PIECES

Spago's crispy flatbread has been a longtime favorite with our guests, and I introduced this new, healthier, incredibly flavorful multigrain version after we remodeled our flagship Beverly Hills location in the autumn of 2012. To roll out the dough to the necessary thinness, you'll need a hand-cranked or electric pasta rolling machine, widely and inexpensively available in housewares and kitchen supply stores.

Dough:

¾ cup cool (60°F) water, plus more as needed

2 teaspoons instant espresso powder

1 tablespoon blackstrap molasses

2 teaspoons honey

1 tablespoon extra-virgin olive oil

1½ cups bread flour, plus more for dusting

¾ cup medium rye flour

⅓ cup teff flour

⅓ cup whole wheat flour

1 tablespoon black cocoa powder

1½ teaspoons sugar

1½ teaspoons kosher salt

Toppings:

2 large egg whites

½ cup shelled raw pumpkin seeds

½ cup shelled raw sunflower seeds

1 tablespoon extra-virgin olive oil

2 tablespoons caraway seeds

2 tablespoons poppy seeds

2 tablespoons sesame seeds

1 large shallot, finely diced

Sea salt

Freshly ground black pepper

Prepare the Dough: In a bowl, whisk together ½ cup of the water and the espresso powder until the powder dissolves. Whisk in the molasses, honey, and olive oil.

In the bowl of a stand mixer fitted with the dough hook, combine the bread flour, rye flour, teff flour, whole wheat flour, cocoa powder, sugar, and salt. Mix on low speed for 2 minutes.

Add the espresso mixture. Continue mixing until the mixture resembles coarse flour, about 2 minutes. With the mixer running, very slowly pour in the remaining ¼ cup water. Don't worry if the mixture looks dry. Continue mixing about 8 minutes more, until the dough—when the mixer is stopped—registers 90°F on an instant-read thermometer.

If the dough still looks dry after 8 minutes of mixing, continue mixing while adding a little more water, 1 teaspoon at a time, until the dough comes together.

Turn out the dough onto a clean, lightly floured work surface. With clean hands, pat it into a square about 1 inch thick. Wrap the square of dough in plastic wrap and refrigerate for at least 12 hours.

Remove the dough from the refrigerator and leave it at room temperature for 1 hour. Then, with a sharp knife or dough cutter, cut it into four equal pieces. Lightly dust a piece with flour and, with

a rolling pin, roll it out into a rectangle about 4 by 6 inches and thin enough to pass through a pasta machine set at the thickest setting. Repeat with the remaining pieces.

Lightly dust a rectangle of the dough with flour on both sides. Crank it through a pasta machine at the thickest setting. Then, decrease the setting by 2, dust the piece with flour, and pass it through again. Continue until you pass the dough through at the machine's narrowest setting, and then pass it through once more.

Cut the sheet of dough in half lengthwise, and then cut each piece lengthwise into two triangles. Line a baking sheet with parchment paper and place two triangles on top, not touching. Lightly dust them with bread flour. Top with a double layer of parchment and then two more triangles, lightly dusting them, too.

Repeat the rolling, cutting, layering, and dusting with the three remaining rectangles of dough and more parchment paper in double layers. Cover the top layer with parchment and refrigerate until ready to bake.

Place a sheet pan upside down on the middle rack of the oven. Preheat the oven to 450°F.

To top the dough: Remove the dough from the refrigerator. Working with one layer of dough (two pieces) at a time, lightly dust them with bread flour; then, leaving them on the parchment, flip them over and dust the other sides with flour. Repeat with the remaining pieces, leaving them on their parchment.

Put the egg whites in a mixing bowl and lightly whisk them until frothy. Brush the tops of all the pieces of dough with the egg whites.

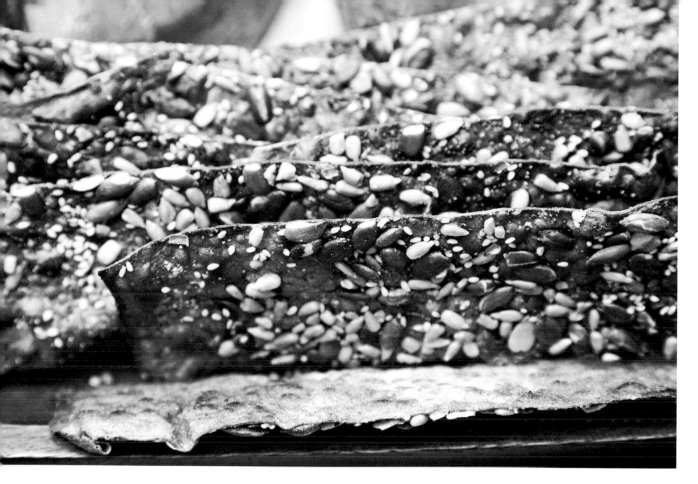

In a small bowl, stir together the pumpkin seeds, sunflower seeds, and olive oil. Evenly scatter the seed-and-oil mixture and the caraway seeds, poppy seeds, sesame seeds, and shallot over the pieces of dough.

With a small rolling pin, lightly roll over the toppings, pressing them into each piece of dough. Sprinkle with salt and pepper to taste.

To bake the flatbreads: Carefully slide the rack out of the oven and lightly dust the sheet pan with flour. Lifting each piece of dough from opposite ends, carefully place as many pieces of dough as will fit on the sheet pan. Gently slide the rack back into the oven, close the oven door, and bake the flatbreads until dark golden brown and crispy, 5 to 6 minutes.

Use a spatula to transfer the baked flatbreads from the pan to a wire rack to cool. Repeat with any unbaked triangles.

Serve at room temperature within 1 to 2 hours of baking.

Nutrition Facts Per 1-Piece Serving: Calories: 164; Calories from Fat: 60; Total Fat: 6.70g; Saturated Fat: 0.96g; Monounsaturated Fat: 2.51g; Polyunsaturated Fat: 3.06g; Cholesterol: 0mg; Sodium: 35mg; Total Carbohydrate: 21.16g; Dietary Fiber: 2.98g; Sugars: 2.08g; Protein: 5.52g

WOLFGANG'S HEALTHY TIPS

→ The oil-rich seeds and the olive oil in this recipe, all healthy fats, push the fat calories just a bit above one-third. Enjoy this with a light salad or soup, though, and you have a low-fat and very satisfying combination.

→ I also love to serve this with hors d'oeuvre dips or spreads, and it's excellent topped with some good smoked salmon or lean, thinly sliced ham in the morning.

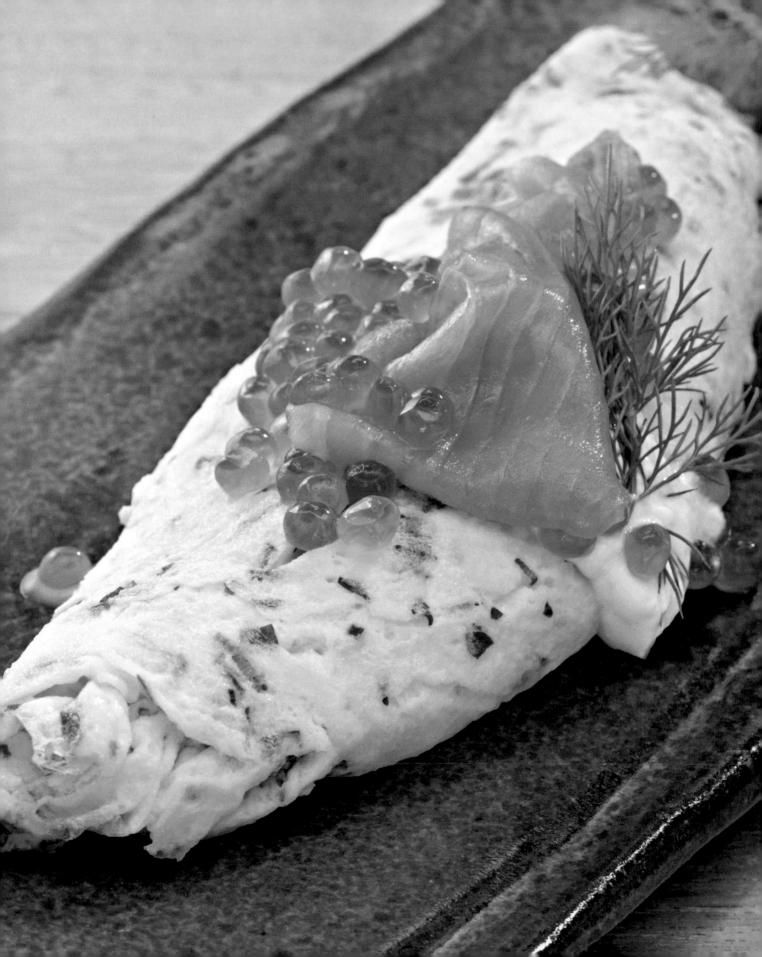

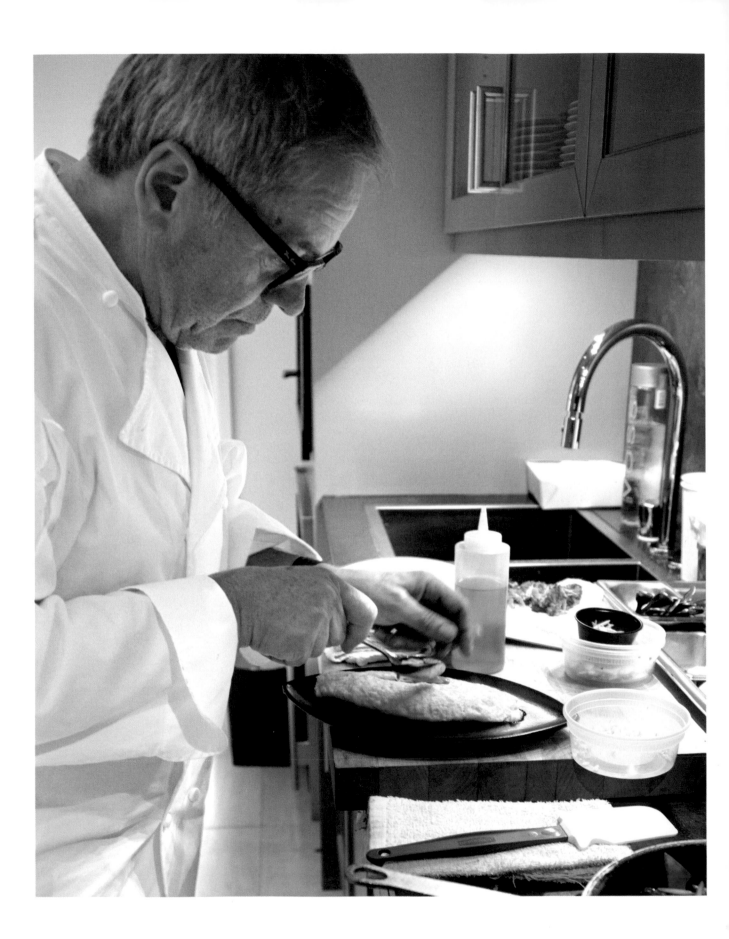

BREAKFAST AND BRUNCH

We all grew up hearing that the first meal of the day is the most important one. Guess what: Our mothers were right! If you eat a good, nutritious, balanced, healthy breakfast, you'll start your day feeling as energetic as you can be. You'll also be less likely to feel your energy dropping midmorning, a time when too many people have unwise coffee break treats; and you'll feel more willpower to eat a smart lunch as well. And the benefits keep adding up through the rest of your day.

I've developed all of the breakfast and brunch dishes in this chapter with the idea that morning foods can be both healthy *and* exciting. Whether you want just a quick bowl of granola that you've prepared in advance over the weekend or an egg white omelet made to order for one, wholesome pancakes or a robust savory bread pudding you've whipped up to entertain late on a Sunday morning, you'll find inspiration and solutions here to make your morning meals as good to eat as they are good for you.

These recipes are so delicious, in fact, that there's no reason you should confine them to the morning alone. Try them for dinner, too!

→ Oat and Nut Granola with Dried Fruit

  ★ Granola Bars

→ Granola and Yogurt Parfaits with Fresh Berries

→ Buttermilk French Toast with Fresh Berry Compote

→ Whole Wheat and Walnut Buttermilk Pancakes

→ Baked Vegetable Frittata with Yogurt and Parmesan

→ French-Style Egg White Omelet with Vegetables

→ Spanish-Style Flat Omelet with Bell Peppers and Ham

→ Italian Strata with Tomatoes, Bell Pepper, and Swiss Cheese

→ Yogurt Oatmeal Muffins

→ Spelt Coconut Scones

Oat and Nut Granola with Dried Fruit

MAKES ABOUT 24 CUPS; TWENTY-FOUR 1-CUP SERVINGS

I like my granola filled with crunchy nuts and chewy dried fruit. Serve this as a breakfast cereal with low-fat or nonfat milk, enjoy it as a healthy snack, turn it into granola bars (see Variation, page 219), or use it to make Granola and Yogurt Parfaits (page 220) for a special brunch. Note that you'll need more than one large baking pan to oven-toast the granola easily.

1½ ounces shredded unsweetened coconut

1 pound rolled oats (about 5 cups)

¼ pound sliced blanched almonds

¼ pound raw shelled cashews

¼ cup packed dark brown sugar

1 tablespoon grated orange zest

1½ teaspoons kosher salt

1 teaspoon ground cinnamon

½ teaspoon freshly grated nutmeg

1 cup pure maple syrup

Butter-flavored nonstick cooking spray

1 cup seedless raisins

1 cup dried cherries or dried cranberries

Preheat the oven to 325°F.

Spread the coconut evenly in a thin layer on a rimmed baking sheet or in a baking pan. Toast in the oven until golden brown, 5 to 7 minutes, keeping careful watch to ensure that it doesn't burn. Immediately transfer the toasted coconut to a bowl to cool. Raise the oven temperature to 350°F.

In a very large bowl, combine the oats, almonds, and cashews. Add the brown sugar, orange zest, salt, cinnamon, and nutmeg and stir well to combine them with the other ingredients.

In a small saucepan, heat the syrup over low heat until hot but not yet boiling. Pour it evenly over the dry ingredients and stir well with a large, sturdy metal spoon to coat the dry ingredients evenly with the syrup.

Spray one or two large rimmed baking sheets or baking pans with nonstick cooking spray. Empty the mixture onto the sheet or sheets and, with a large spoon or spatula, spread it and press it down to an even thickness of about ½ inch.

Bake for about 30 minutes, then very carefully invert the mixture onto another nonstick-sprayed sheet or pan and bake until it reaches a deep golden brown color, about 20 to 30 minutes more.

Remove from the oven and transfer the sheet or sheets to wire racks, leaving them to cool completely. By hand, break the sheets of granola into bite-size chunks, transferring them to a clean bowl. Add the raisins and dried cherries or cranberries and the toasted coconut and toss well to combine. Transfer to airtight containers or sealable heavy-duty food-storage bags and store at cool room temperature; the granola will keep for up to several weeks.

WOLFGANG'S HEALTHY TIPS

→ Most granola recipes contain a lot of butter or oil, which can make the results surprisingly high in fat and calories for what most people think of as a healthy breakfast or snack food. I've eliminated virtually all of the added fat in this version, leaving only that present in the nuts, coconut, and what little there is in the oats.

→ Yes, this recipe yields a lot of granola. There's enough (easy) work involved, though, that it makes sense to prepare it in large quantities, and the granola will keep well for a few weeks stored in an airtight container. But, if you like, prepare just half or a fourth of the given quantities.

Nutrition Facts Per Serving: Calories: 239; Calories from Fat: 59; Total Fat: 6.57g; Saturated Fat: 1.85g; Monounsaturated Fat: 3.25g; Polyunsaturated Fat: 1.47g; Cholesterol: 0mg; Sodium: 22mg; Total Carbohydrate: 43.55g; Dietary Fiber: 3.82g; Sugars: 24.89g; Protein: 4.43g

Variation: Granola Bars

To turn my granola into a portable snack, use one-half of the total dry ingredients and ¾ cup of the maple syrup in the main recipe. Do not toast the coconut. Put the 2½ cups of oats in a food processor with the stainless-steel blade and process until ground to a fine meal. Stir them into ¾ cup of the hot maple syrup along with the sugar and spices, and then combine with all the remaining ingredients as directed in the main recipe. Transfer the mixture to a 9-by-12-inch rimmed baking pan lined with foil and sprayed with nonstick cooking spray, and use the underside of a sturdy spatula to press it down firmly and evenly. Bake on one side as directed; then invert the pan onto a large cutting board and, while still warm, cut the sheet into 12 equal rectangles, making five cuts every 2 inches across its width and one length-wise cut down the middle. Carefully separate the bars, place on a larger foil-lined baking sheet sprayed with nonstick cooking spray, and continue baking as directed, until golden brown, firm, and crisp, about 20 minutes longer, checking to make sure they don't overbrown. Transfer to a wire rack to cool, then store in an airtight container at room temperature.

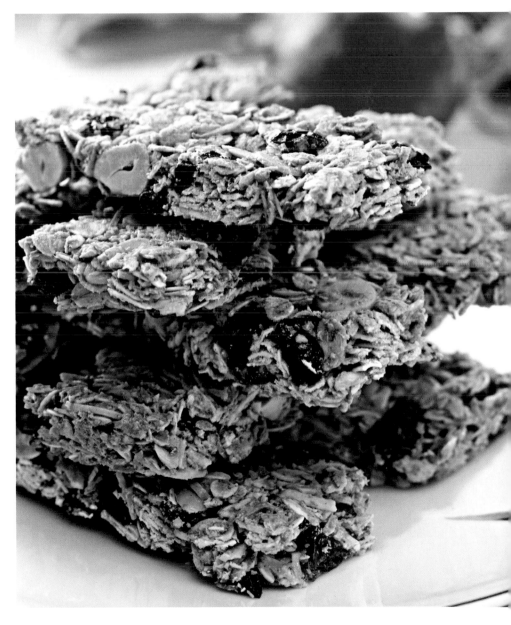

Granola and Yogurt Parfaits with Fresh Berries

SERVES 4

Try this refreshing breakfast or brunch main dish when peak-of-season berries are at the market. Use my recipe for Oat and Nut Granola (page 218) or a healthy low-fat granola from the market.

2 cups nonfat plain yogurt

2 cups fresh raspberries or other berries

4 cups Oat and Nut Granola with Dried Fruit (page 218) or good-quality low-fat store-bought granola

4 sprigs fresh mint, for serving

Put the yogurt in a food processor fitted with the stainless-steel blade. Add 1 cup of the berries and process until pureed.

Spoon ½ cup of the Oat and Nut Granola into each of four large wine glasses, parfait glasses, or other decorative serving glasses. Divide half of the yogurt among the glasses, and then half of the remaining berries. Add another ½ cup granola per glass, and then another layer each of the yogurt and berries.

Serve immediately, garnished with fresh mint sprigs.

WOLFGANG'S HEALTHY TIPS

→ Other juicy seasonal fruits would work well in this recipe, too. Try pitted fresh cherries or thin slices of ripe peach, nectarine, or plum.

→ If you'd like the granola to be a little softer, cover each filled glass with plastic wrap and refrigerate for at least 1 hour or as long as overnight before serving.

Nutrition Facts Per Serving: Calories: 341; Calories from Fat: 63; Total Fat: 7.09g; Saturated Fat: 2.01g; Monounsaturated Fat: 3.35g; Polyunsaturated Fat: 1.73g; Cholesterol: 2mg; Sodium: 118mg; Total Carbohydrate: 60.78g; Dietary Fiber: 8.21g; Sugars: 37.02g; Protein: 7.94g

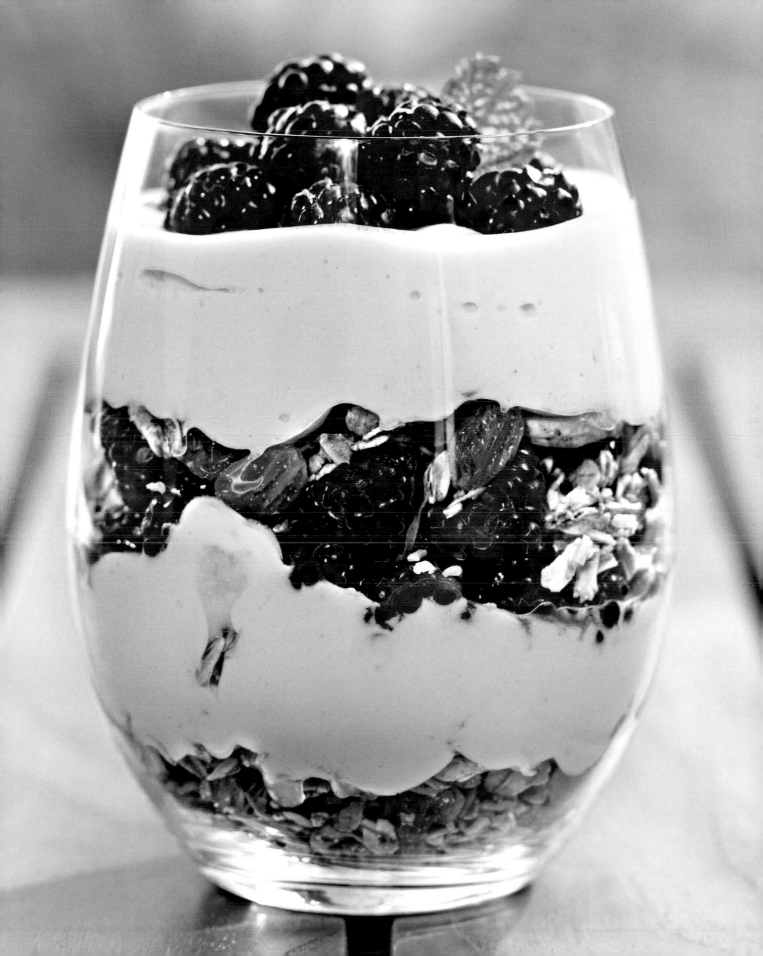

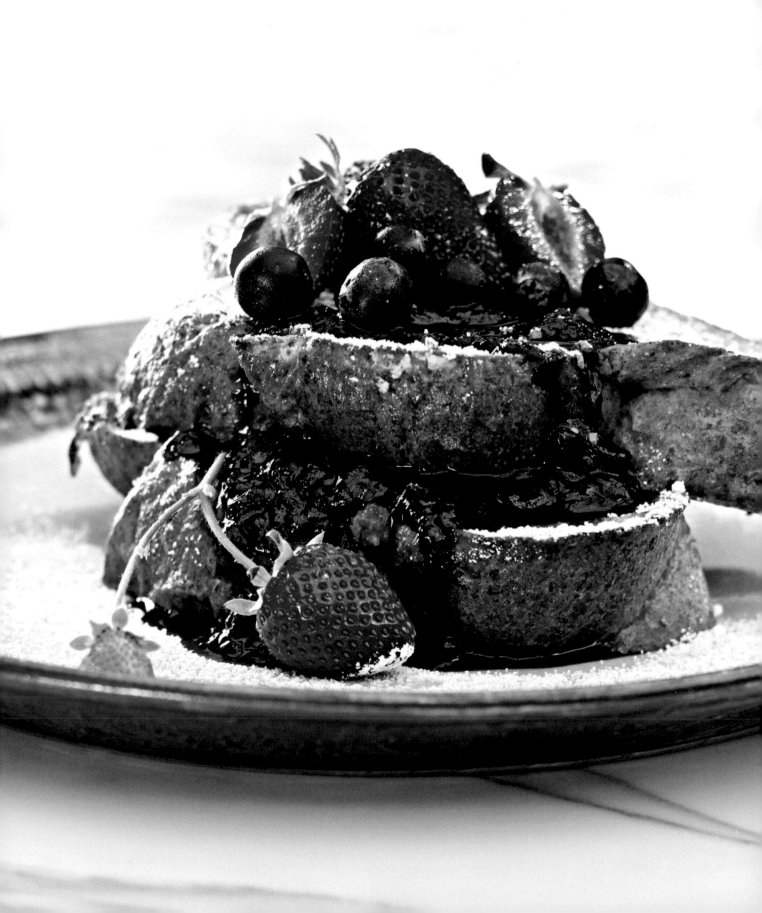

Buttermilk French Toast with Fresh Berry Compote

SERVES 4

A family-style Sunday morning favorite takes a very healthy turn while losing none of its appeal to the eye or its delicious flavor. If you can, use a good artisanal whole-grain but light-textured loaf from the bakery, slicing it yourself.

French Toast:

2 large eggs, lightly beaten

2 large egg whites

2 cups buttermilk

1 tablespoon honey

1 teaspoon pure vanilla extract

1 teaspoon ground cinnamon

1 teaspoon ground ginger

⅛ teaspoon freshly grated nutmeg

¼ teaspoon kosher salt

8 slices good-quality whole wheat bread, each about 1 inch thick, halved diagonally

Butter-flavored nonstick cooking spray

Fresh Berry Compote:

¾ cup fresh blueberries

¾ cup fresh raspberries

3 tablespoons honey

1 tablespoon grated orange zest

3 ounces fresh orange juice (from about 1 large orange)

Pinch of kosher salt

To Assemble:

Confectioners' sugar, for dusting (optional)

Fresh berries (optional)

For the French Toast: In a large, wide bowl, whisk together the eggs, egg whites, buttermilk, honey, vanilla, cinnamon, ginger, nutmeg, and salt.

Over medium heat, heat a heavy nonstick skillet, or a pair of skillets, large enough to hold all the French toast slices in a single layer without crowding. Dip the bread slices into the egg mixture, turning them and making sure they are completely saturated.

Spray the heated skillet or skillets with nonstick cooking spray. Add the soaked bread pieces and cook until golden brown on both sides, 5 to 7 minutes total.

Meanwhile, prepare the Fresh Berry Compote: In a nonreactive saucepan, combine the blueberries, raspberries, honey, orange zest, orange juice, and salt. Bring to a simmer over medium heat, stirring occasionally, and continue simmering just until the berries have given up some of their juices and have turned slightly syrupy, 3 to 4 minutes. Transfer to a serving bowl and keep warm.

Assemble the dish: Arrange 2 slices of the French toast on each of four heated serving plates. Spoon some of the compote over each serving. If you like, spoon a little confectioners' sugar into a small, fine-mesh sieve held over each plate and tap the sieve lightly to dust the French toast; then, garnish with fresh berries. Serve immediately, passing more Fresh Berry Compote at the table.

WOLFGANG'S HEALTHY TIPS

→ In place of the usual soaking mixture of whole eggs and whole milk or cream for French toast, this recipe uses a mixture of whole eggs, egg whites, and low-fat buttermilk to cut the fat without loss of rich flavor. Butter-flavored nonstick cooking spray replaces the butter in which French toast is usually cooked.

→ A beautiful, light, quick, very flavorful compote of fresh berries replaces the usual melted butter and sugary syrup to complement each serving. Feel free to substitute any seasonal berries you like. Or try a mixture of other fresh, juicy fruit, such as chunks of peaches, nectarines, or plums, or pitted and halved cherries.

Nutrition Facts Per Serving: Calories: 329; Calories from Fat: 51; Total Fat: 5.68g; Saturated Fat: 1.87g; Monounsaturated Fat: 1.80g; Polyunsaturated Fat: 2.01g; Cholesterol: 97mg; Sodium: 372mg; Total Carbohydrate: 57.51g; Dietary Fiber: 5.59g; Sugars: 30.86g; Protein: 13.65g

Whole Wheat and Walnut Buttermilk Pancakes

MAKES ABOUT 12 PANCAKES, 4 SERVINGS

I love to make pancakes for my family—especially when they're healthy ones like these. Preparing the batter with a mixture of soft pastry flour and whole wheat flour, more egg whites than yolks, and low-fat buttermilk produces flavorful, tender-but-hearty pancakes that are good for you.

4 large egg whites

2 large egg yolks

1 cup buttermilk

2 tablespoons canola oil

½ cup pastry flour

½ cup whole wheat flour

1 tablespoon sugar

½ teaspoon baking powder

½ teaspoon kosher salt

½ teaspoon ground cinnamon

½ teaspoon ground ginger

¼ cup walnut pieces, toasted (see page 289)

Fresh Berry Compote (page 223)

Butter-flavored nonstick cooking spray

1 cup fresh blueberries (optional)

In a bowl, use a hand mixer on medium speed or a wire whisk to beat the egg whites until they form soft peaks that droop slightly when the beaters or whisk are lifted out. Set aside.

In a separate bowl, whisk the egg yolks until smooth and slightly frothy. Whisk in the buttermilk and oil.

In a large mixing bowl, sift together the pastry and whole wheat flours, sugar, baking powder, salt, cinnamon, and ginger. Make a well in the center, pour the egg yolk mixture into the well, and whisk just enough to incorporate it into the dry ingredients. Fold in the walnuts. With a rubber spatula, gently fold about one-quarter of the egg whites into this batter to lighten it. Then, in two more batches, lightly fold in the remaining egg whites until fully incorporated. Cover the bowl with plastic wrap and refrigerate at least 30 minutes or, better, overnight.

Prepare the Fresh Berry Compote and keep it warm.

Heat a large nonstick griddle over medium heat.

Spray the hot griddle with nonstick cooking spray. Using a ¼-cup ladle or measure, pour the batter onto the griddle to form pancakes, spacing them about 1 inch apart. If you like, scatter some blueberries onto the surface of each pancake as it is formed. Cook until the undersides of the pancakes are golden brown and the surface is covered with small bubbles, 3 to 4 minutes. With a spatula, turn the pancakes over and continue cooking until the other sides are browned, about 3 minutes more. As the pancakes are done, transfer them to a heated platter. Repeat with any remaining batter.

To serve, present the pancakes on the platter or arrange them slightly overlapping on individual heated plates.

Transfer the berry compote to a sauceboat or serving bowl and pass it at the table.

WOLFGANG'S HEALTHY TIPS

→ Many pancake batters benefit from sitting overnight in the refrigerator, which lets the flavors develop and the flour soften. That's especially true for the hardier whole wheat flour.

→ If you want to make the pancakes even more low fat, leave out the walnuts, which contribute 49 calories per serving, 38 of those from fat (although it's a fat high in heart-healthy omega-3 fatty acids).

→ For a change of pace and a slight indulgence, serve the pancakes with a light drizzle of pure maple syrup instead of the berry compote. A 3-tablespoon serving of the syrup is less than 100 calories.

Nutrition Facts Per Serving (including Fresh Berry Compote): Calories: 392; Calories from Fat: 129; Total Fat: 14.35g; Saturated Fat: 2.04g; Monounsaturated Fat: 5.68g; Polyunsaturated Fat: 2.73g; Cholesterol: 94mg; Sodium: 224mg; Total Carbohydrate: 54.69g; Dietary Fiber: 5.03g; Sugars: 25.24g; Protein: 12.99g

Baked Vegetable Frittata with Yogurt and Parmesan

SERVES 4 TO 8

Serve this hearty vegetarian Italian-style flat omelet with whole-grain toast for a filling yet healthy breakfast or brunch. It serves four generously as the main dish in a sit-down meal, or up to eight on a buffet. The frittata is also good at room temperature or cold.

Olive oil–flavored nonstick cooking spray

1 teaspoon extra-virgin olive oil

1 large gold-fleshed potato, such as Yukon gold, peeled and cut into ¼-inch dice

1 medium yellow onion, thinly sliced

1 medium zucchini, cut crosswise into ¼-inch-thick slices

½ green bell pepper, stemmed, seeded, deveined, and thinly sliced

1 teaspoon minced garlic

3 large eggs

8 large egg whites

⅓ cup nonfat plain yogurt

2 tablespoons freshly grated Parmesan

Kosher salt

Freshly ground black pepper

Chopped fresh chives or basil, for garnish

Preheat the oven to 500°F.

Heat an 8-inch ovenproof nonstick skillet over medium heat. Spray with nonstick cooking spray, add the olive oil, and swirl it around the pan. Add the potato, onion, zucchini, and bell pepper. Sauté, stirring occasionally, until the vegetables have softened and begun to turn a light golden color, about 5 minutes. Stir in the garlic, remove the skillet from the heat, and set aside.

Put the eggs, egg whites, yogurt, Parmesan, and salt and pepper to taste in the bowl of a food processor fitted with the stainless-steel blade. Process until smooth, stopping once or twice to scrape down the bowl with a rubber spatula. (Alternatively, combine the ingredients in a bowl and stir together thoroughly with a wire whisk.)

Spread the sautéed vegetables evenly in the skillet and pour the egg-yogurt mixture evenly over them. Transfer the skillet to the preheated oven and cook just until the eggs are set, 15 to 20 minutes.

If the eggs on top still look a little moist for your liking, switch the oven to the broil setting, or preheat a separate broiler, and pop the pan under the broiler for 1 to 2 minutes until they are set and light golden.

Set the skillet aside to let the frittata settle for about 5 minutes. Carefully invert a serving platter over the skillet and, using a potholder to hold the platter and skillet securely together, invert them and lift away the skillet to unmold the frittata. (Alternatively, serve directly from the skillet.) Cut into wedges and serve hot, lukewarm, or even cold, garnished with fresh herbs.

WOLFGANG'S HEALTHY TIPS

→ Take a look at the calories from fat, less than 25 percent of the total, and you'll see what a difference you can make by substituting egg whites for some of the whole eggs in a recipe, while keeping just enough yolks to give flavor and color.

→ The yogurt included in the frittata mixture adds healthy protein and calcium while enriching the flavor and adding a pleasant tanginess.

→ Change up the vegetables as you like, adding whatever is best from the farmers' market and cutting it up into pieces that sauté quickly.

Nutrition Facts Per Serving (based on 4 servings): Calories: 195; Calories from Fat: 47; Total Fat: 5.30g; Saturated Fat: 1.89g; Monounsaturated Fat: 2.43g; Polyunsaturated Fat: 0.98g; Cholesterol: 141mg; Sodium: 227mg; Total Carbohydrate: 19.24g; Dietary Fiber: 2.50g; Sugars: 6.63g; Protein: 16.78g

French-Style Egg White Omelet with Vegetables

SERVES 1

A French-style folded omelet—perfectly cooked with a light golden exterior and still slightly moist within—is one of the classic tests of a cook's skill, whether in a professional kitchen or at home. A nonstick omelet pan helps, as I hope my detailed instructions will! Follow the classic chef's technique I describe for using the flat underside of the tines of an ordinary table fork to stir and help fold the omelet, and you'll become a master in no time.

4 large egg whites

1 large egg

Kosher salt

Freshly ground white pepper

Butter-flavored nonstick cooking spray

¼ cup thinly sliced asparagus

¼ cup thinly sliced snow peas

1 teaspoon minced shallot

½ tablespoon chopped fresh chives, fresh flat-leaf parsley, or other fresh herbs, for garnish

In a bowl, whisk together the egg whites, egg, and a little salt and pepper to taste until well blended and slightly frothy. Set aside.

Heat a 10-inch nonstick omelet pan over medium-high heat. Spray lightly with nonstick cooking spray. Add the asparagus, snow peas, and shallot and sauté, stirring continuously, until the vegetables are bright green and tender-crisp, 2 to 3 minutes. Transfer to a bowl, cover, and keep warm.

Wipe the pan clean with a paper towel. Return it to medium heat and spray again with nonstick cooking spray. Add the egg mixture and grasp the pan by its handle. Start shaking the pan back and forth while stirring the eggs slowly with the back of a fork, gently lifting and moving the cooked egg so that the liquid egg slips beneath it. After about 30 seconds, the egg will have formed a uniformly cooked but still fairly moist pancake shape.

To fold the omelet, immediately tilt the pan to about a 45-degree angle by

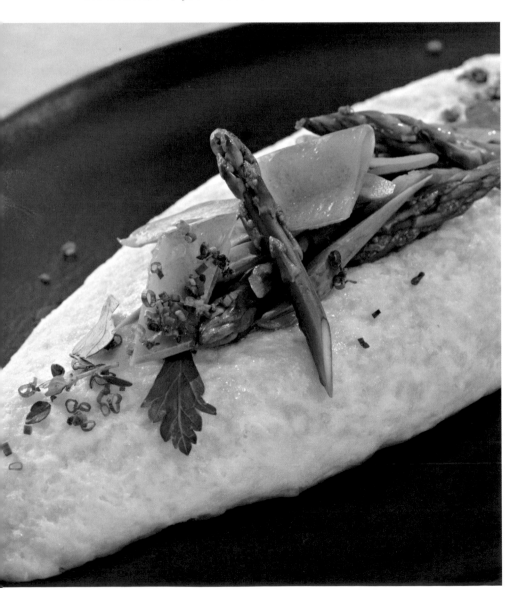

raising the handle, so that the cooked eggs nearest the handle begin to fall and fold; you may use the fork or a spatula to help this happen. Hold the far edge of the pan over a heated serving plate and continue tipping the handle up, so that the omelet folds over on itself and rolls out of the pan onto the plate.

To fill the omelet, use a small, sharp knife to cut a shallow slit lengthwise through the top of the omelet through the upper layer of egg. Spoon the reserved sautéed vegetables into and spilling out of the slit. Serve immediately, garnished with the fresh herbs.

WOLFGANG'S HEALTHY TIPS

→ Using only 1 egg yolk mixed with egg whites, plus the nonstick pan and nonstick cooking spray, turns the omelet into a low-fat main dish that still has a sunny yellow color and a welcome touch of richness.

→ You can add any filling you like to the omelet. The combination of vegetables here is just one suggestion (see variation, right).

Nutrition Facts Per Serving: Calories: 157; Calories from Fat: 39; Total Fat: 4.42g; Saturated Fat: 1.59g; Monounsaturated Fat: 1.84g; Polyunsaturated Fat: 1.00g; Cholesterol: 186mg; Sodium: 290mg; Total Carbohydrate: 5.10g; Dietary Fiber: 1.38g; Sugars: 2.76g; Protein: 22.22g

Variation: French-Style Egg White Omelet with Smoked Salmon and Salmon Caviar

For a luxury version of the omelet, whisk 1 tablespoon finely chopped fines herbes (mixed parsley, chives, tarragon, and chervil, or any combination of these) into the egg mixture. After cooking as described in the recipe opposite, cut a slit in the top of the omelet and fill with 1 tablespoon nonfat plain Greek yogurt, ½ ounce thinly sliced smoked salmon, and 1 tablespoon salmon roe. Garnish with a fresh dill sprig.

Nutrition Facts Per Serving: Calories: 237; Calories from Fat: 75; Total Fat: 8.38g; Saturated Fat: 2.59g; Monounsaturated Fat: 3.15g; Polyunsaturated Fat: 2.65g; Cholesterol: 301mg; Sodium: 542mg; Total Carbohydrate: 2.82g; Dietary Fiber: 0.09g; Sugars: 1.73g; Protein: 34.83g

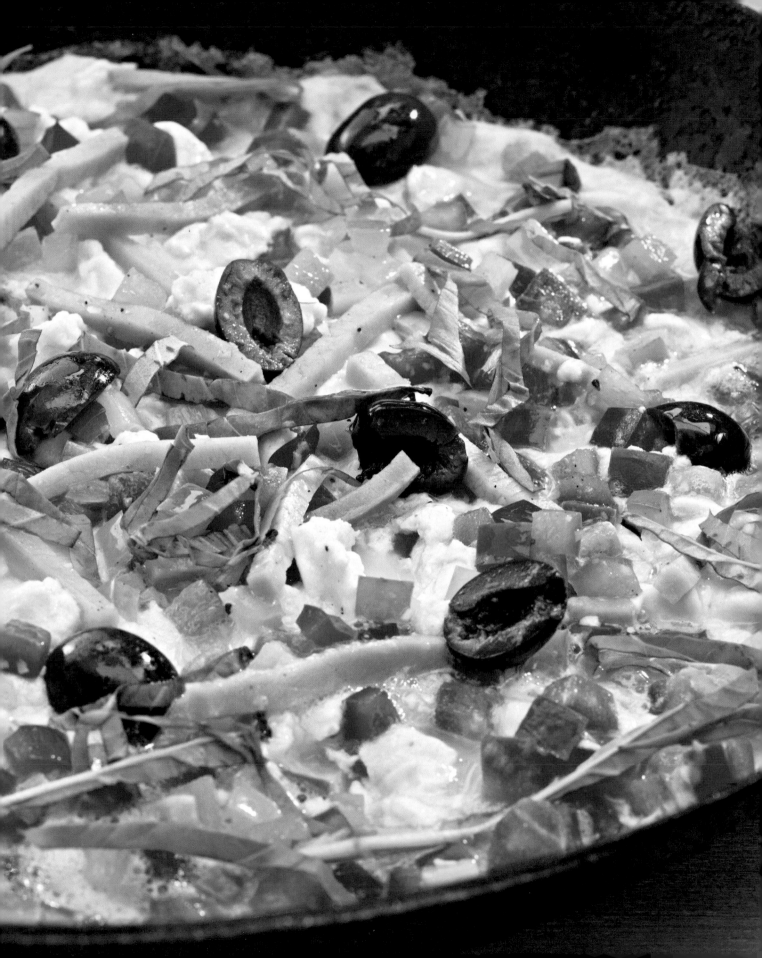

Spanish-Style Flat Omelet with Bell Peppers and Ham

SERVES 4 TO 8

The thick, flat omelets of Spain, called *tortillas*, make a perfect brunch or breakfast dish, especially considering that you can prepare them easily with an eye toward cutting the fat while including lots of vegetables. For the best texture and even cooking, cut the bell peppers and tomato into uniform ¼-inch dice.

Olive oil–flavored nonstick cooking spray

½ cup diced red bell pepper

½ cup diced yellow bell pepper

½ cup diced green bell pepper

1 garlic clove, finely chopped

½ jalapeño, stemmed, seeded, deveined, and finely chopped (optional)

Kosher salt

Freshly ground black pepper

½ cup peeled, seeded (see page 288), and diced tomato

2 large eggs

12 large egg whites

¼ cup pitted Kalamata olives, sliced

3 ounces thinly sliced lean cured ham, cut into thin ribbons

6 fresh basil leaves, cut into fine strips

Preheat the oven to 400°F.

Heat an 8-inch ovenproof nonstick skillet over medium heat. Spray with nonstick cooking spray. Add the peppers and sauté, stirring occasionally, until they have softened and their edges begin to turn golden, about 5 minutes. Add the garlic and jalapeño (if using) and sauté until fragrant, about 30 seconds more. Season to taste with salt and pepper. Add the tomatoes and cook for 2 minutes more.

Put the eggs and egg whites in a large bowl. Season to taste with salt and pepper and whisk until thoroughly blended. Add the egg mixture to the skillet with the vegetables and stir constantly over medium heat until curds start to form. Continue cooking until the mixture has begun to set but is still fairly moist.

Remove the skillet from the heat and scatter the olives and ham evenly over the top. Put the skillet in the oven and bake until the omelet is completely set but still slightly moist, about 5 minutes.

If the eggs on top still look a little moist for your liking, switch the oven to the broil setting, or preheat a separate broiler, and pop the pan under the broiler for 1 to 2 minutes until they are set and light golden.

Set the skillet aside to let the omelet settle for about 5 minutes. Sprinkle with the basil. Cut it into wedges and serve hot, lukewarm, or even cold.

WOLFGANG'S HEALTHY TIPS

→ I've used one fewer whole egg in this flat omelet than in the Baked Vegetable Frittata (page 225), replacing it with even more egg whites, to allow for the fact that I've introduced a little more fat and richness into the recipe with the ham and olives. But you'll taste how rich and flavorful the results still are.

→ You could make this a vegetarian omelet by substituting some sliced or crumbled and precooked chorizo-style vegetarian sausage that you can find in well-stocked supermarkets and health food stores.

Nutrition Facts Per Serving (based on 4 servings):
Calories: 150; Calories from Fat: 43; Total Fat: 4.82g; Saturated Fat: 1.54g; Monounsaturated Fat: 2.50g; Polyunsaturated Fat: 0.78g; Cholesterol: 104mg; Sodium: 537mg; Total Carbohydrate: 6.47g; Dietary Fiber: 1.93g; Sugars: 3.41g; Protein: 18.27g

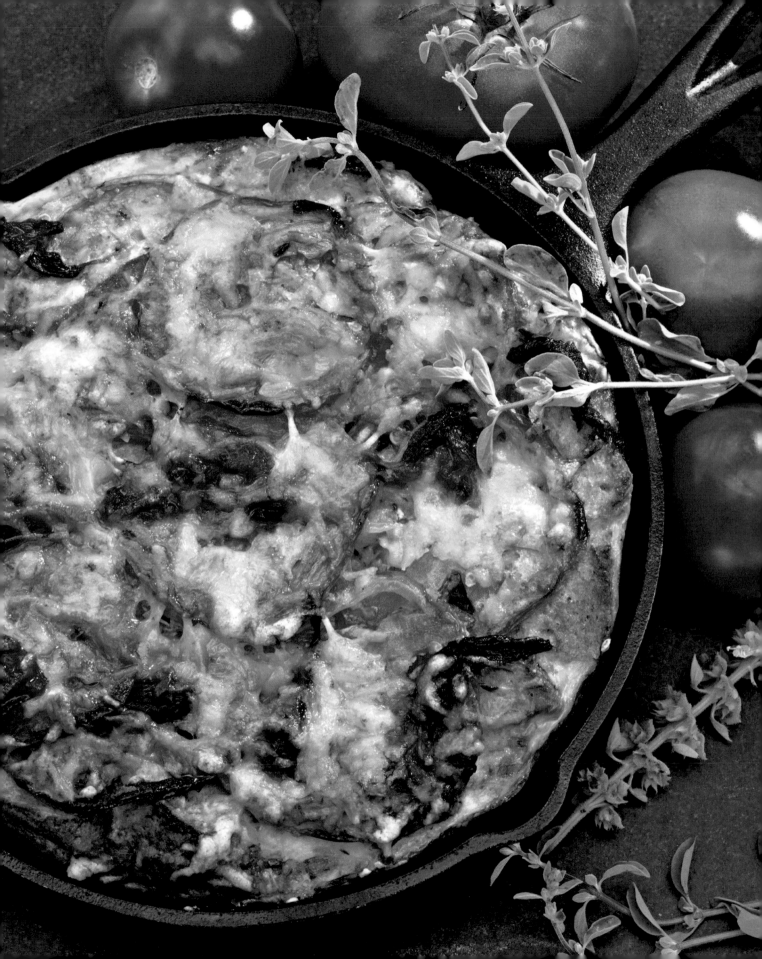

Italian Strata with Tomatoes, Bell Pepper, and Swiss Cheese

SERVES 8

Somehow, enjoying the flavors of a pizza in the morning—as you'll find in this savory, eggy bread pudding—doesn't feel like you're eating a low-fat dish. But that's exactly the experience this recipe offers. For convenience, assemble the strata completely the night before; then, the next morning, uncover and bake as directed.

½ pound stale country-style whole wheat or multigrain bread

1 garlic clove, halved

Olive oil–flavored nonstick cooking spray

1 cup finely shredded reduced-fat Swiss cheese

1 large red bell pepper, roasted, peeled, seeded (see page 289), and torn into thin strips

2 large ripe tomatoes, cored and thinly sliced

3 large eggs

3 large egg whites

2 cups buttermilk

½ teaspoon red pepper flakes

½ teaspoon dried oregano

½ teaspoon sea salt

Freshly ground black pepper

Preheat the oven to 350°F.

With a sharp bread knife, cut the bread into slices ¾ inch thick. Rub one or both sides of each bread slice with the cut sides of the garlic clove halves, using more or less depending on how garlicky you want the strata to be. Then, cut the bread into ¾-inch cubes.

Lightly coat the inside of a 12-by-10-inch baking dish, gratin dish, or a heavy nonstick 10-inch skillet with nonstick cooking spray.

Place the bread cubes in the dish in a single, even layer. Evenly sprinkle half of the cheese over the bread. Evenly layer the bell pepper strips and tomato slices on top, and then sprinkle the remaining cheese evenly over the peppers and tomatoes.

Put the eggs and egg whites in a mixing bowl and beat them lightly with a fork. Add the buttermilk, red pepper flakes, oregano, and salt and pepper to taste and beat until thoroughly combined. Pour the egg mixture evenly over the layered ingredients in the baking dish.

Bake the strata until it looks slightly puffed up and the top is golden brown, 45 minutes to 1 hour. Remove the dish from the oven and let it set at room temperature for at least 10 minutes before using a large serving spoon to scoop it onto individual serving plates.

WOLFGANG'S HEALTHY TIPS

→ This is a good example of how a few smart, small decisions can transform a too-rich dish into something that's good for you and still tastes great. Substituting egg whites for some of the whole eggs, using reduced-fat cheese and low-fat buttermilk, and choosing whole-grain bread instead of white bread together have a big impact.

→ If you like, for a hint of meaty flavor, add 3 or 4 ounces lean ham or Canadian bacon, trimmed of any visible fat and cut into thin julienne strips, and toss with the bread cubes.

→ The quantities here yield eight servings, making this a great dish to offer as part of a brunch party buffet. If you'd like to make only four servings, use half the quantity for each ingredient and a baking dish measuring approximately 10 by 6 inches.

Nutrition Facts Per Serving: Calories: 180; Calories from Fat: 38; Total Fat: 4.27g; Saturated Fat: 1.61g; Monounsaturated Fat: 1.37g; Polyunsaturated Fat: 1.29g; Cholesterol: 76mg; Sodium: 267mg; Total Carbohydrate: 21.46g; Dietary Fiber: 2.71g; Sugars: 6.50g; Protein: 13.93g

Yogurt Oatmeal Muffins

MAKES 24

My thanks go to baker Christine Beard, who worked with me at my catering company, for coming up with this great fiber-rich muffin. You won't believe how tender, rich, and flavorful it tastes for something so healthy. Starting with frozen berries helps keep the fruit intact during baking, but fresh berries will give fine results, too. For convenience, prepare the batter the night before up to the point at which you combine the egg and oat mixtures; then, the next morning, add the flour–baking soda mixture and bake.

2¼ cups old-fashioned rolled oats

2 cups nonfat plain yogurt

2 large eggs

1¼ cups packed dark brown sugar

1 cup canola oil

2½ cups all-purpose flour

2½ teaspoons baking soda

2 cups frozen unsweetened raspberries, or fresh raspberries

In a large bowl, stir together the oats and yogurt. Cover and refrigerate for 1 hour to soften the oats. (If you mix the batter the night before, there's no need to do this.)

Preheat the oven to 350°F.

In a separate bowl, whisk together the eggs, sugar, and oil. With a rubber spatula or large spoon, stir the egg mixture into the oat mixture.

In a separate bowl, stir together the flour and baking soda. Stir the flour mixture into the egg-oat mixture until just combined.

Just before baking, fold the frozen berries into the batter. (If using fresh raspberries, stir carefully to avoid breaking or crushing them.)

Line 2 dozen muffin tin cups with paper muffin cups. Scoop batter evenly into the muffin cups.

Bake until the muffins are golden brown and spring back when pressed lightly with a fingertip, 30 to 40 minutes.

Transfer the muffin tins to a wire rack to cool. Serve the muffins warm or at room temperature.

WOLFGANG'S HEALTHY TIPS

→ Be sure to include this as part of a well-rounded breakfast, complementing a low-fat egg dish, some fresh fruit, and your favorite morning beverage.

→ Use this recipe as a base for coming up with all sorts of healthy muffins of your own. Use blueberries or pitted cherries in place of the raspberries. Add chopped walnuts or pecans for a little crunch.

Nutrition Facts Per Serving (1 muffin): Calories: 221; Calories from Fat: 88; Total Fat: 9.87g; Saturated Fat: 0.90g; Monounsaturated Fat: 6.07g; Polyunsaturated Fat: 2.90g; Cholesterol: 15mg; Sodium: 148mg; Total Carbohydrate: 28.32g; Dietary Fiber: 1.72g; Sugars: 12.47g; Protein: 5.03g

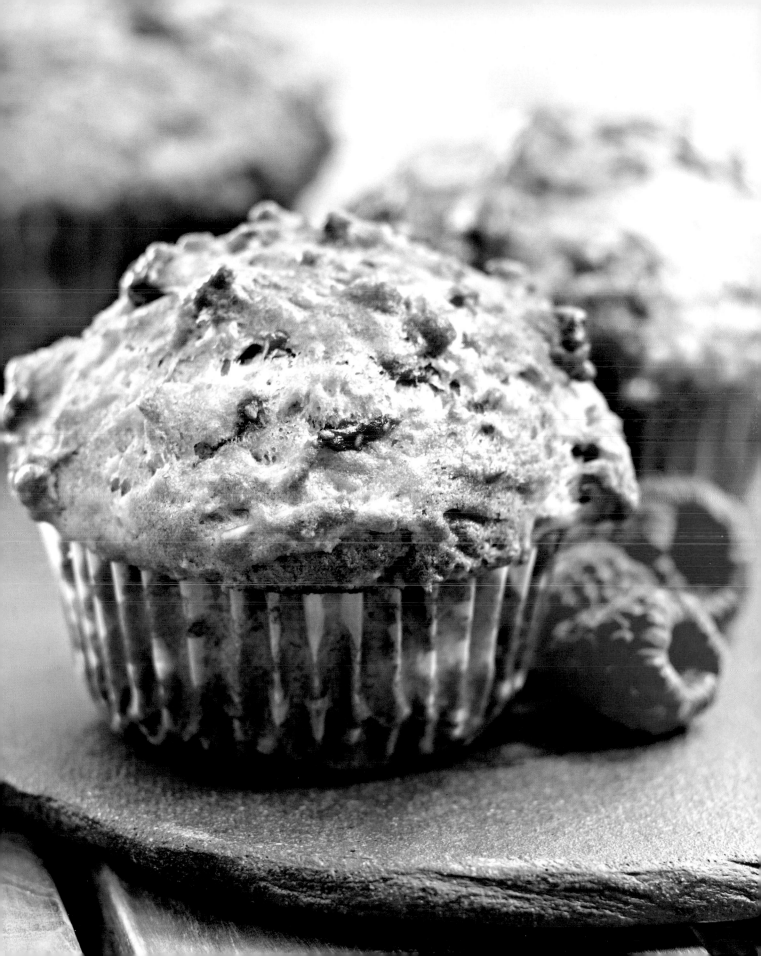

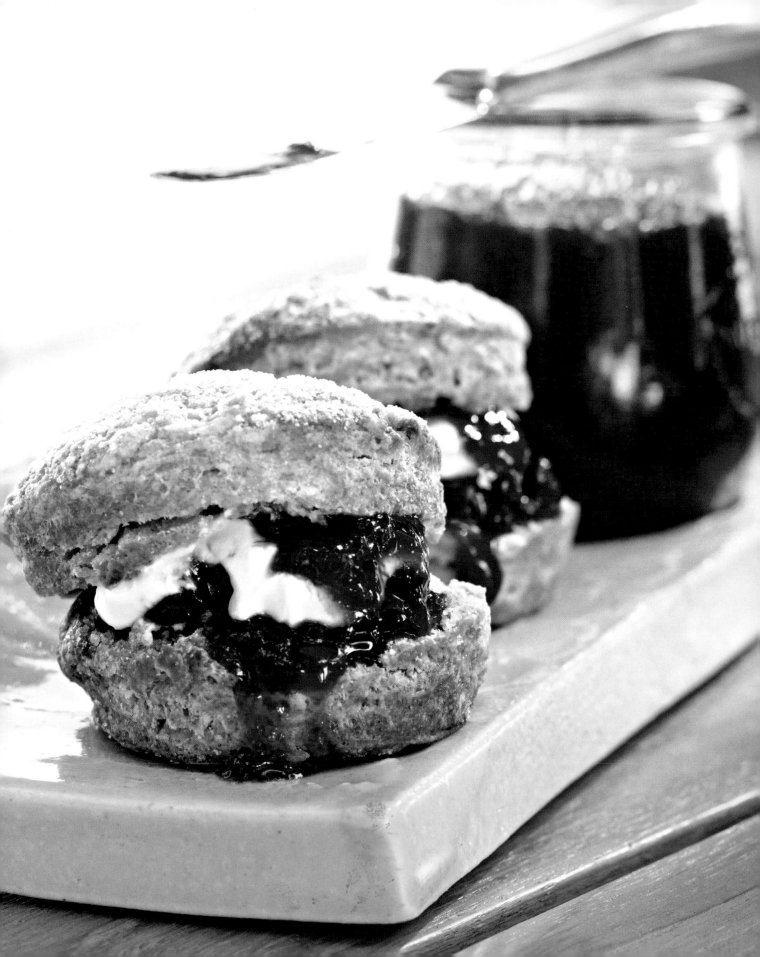

Spelt Coconut Scones

MAKES ABOUT 15

Serve these tender, flavorful, healthy scones as a special weekend brunch treat. Or offer them with your morning coffee or at teatime, accompanied by your favorite fruit spread or fresh berries and yogurt. I love them split and filled with jam and nonfat yogurt.

3 cups white spelt flour

¾ cup whole-grain spelt flour

¼ cup granulated sugar, plus more for sprinkling, if desired

1½ tablespoons baking powder

½ teaspoon kosher salt

⅓ cup coconut oil, at cool room temperature (cool enough to be solid), cut into ½-inch pieces

1 large egg

1 cup nonfat plain yogurt

½ cup nonfat milk

6 tablespoons heavy cream (optional)

In the bowl of a stand mixer fitted with the paddle attachment, combine the spelt flours, sugar, baking powder, and salt. Mix briefly on low speed. Add the coconut oil and continue mixing on low speed, watching carefully, just until the coconut oil forms pea-size pieces.

In a separate bowl, lightly whisk the egg. Add the yogurt and milk and whisk just until blended.

Add the egg mixture to the flour mixture. Mix briefly on low speed, just until a soft dough forms.

Turn out the dough onto a floured work surface. With floured hands, pat it down into a rough rectangle and fold in half. Pat down and fold again 2 or 3 times more. Wrap the dough in plastic wrap and refrigerate for 20 minutes.

Preheat the oven to 350°F.

With a rolling pin on a floured work surface, roll out the chilled dough to a 1¼-inch thickness. With a 2-inch round cutter, cut out rounds of dough, placing them on a nonstick baking sheet. Gather up any scraps, knead them briefly, and roll them out and cut into rounds. If desired, lightly brush the tops with cream and sprinkle with a little sugar.

Bake until lightly browned, 15 to 20 minutes.

WOLFGANG'S HEALTHY TIPS

→ Spelt, an ancient cousin of wheat, has a nutty flavor and generous fiber content. You can find both white and whole-grain spelt flours in the baking sections of well-stocked markets and health food stores.

→ Rich, sweet-tasting coconut oil has been found by some studies to help lower cholesterol and reduce belly fat. Well-stocked markets will carry it. The oil tends to solidify at cool room temperatures, but, for the purpose of this recipe, transfer the amount you need to a bowl and chill it in the refrigerator before cutting it into cubes.

Nutrition Facts Per Serving (1 scone): Calories: 188, Calories from Fat: 72; Total Fat: 8.10g; Monounsaturated Fat: 0.55g; Polyunsaturated Fat: 0.20g; Cholesterol: 12mg; Sodium: 239mg; Total Carbohydrate: 26.12g; Dietary Fiber: 3.80g; Sugars: 4.37g; Protein: 6.11g

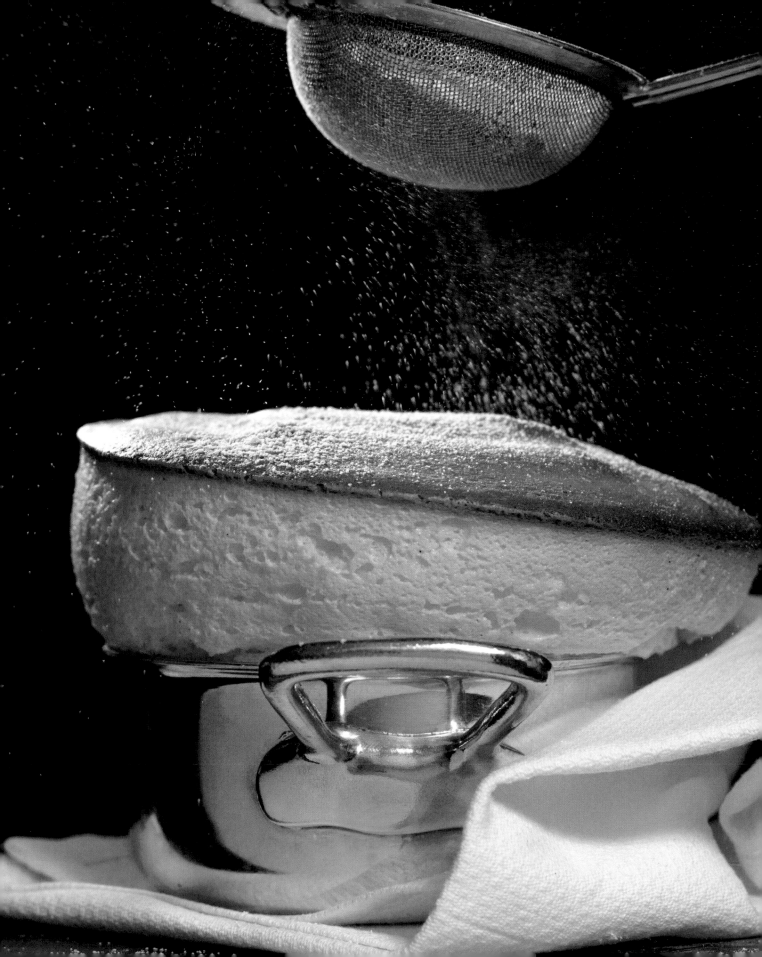

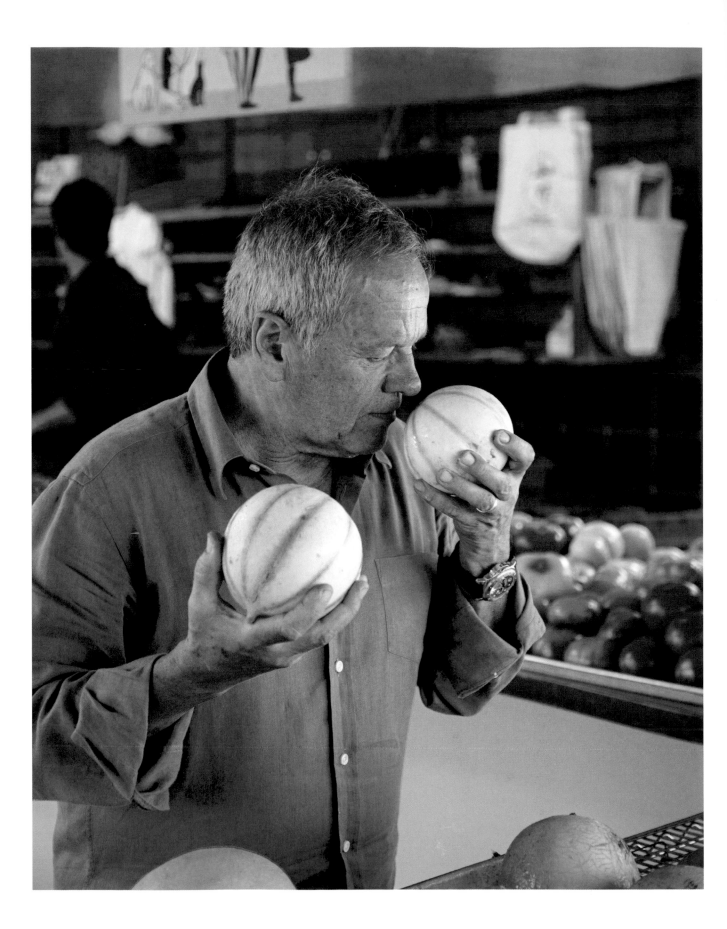

DESSERTS

Many people live for dessert. Which is why embarking on a new path of healthy eating can make some feel as if life as they know it has come to an end. I'm happy to share the news that, as the recipes in this chapter demonstrate, you can dedicate yourself to eating healthy meals and still enjoy fabulous desserts. It's easy to do if you choose the right ingredients, make smart cooking choices, and exercise a little portion control.

Start with the best fresh fruit and you're already doing well, making the most of its natural sweetness as well as benefiting from the great flavor, texture, and nutrients of in-season produce. Substitute low-fat or nonfat choices for the dairy products that figure in many dessert recipes, and you make the desserts leaner without sacrificing rich flavor. And preparing dessert recipes to maximize flavor amps up the pleasure they deliver, so you'll find it easy to slow down, savor every bite, and feel satisfied with less.

As you flip through the following pages, you'll be surprised by how many great healthy dessert choices there are, just waiting to reward you at the end of a day of smart eating and exercise.

→ Honeydew Melon Soup with Fresh Berries and Crystallized Mint

→ Berries and Cherries Jubilee

→ Fresh Peach Melba with Yogurt Sherbet and Fresh Raspberry Sauce

→ Buttermilk Panna Cotta "Martinis" with Stone Fruit Compote

→ Raspberry Sorbet

→ Zesty Vanilla Nonfat Yogurt Sherbet

→ Individual Baked Alaskas

→ Raspberry Soufflés with Raspberry Sauce

→ Banana–Passion Fruit Soufflés

→ Chocolate Soufflés with Orange Marmalade

→ Chocolate Bread Pudding with Dried Cherries

→ Cherry Cobbler with Just a Little Shortcake Crust

→ Teff Pie Dough

   ★ Apple Pie with Teff Pastry Crust

   ★ Blueberry Pie with Teff Pastry Crust

   ★ Cherry Pie with Teff Pastry Crust

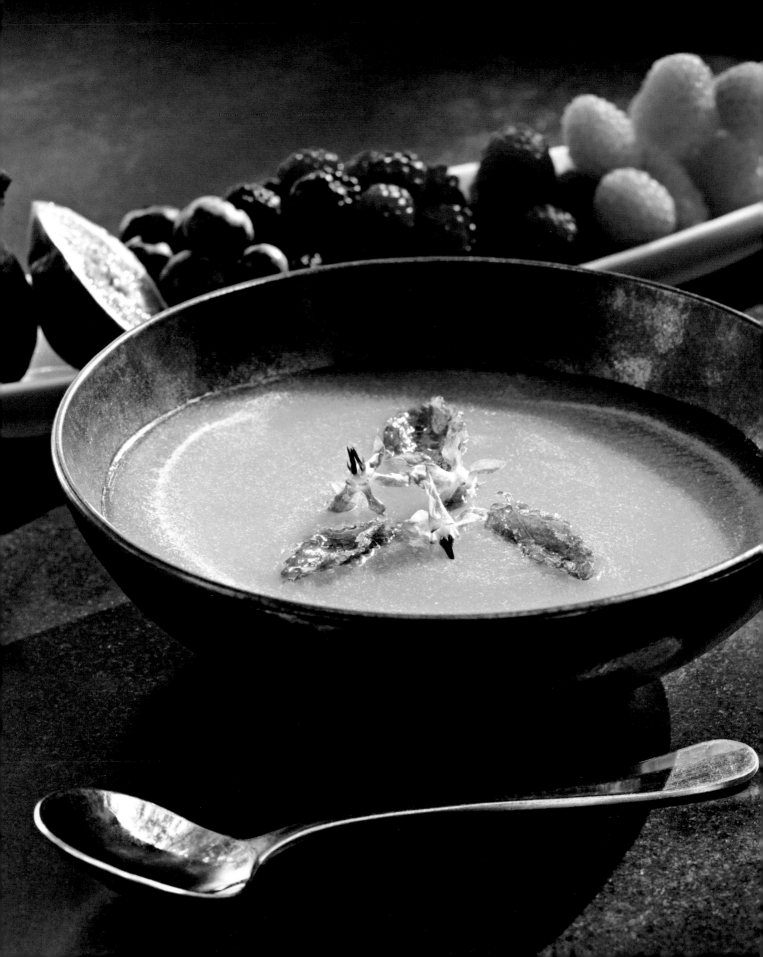

Honeydew Melon Soup with Fresh Berries and Crystallized Mint

SERVES 4

It's so easy to turn sweet, juicy seasonal fruit into a beautiful chilled soup to enjoy for a light dessert. Garnish each serving with fresh berries as you might garnish a warm first-course soup with sautéed vegetables.

Crystallized Mint:

2 tablespoons superfine sugar

12 fresh mint leaves, rinsed and patted dry

1 egg white, lightly beaten with 1 tablespoon water

Honeydew Melon Soup:

6 cups ripe sweet honeydew melon pieces, well chilled

2 tablespoons fresh lemon juice

Superfine sugar (optional)

1 cup Moscato d'Asti or other sweet sparkling wine, well chilled

To Assemble:

2 cups mixed fresh berries or pieces of other juicy fresh fruit

At least 6 hours before serving the soup, prepare the Crystallized Mint: Put the superfine sugar in a bowl. With a pastry brush, lightly brush the mint sprigs all over with the egg white mixture. Put them in the bowl with the sugar and toss lightly to coat them evenly, then transfer to a wire rack to dry at room temperature for at least 6 hours. Store in an airtight container until ready to use.

Prepare the Honeydew Melon Soup: Put the melon pieces and lemon juice in a blender or food processor fitted with the stainless-steel blade. Blend or process until finely pureed. Taste the puree and, only if needed, pulse in a little superfine sugar to sweeten it to your liking. Strain the puree through a fine-mesh sieve set over a nonreactive bowl, pressing it through with a rubber spatula. Discard the solids left in the sieve. Cover the bowl with plastic wrap and refrigerate for at least 1 hour.

Before serving, stir the sparkling wine into the melon puree.

Assemble the dish: Ladle the soup into chilled shallow soup plates. Serve the berries or other fresh fruit on the side, for guests to add to their own servings. Place 3 Crystallized Mint leaves in each bowl and serve immediately.

WOLFGANG'S HEALTHY TIPS

→ In addition to honeydew or cantaloupe, look for other related sweet melon varieties, such as Persian melons or Sharlyn melons, at your farmers' market.

→ Instead of the berry garnish, use any other small pieces of fresh fruit you like, including figs, cherries, peaches, nectarines, Asian pear, and kiwifruit.

→ If you like, add a ¼-cup scoop of Zesty Vanilla Nonfat Yogurt Sherbet (page 249) to each bowl before garnishing with the mint and fresh fruit.

Nutrition Facts Per Serving: Calories: 252; Calories from Fat: 4; Total Fat: 0.48g; Saturated Fat: 0.12g; Monounsaturated Fat: 0.05g; Polyunsaturated Fat: 0.32g; Cholesterol: 0mg; Sodium: 65mg; Total Carbohydrate: 47.19g; Dietary Fiber: 4.96g; Sugars: 36.88g; Protein: 3.07g

Berries and Cherries Jubilee

SERVES 4

Most people have heard of the dessert called Cherries Jubilee. So I thought it would be fun to come up with a variation that wasn't limited just to cherry season, since fresh berries of all kinds are widely available year round and can star on their own when cherries are not in season.

2 pints mixed fresh berries and halved and pitted cherries, larger berries cut in half

2 cups Zesty Vanilla Nonfat Yogurt Sherbet (page 249) or good-quality store-bought vanilla nonfat frozen yogurt

1½ tablespoons unsalted butter

⅓ cup packed dark brown sugar

1 teaspoon grated orange zest

Juice of 1 orange

¼ cup Grand Marnier

Fresh mint sprigs, for garnish

Reserve several perfect-looking pieces of fruit as garnishes, if you like.

Scoop the Zesty Vanilla Nonfat Yogurt Sherbet or frozen yogurt attractively into four serving bowls. Put the bowls in the freezer.

In a medium sauté pan, melt the butter over medium heat. Sprinkle in the sugar and stir until it combines with the butter and begins to melt. Continue cooking until the syrup thickens, 1 to 2 minutes more.

Add the fruit to the pan. Sauté, stirring frequently but gently, just until they begin to soften and give up some of their juices, 3 to 4 minutes. Stir in the orange zest and juice. Remove from the heat.

Remove the bowls from the freezer.

If you don't want to flambé the Berries and Cherries Jubilee, remove the pan from the stove. Add the Grand Marnier and gently stir it into the mixture before spooning or ladling the fruit over the frozen yogurt.

If you would like to flambé the fruit mixture, carefully sprinkle the Grand Marnier over the sautéed fruit. Light a long wooden kitchen match or fireplace match. Keeping the match and the sauté pan safely clear of any flammable objects, carefully hold the burning tip of the match just above the surface of the pan's contents to ignite the vapors.

While the blue flames are still visible in the pan, carefully spoon or ladle the fruits and their sauce over the frozen yogurt in each bowl and present the bowls to your guests. As soon as the flames vanish, garnish each serving with some reserved fruit and a mint sprig.

WOLFGANG'S HEALTHY TIPS

→ The nonfat yogurt–based sherbet replaces the usual vanilla ice cream for a dramatic reduction in fat and calories without any drop in the pleasure that the dessert delivers.

→ Try this recipe with any other combination of berries you like.

Nutrition Facts Per Serving (including Zesty Vanilla Nonfat Yogurt Sherbet): Calories: 315; Calories from Fat: 40; Total Fat: 4.55g; Saturated Fat: 2.88g; Monounsaturated Fat: 1.25g; Polyunsaturated Fat: 0.42g; Cholesterol: 12mg; Sodium: 97mg; Total Carbohydrate: 62.43g; Dietary Fiber: 4.58g; Sugars: 55.35g; Protein: 8.15g

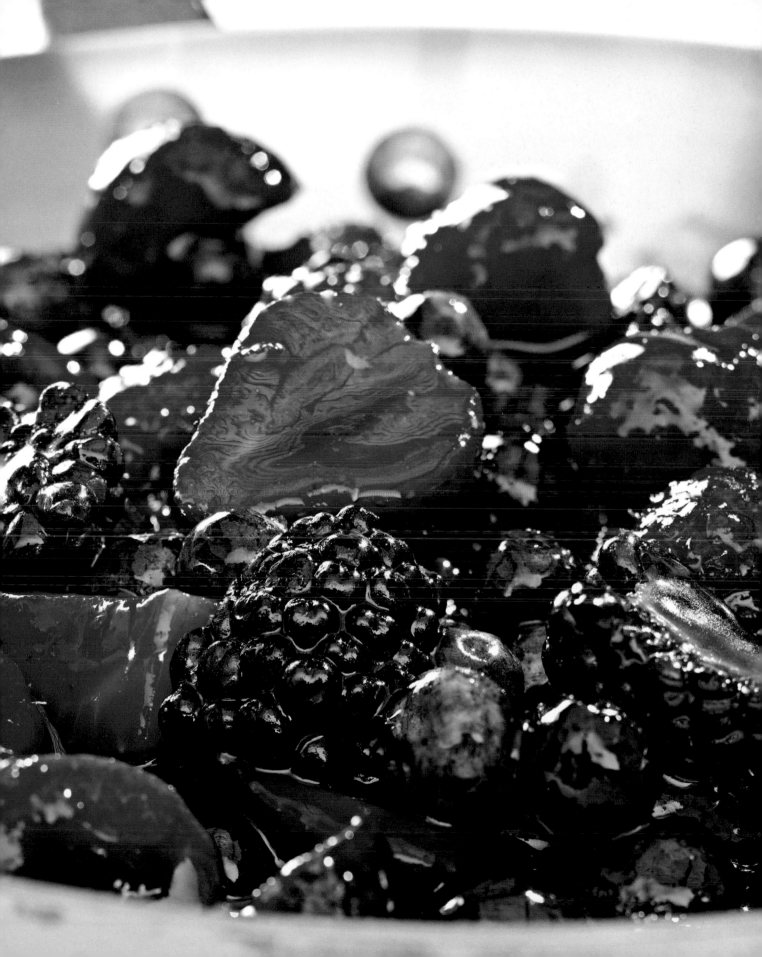

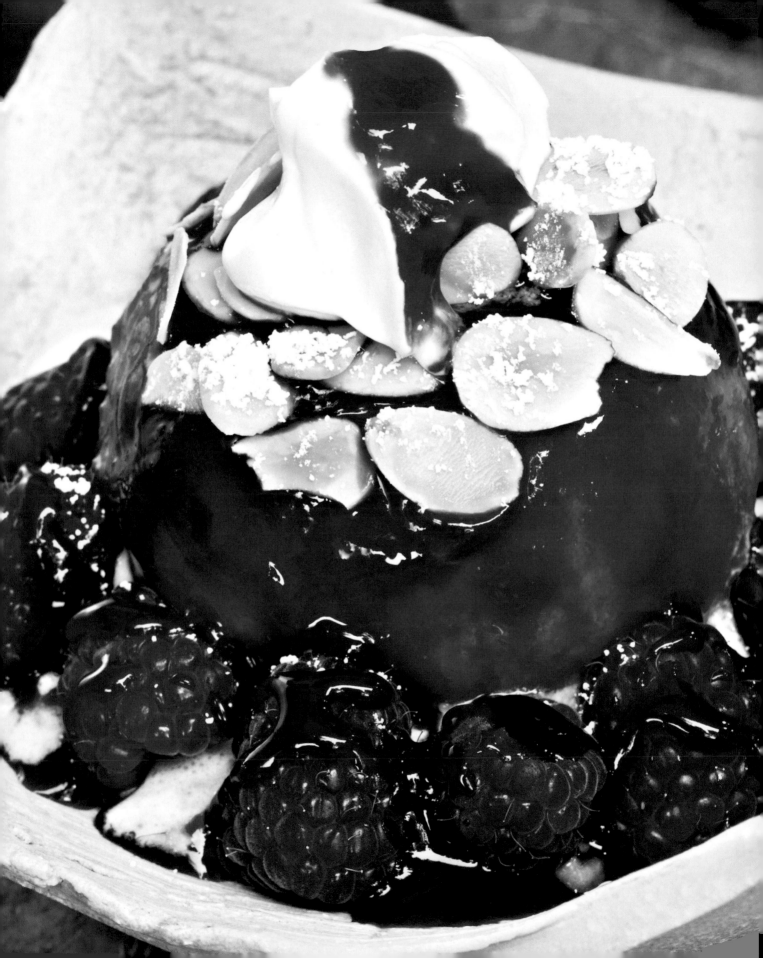

Fresh Peach Melba with Yogurt Sherbet and Fresh Raspberry Sauce

SERVES 4

Peach Melba has been a popular special-occasion dessert since the late nineteenth century, when it was created in honor of the great Australian soprano Nellie Melba. This low-fat version brings it up to date for health-conscious eaters.

Poached Peaches:

2 large ripe, firm, freestone peaches

⅔ cup granulated sugar

1 teaspoon grated lemon zest

1½ tablespoons fresh lemon juice

Fresh Raspberry Sauce:

⅔ cup fresh raspberries

3 tablespoons granulated sugar

4 teaspoons fresh lemon juice

To Assemble:

2 cups Zesty Vanilla Nonfat Yogurt Sherbet (page 249), or good-quality store bought vanilla nonfat frozen yogurt

2 tablespoons sliced almonds, toasted (see page 289)

4 tablespoons nonfat plain yogurt

1 cup fresh raspberries

Confectioners' sugar, for dusting (optional)

Prepare the Poached Peaches: Bring a saucepan of water to a boil. Fill a bowl with ice cubes and water and set it nearby. With a small, sharp knife, score a shallow X in the skin at the blossom end of each peach. Carefully place the peaches in the boiling water and boil until their skins wrinkle, about 20 seconds. With a slotted spoon, lift them from the boiling water and immerse in the ice water. When they are cool enough to handle, drain well. Starting at the X, peel off the skin. Cut each peach in half along its seam. Remove the pits.

In a small saucepan, stir together the granulated sugar, lemon zest, lemon juice, and ⅔ cup water. Bring to a boil over medium-high heat, then reduce the heat to low. Add the peeled peach halves and simmer until tender, 5 to 7 minutes. Remove the pan from the heat and leave the peaches to cool in the syrup at room temperature. Transfer the peaches and syrup to a nonreactive bowl, cover with plastic wrap, and refrigerate.

Prepare the Fresh Raspberry Sauce: In a blender or food processor, combine the berries, sugar, and lemon juice and process until pureed. Strain the puree through a fine-mesh strainer into a nonreactive bowl, pressing it through with a rubber spatula. Discard the solids left in the strainer. Cover the bowl with plastic wrap and refrigerate.

Assemble the dish: Scoop the Zesty Vanilla Nonfat Yogurt Sherbet into individual chilled serving bowls. Place a peach half cut side down on top of the yogurt sherbet. Sprinkle the almonds over the peach and place 1 tablespoon of plain yogurt on top. Scatter the fresh raspberries around the peach. Drizzle with the raspberry sauce. If you like, dust each serving with a little confectioners' sugar, spooning it into a small fine-mesh sieve held over each serving and then tapping the side of the sieve.

WOLFGANG'S HEALTHY TIPS

→ For a change, try making the dessert with nectarines; or with a sauce featuring different kinds of berries; or with Raspberry Sorbet (page 248).

→ You could also serve it with a more casual presentation of your choice, such as scooping the sherbet into the serving bowls and topping them with sliced peach halves and the sauce and garnishes.

Nutrition Facts Per Serving (including Zesty Vanilla Nonfat Yogurt Sherbet): Calories: 383; Calories from Fat: 16; Total Fat: 1.95g; Saturated Fat: 0.26g; Monounsaturated Fat: 1.05g; Polyunsaturated Fat: 0.65g; Cholesterol: 1mg; Sodium: 97mg; Total Carbohydrate: 85.12g; Dietary Fiber: 5.53g; Sugars: 79.21g; Protein: 9.28g

Buttermilk Panna Cotta "Martinis" with Stone Fruit Compote

SERVES 4

I've always loved the way the Italian dessert *panna cotta* ("cooked cream") achieves the consistency of pudding by using gelatin instead of egg yolks. Here, replacing the cream with buttermilk reduces the fat even more dramatically.

Buttermilk Panna Cotta:

2 cups buttermilk

2 teaspoons powdered gelatin

1 vanilla bean

3 tablespoons sugar

½ teaspoon lemon juice

Stone Fruit Compote:

1½ tablespoons sugar

1 cup mixed pitted and sliced fresh nectarines and apricots

Prepare the Buttermilk Panna Cotta: Pour 1 cup of the buttermilk into a small bowl and sprinkle the gelatin on top. Set aside to soften.

With a small, sharp knife, split the vanilla bean lengthwise. With the back of the blade, scrape the seeds from inside each bean half and put them in a small saucepan along with the bean pod halves. Add the remaining buttermilk and the sugar and set the pan over low heat. Gently warm the mixture, stirring, until the sugar has dissolved, taking care not to let the buttermilk boil. Remove from the heat and stir in the reserved buttermilk-gelatin mixture. Leave the mixture to cool to room temperature, stirring occasionally. Remove the vanilla bean pod. Stir in the lemon juice.

Spoon the room-temperature panna cotta mixture evenly among four large martini glasses. Cover each glass with plastic wrap. Place them on a tray and refrigerate until the panna cotta has set, at least 3 hours.

As soon as you put the panna cotta in the refrigerator, prepare the Stone Fruit Compote: In a small saucepan, combine the sugar and 3 tablespoons water. Stir with a wooden spoon over medium heat until the sugar dissolves. Add half of the sliced fruit. Cook for 2 to 3 minutes, stirring and lightly pressing down on the fruit, until the mixture has a jam-like consistency. Remove the pan from the heat and gently stir in the remaining fruit.

Transfer to a bowl, cover with plastic wrap, and refrigerate.

To serve, gently stir the Stone Fruit Compote and then spoon it evenly into the four glasses of panna cotta.

WOLFGANG'S HEALTHY TIPS

→ Notice how the thick consistency of low-fat buttermilk gives you the richness of cream without all the fat. And the buttermilk's tanginess works perfectly with the other flavors in this recipe.

→ If you want to reduce the sugar in the recipe, replace the compote with a simple salad of the sweetest, juiciest in-season fruit you can find. I also like this dessert made with the same amount of other summer stone fruit such as pitted cherries or sliced peaches or plums, or with a mixture of fresh berries.

→ The compote also makes a delicious topping for my Zesty Vanilla Nonfat Yogurt Sherbet (page 249).

Nutrition Facts Per Serving: Calories: 130; Calories from Fat: 10; Total Fat: 1.12g; Saturated Fat: 0.68g; Monounsaturated Fat: 0.36g; Polyunsaturated Fat: 0.08g; Cholesterol: 4mg; Sodium: 131mg; Total Carbohydrate: 24.44g; Dietary Fiber: 0.72g; Sugars: 23.50g; Protein: 6.04g

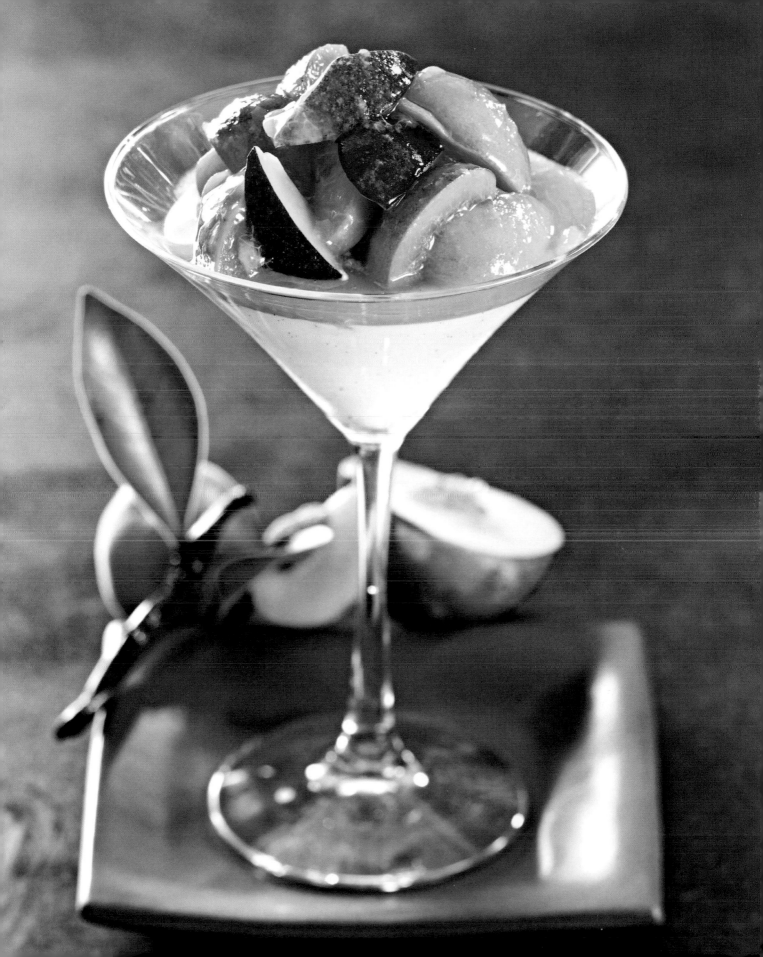

Raspberry Sorbet

MAKES ABOUT 1 QUART; EIGHT ½-CUP SERVINGS

Fresh berries are among my favorite desserts. But when I want something sweeter and even more refreshing, I'll often choose a sorbet made from ripe, sweet, peak-of-season fruit from the farmers' market.

2 pounds fresh raspberries

1 cup sugar

Juice of 1 medium lemon

Put the raspberries in a blender or a food processor fitted with the stainless-steel blade. Blend or process until pureed. Add the sugar and lemon juice and pulse until combined.

Strain the puree through a fine-mesh sieve over a bowl, pressing it through with a rubber spatula. Discard the solids left in the sieve.

Put the strained puree in an ice cream maker and freeze according to the manufacturer's instructions. Transfer to a covered container and store in the freezer for at least 2 hours before serving. Let soften at room temperature for 15 to 30 minutes before scooping.

WOLFGANG'S HEALTHY TIPS

→ This low-fat, low-calorie recipe is ideal for people craving a little bit of something sweet to end a meal. But, obviously, it should be avoided by anyone who is restricting sugar intake for health reasons. Rather than sweetening it artificially, I would prefer simply to eat fresh berries on their own.

→ The recipe works very well with other ripe, juicy, sweet summertime berries. I especially like it with blackberries, boysenberries, or golden raspberries.

→ Try this in desserts calling for fresh sorbet, such as my Individual Baked Alaskas (page 250).

Nutrition Facts Per Serving: Calories: 161; Calories from Fat: 5; Total Fat: 0.57g; Saturated Fat: 0.03g; Monounsaturated Fat: 0.08g; Polyunsaturated Fat: 0.47g; Cholesterol: 0mg; Sodium: 1mg; Total Carbohydrate: 40.10g; Dietary Fiber: 8.01g; Sugars: 30.54g; Protein: 1.50g

Zesty Vanilla Nonfat Yogurt Sherbet

MAKES ABOUT 1 QUART; EIGHT ½-CUP SERVINGS

Unlike the store-bought frozen yogurt you may be used to, this has a very light, velvety consistency thanks to beaten egg whites folded into the mixture before freezing.

3 large egg whites

⅔ cup sugar

3 cups nonfat plain yogurt

1 teaspoon grated lemon zest

2 teaspoons pure vanilla extract

In the bowl of a stand mixer fitted with the wire whip, or in a bowl using a hand mixer, beat the egg whites at medium speed until foamy. Increase the speed to high and slowly stream in the sugar, continuing to beat until the whites form stiff peaks that hold their form when the beaters are lifted out.

In a separate bowl, combine the yogurt, lemon zest, and vanilla extract and whisk until smooth. In three batches, use a rubber spatula to gently fold the egg whites into the yogurt mixture.

Transfer the mixture to an ice cream maker and freeze according to the manufacturer's instructions. Transfer to a covered container and freeze for at least 2 hours before serving, and serve within 2 to 3 days. Let soften at room temperature for 15 to 30 minutes before scooping.

WOLFGANG'S HEALTHY TIPS

→ Enjoy this recipe simply on its own, or topped with some juicy fresh seasonal fruit or a few chopped oven-roasted nuts—or even a spoonful of good-quality chocolate chips.

→ It's also excellent used in healthy versions of the sorts of desserts that might ordinarily call for richer ice creams, such as my Berries and Cherries Jubilee (page 242) or Fresh Peach Melba (page 245).

→ Once you've tried the recipe this way, feel free to vary it by using different citrus zests instead of the lemon; or by leaving out the zest entirely and using different flavors of store-bought baking extracts such as coffee, peppermint, almond, banana, or maple.

Nutrition Facts Per Serving: Calories: 125; Calories from Fat: 1; Total Fat: 0.16g; Saturated Fat: 0.11g; Monounsaturated Fat: 0.05g; Polyunsaturated Fat: 0g; Cholesterol: 1mg; Sodium: 91mg; Total Carbohydrate: 23.99g; Dietary Fiber: 0.03g; Sugars: 23.93g; Protein: 6.62g

Individual Baked Alaskas

MAKES 4 BAKED ALASKAS

For a special occasion, make this beautiful, delicious, yet easy dessert—a fine-dining favorite for more than a century and a half—and no one will feel deprived. In fact, your guests might not even suspect that it's incredibly low in fat. If you like, just before serving use a sharp knife to cut each individual portion carefully in half to reveal the beautiful surprise inside.

4 thin slices (about ¼ inch thick) store-bought or homemade pound cake

1 cup Zesty Vanilla Nonfat Yogurt Sherbet (page 249) or good-quality store-bought vanilla nonfat frozen yogurt

1 cup Raspberry Sorbet (page 248) or good-quality store-bought fruit sorbet

4 large egg whites

¼ teaspoon cream of tartar

½ cup sugar

Use a 3-inch round cookie cutter to cut a circular piece from each slice of pound cake. Place the circles of pound cake about 2 inches apart on a baking sheet.

Using a small bowl about 2½ inches in diameter, scoop in ¼ cup of the Zesty Vanilla Nonfat Yogurt Sherbet or frozen yogurt; with the back of a spoon, spread it in an even layer all over the bowl's interior surface. Then, scoop in ¼ cup of the Raspberry Sorbet, packing it in firmly and smoothing the surface. Unmold the bowl onto the center of one of the cake rounds, leaving a ¼-inch rim of cake all around the scoop. Repeat with the remaining sherbet and sorbet and cake slices. Immediately put the baking sheet in the freezer and freeze until very hard, at least 1 hour.

Preheat the broiler, positioning the broiler rack 8 inches away from the heat source.

In the bowl of a stand mixer fitted with the wire whip, or in a bowl using a hand mixer, beat together the egg whites and cream of tartar at medium speed until they hold soft peaks that droop slightly when you lift out the beaters. With the mixer running, 1 tablespoon at a time, slowly stream in the sugar. Beat until the meringue reaches stiff peaks that stand up straight when you lift out the beaters. Spoon the meringue into a pastry bag fitted with a large star tip.

Remove the baking sheet from the freezer. Starting at the bottom exposed rim where the sherbet and sorbet meet the cake, and then spiraling upward, quickly pipe a generous coating of meringue over the pound cake and its frozen topping, covering each serving completely in meringue.

Immediately place the baking sheet under the broiler and broil just until the tops of the meringue are browned, about 2 minutes, watching carefully to prevent burning. Remove from the oven and serve immediately.

WOLFGANG'S HEALTHY TIPS

→ Preparing small individual servings like this, instead of a big Baked Alaska that is usually made and sliced into wedges, is a perfect example of portion control. You won't eat as much as you might if you were to prepare a bigger, multiple-serving version.

→ I've cut the fat and calories here by using a much thinner cake base and filling the dessert with nonfat frozen treats instead of the usual ice cream.

→ In spite of its low fat content, this dessert is fairly high in calories and sugar. Bear that in mind when planning the rest of your menu and your meals for the day you plan to serve it.

Nutrition Facts Per Serving: Calories: 315; Calories from Fat: 28; Total Fat: 3.14g; Saturated Fat: 1.80g; Monounsaturated Fat: 0.96g; Polyunsaturated Fat: 0.45g; Cholesterol: 34mg; Sodium: 160mg; Total Carbohydrate: 64.76g; Dietary Fiber: 4.12g; Sugars: 52.43g; Protein: 8.49g

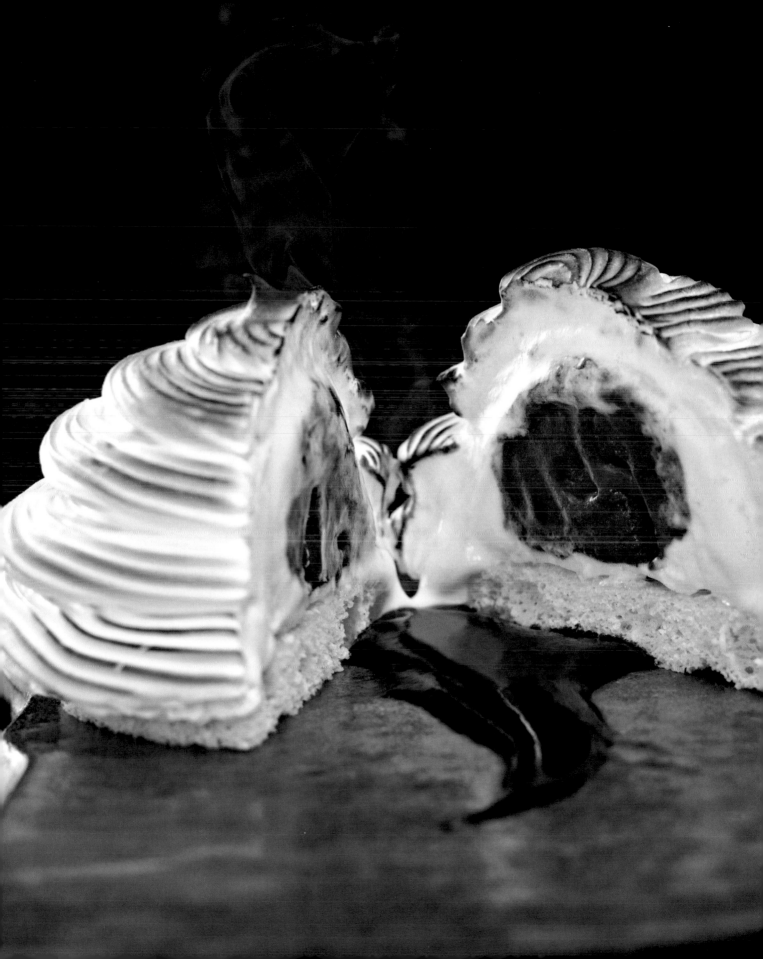

Raspberry Soufflés with Raspberry Sauce

MAKES 8 SOUFFLÉS

Soufflés, like this classic developed by former longtime Spago pastry chef Sherry Yard, feel like the most indulgent of desserts. But, being based on fat-free egg whites, they can be surprisingly light. To get enough volume to beat the whites thoroughly, it works best to prepare this recipe for eight servings, making it appropriate for a special dinner party.

Raspberry Soufflés:

3 cups fresh raspberries

6 tablespoons sugar, plus 1 tablespoon for coating ramekins

1 tablespoon Chambord (raspberry liqueur) (optional)

½ tablespoon fresh lemon juice

¼ teaspoon balsamic vinegar

1 tablespoon unsalted butter, softened

4 large egg whites, at room temperature

Pinch of cream of tartar

¼ cup semisweet chocolate chips (optional)

Raspberry Sauce:

2 cups fresh raspberries

¼ cup sugar

½ teaspoon lemon juice

To Assemble:

1 cup fresh raspberries (optional)

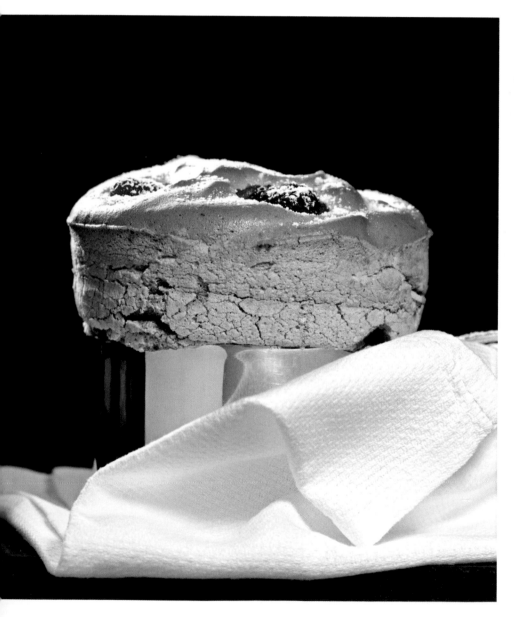

Prepare the Raspberry Soufflés: In a small saucepan, combine ¾ cup of the raspberries, 2 tablespoons of the sugar, the Chambord (if using), the lemon juice, and the vinegar. Bring to a boil over medium heat. Cook, stirring occasionally, until the liquid has reduced and the raspberries have a jam-like consistency, 4 to 5 minutes. Strain the mixture through a fine-mesh sieve set over a heatproof bowl, pressing it through with a rubber spatula. Discard the solids left in the sieve. Set aside to cool to room temperature.

Measure out ½ cup of this mixture and transfer to a large bowl, leaving the rest in the pan. Set aside.

Position a rack in the lowest level of the oven. Preheat the oven to 425°F.

With the butter, coat the insides of eight ½-cup ramekins. Lightly dust the butter with the 1 tablespoon of sugar. Place the ramekins on a baking tray.

Divide half of the remaining raspberries for the soufflés among the ramekins. Drizzle the raspberry sauce left in the pan evenly over the raspberries in the ramekins.

In the bowl of a stand mixer fitted with the wire whip, or in a clean mixing bowl using a hand mixer, beat the egg whites on low speed until foamy, about 1 minute. Add the cream of tartar and continue beating at low speed for 1 minute more. Increase the speed to medium and, with the mixer running, slowly sprinkle in the remaining 4 tablespoons sugar. Continue beating until the whites form firm peaks that stand up when the beaters are lifted out.

With a wire whisk, gently stir about one-third of the beaten egg whites into the reserved ½ cup of raspberry sauce, until combined and lightened. Then, with the whisk, fold in the remaining egg whites. If you like, sprinkle the chocolate chips into the egg whites and gently fold them in with a rubber spatula. Fold in the remaining reserved whole raspberries.

Spoon the egg white mixture into the prepared ramekins, mounding it in peaks resembling cotton candy.

Bake until well puffed and dark golden, 7 to 10 minutes. (The soufflés will still have a pudding-like consistency inside.)

While the soufflés are baking, prepare the Raspberry Sauce: In a small, non-reactive saucepan, combine the raspberries, sugar, and lemon juice. Cook over medium heat, stirring occasionally, until the berries have given up their juices, 3 to 4 minutes. Bring to a boil and continue cooking, stirring frequently, until the mixture is syrupy, 2 to 3 minutes more. Strain the mixture through a fine-mesh sieve over a heatproof bowl, pressing down on it with a rubber spatula. Discard the solids left in the sieve.

Assemble the dish: As soon as the soufflés are done, transfer the ramekins to individual plates and serve immediately, garnished with a few fresh berries, if you like. Pass the Raspberry Sauce on the side, suggesting that guests use their spoons to gently break into the soufflés and spoon the sauce inside.

WOLFGANG'S HEALTHY TIPS

→ If you love chocolate and are looking for an extra little splurge, the optional chocolate chips add only 25 calories (14 from fat) and just under 3 grams more sugar per serving.

→ The fresh raspberry sauce, spooned into each serving at the table, adds only a few extra calories while making the dessert feel extra special. But, if you prefer, leave it out.

→ Try this recipe with other sweet, juicy, in-season berries, such as blackberries or strawberries.

Nutrition Facts Per Serving: Calories: 127; Calories from Fat: 15; Total Fat: 1.69g; Saturated Fat: 0.93g; Monounsaturated Fat: 0.42g; Polyunsaturated Fat: 0.34g; Cholesterol: 3mg; Sodium: 28mg; Total Carbohydrate: 26.61g; Dietary Fiber: 5.00g; Sugars: 20.73g; Protein: 2.74g

Banana–Passion Fruit Soufflés

SERVES 8

The tropical flavors of banana and passion fruit go together harmoniously, giving these soufflés a wonderful combination of richness and exotic perfume.

Banana–Passion Fruit Base:

2 tablespoons unsalted butter

2 tablespoons plus 2 teaspoons dark brown sugar

2 tablespoons granulated sugar

4 ounces very ripe peeled banana, cut into ½-inch pieces

¼ cup passion fruit puree
(see Tip, right)

Soufflés:

1 tablespoon unsalted butter, at room temperature

6 tablespoons granulated sugar, plus 2 teaspoons for coating ramekins

6 large egg whites

Confectioners' sugar, for dusting

Prepare the Banana–Passion Fruit Base: In a small saucepan, melt the butter over high heat and cook it until it turns nut brown, watching carefully to make sure it doesn't burn. Stir in the brown and granulated sugars and continue to cook, stirring constantly, until the mixture turns caramel-colored, about 5 minutes. Add the banana and stir until well coated. Continue cooking for 2 minutes more. Remove the pan from the heat and stir in the passion fruit puree. Transfer the mixture to a food processor and pulse until smooth. Transfer to a bowl and set aside to cool to room temperature.

Preheat the oven to 425°F.

Prepare the Soufflés: Brush the insides of eight individual ½-cup ramekins with the softened butter. Sprinkle the inside bottom and sides of the ramekins evenly with 2 table-spoons plus 2 teaspoons of the sugar.

Put the egg whites in a clean bowl. Beat with a hand mixer at medium-high speed while pouring in the remaining 4 tablespoons sugar in a slow, steady stream. Continue beating until the egg whites form moderately stiff peaks that barely stand up straight when the beaters are lifted out.

With a rubber spatula, gently fold half of the beaten egg whites into the cooled banana–passion fruit mixture. Then, fold in the rest of the egg whites until just a few streaks of white remain. Spoon the soufflé mixture evenly among the prepared ramekins, mounding it above

their rims. Place the ramekins on a baking sheet and bake in the center of the oven until they are nicely risen and their tops are golden brown, 7 to 10 minutes.

Carefully transfer the ramekins to individual serving plates. Serve immediately, dusted with confectioners' sugar.

WOLFGANG'S HEALTHY TIPS

→ This is a good example of how a rich texture and flavor—here, from ripe bananas—can make you feel you're eating something richly indulgent, even though it is low in fat and calories.

→ Look for frozen passion fruit puree in well-stocked supermarkets. Or, to make your own, buy ripe passion fruits, cut them in half, and scoop the pulp into a strainer set over a bowl. Press down on the pulp with a rubber spatula to force it through the strainer, holding back the black seeds. Store any extra passion fruit puree in a container in the freezer.

→ For an extra treat that won't make the dessert too indulgent, gently fold 1 ounce semisweet chocolate chips into the soufflé mixture before putting it into the ramekins.

Nutrition Facts Per Serving: Calories: 140; Calories from Fat: 36; Total Fat: 4.09g; Saturated Fat: 2.76g; Monounsaturated Fat: 1.13g; Polyunsaturated Fat: 0.20g; Cholesterol: 11mg; Sodium: 44mg; Total Carbohydrate: 23.28g; Dietary Fiber: 1.13g; Sugars: 20.81g; Protein: 3.06g

Chocolate Soufflés
with Orange Marmalade
SERVES 8

When you're really craving an intensely chocolaty dessert, here's a good choice: a light soufflé that delivers rich chocolate flavor in every spoonful. The touch of orange marmalade, spooned into each soufflé just before serving, adds a surprising, zesty contrast.

1 tablespoon unsalted butter, at room temperature

2 tablespoons granulated sugar

4 ounces bittersweet chocolate, cut into small pieces, or bittersweet chocolate chips

2 tablespoons orange liqueur

2 large egg yolks

7 large egg whites

Juice of ½ lemon

½ cup fine-shred orange marmalade

Confectioners' sugar, for dusting (optional)

Preheat the oven to 425°F.

With the butter, coat the insides of eight ½-cup ramekins or soufflé dishes. Lightly dust them with about 1 tablespoon of the granulated sugar. Place them on a baking sheet and refrigerate until needed.

Melt the chocolate in a metal bowl set over a saucepan of gently simmering water. Remove from the heat and stir in the liqueur and egg yolks.

In a clean bowl, beat the egg whites with a hand mixer on medium speed until they form soft peaks. Beat in the lemon juice and the remaining 1 tablespoon sugar. Continue to beat the whites until they are stiff, holding peaks that stand upright when the beaters are lifted out, but still very shiny. With a rubber spatula, gently fold one-quarter of the egg whites into the chocolate mixture, and then gently fold that mixture back into the remaining whites.

Distribute the soufflé mixture evenly among the ramekins. Run your thumb around the inside edge of each ramekin to help the soufflés form "hats" as they rise. Bake for 7 to 10 minutes, or until the edges are set but the middles are still just a little soft.

While the soufflés are baking, gently warm the marmalade in a small saucepan over low heat.

When the soufflés are done, transfer each ramekin to a dessert plate. If you like, spoon a little confectioners' sugar into a fine-mesh sieve and tap its edge over the soufflés to dust them with some sugar. Spoon 1 tablespoon of warm marmalade into the center of each soufflé. Serve immediately.

> **WOLFGANG'S HEALTHY TIPS**
>
> → The percentage of calories from fat here is just slightly higher than 33 percent (about 35 percent). But it would work fine to end a meal featuring lower-fat appetizer and main dishes, or as an occasional almost-guilt-free treat.
>
> → For a nice change of pace, try this with the Raspberry Sauce from the Raspberry Soufflés (page 252) instead of the marmalade.

Nutrition Facts Per Serving: Calories: 191; Calories from Fat: 67; Total Fat: 7.51g; Saturated Fat: 4.45g; Monounsaturated Fat: 2.60g; Polyunsaturated Fat: 0.46g; Cholesterol: 50mg; Sodium: 65mg; Total Carbohydrate: 29.15g; Dietary Fiber: 1.19g; Sugars: 26.02g; Protein: 4.65g

Chocolate Bread Pudding with Dried Cherries

SERVES 8 TO 12

Traditional bread puddings are made with custards that are rich with egg yolks and cream. This version is much lighter, basing its "custard" mixture on low-fat buttermilk and mostly egg whites, while whole wheat bread adds fiber. It's easier to prepare the custard when making a larger number of servings; so make this for a dinner party, or enjoy leftovers cold or reheated the next day.

1 cup buttermilk

⅔ cup bittersweet chocolate chips

½ cup plus 2 tablespoons sugar

3 tablespoons unsweetened cocoa powder

4 large egg whites

2 large eggs

Nonstick cooking spray

4 (½-inch-thick) slices good-quality whole wheat bread, trimmed and cut into 1-inch cubes

6 tablespoons dried cherries or dried cranberries

1 cup nonfat plain Greek yogurt or Zesty Vanilla Nonfat Yogurt Sherbet (page 249), for serving (optional)

Confectioners' sugar, for dusting (optional)

In a saucepan, combine the buttermilk, chocolate chips, ½ cup of the sugar, and the cocoa powder. Heat over medium-low heat, stirring occasionally, until the chocolate and sugar have melted and the mixture is well combined. Remove from the heat.

Fill a large bowl with ice cubes and water.

In a slightly smaller bowl, using a hand mixer or wire whisk, beat together the egg whites and eggs until lightly foamy. Beating continuously, slowly sprinkle in the remaining 2 tablespoons sugar and continue beating until the mixture looks fluffy. Then, whisking continuously, very slowly pour in the chocolate mixture. Set the bowl inside the larger bowl of ice water to chill.

Preheat the oven to 350°F. Fill a pan or kettle with water and bring to a boil.

Spray the inside of a 4-by-9-inch baking dish with nonstick cooking spray. Spread half of the bread cubes in the baking dish. Scatter in the dried cherries or cranberries and then top with more bread cubes. Stir the cooled chocolate-egg mixture and spoon it evenly over the bread cubes. Leave to soak until the oven has reached the desired temperature.

Place the baking dish inside a baking pan with high sides. Pull out an oven rack and place the baking pan on the rack; carefully pour enough of the boiling water into the pan to come halfway up the side of the baking dish; and then carefully slide the rack into the oven.

Bake the bread pudding until the custard has set, about 20 minutes. Carefully remove the pan from the oven and remove the baking dish from the pan to a rack. Serve hot, lukewarm, or cooled and refrigerated, cutting into 8 to 12 portions. If you like, top each portion with a small scoop of nonfat yogurt or Zesty Vanilla Nonfat Yogurt Sherbet and dust with a little confectioners' sugar before serving.

WOLFGANG'S HEALTHY TIPS

→ If you like, substitute other dried fruit such as raisins or diced apricots or pineapple.

→ Try using white chocolate chips in place of the dark chocolate.

Nutrition Facts Per Serving (based on 8 servings): Calories: 267; Calories from Fat: 85; Total Fat: 9.45g; Saturated Fat: 5.52g; Monounsaturated Fat: 3.31g; Polyunsaturated Fat: 0.62g; Cholesterol: 48mg; Sodium: 147mg; Total Carbohydrate: 37.16g; Dietary Fiber: 4.00g; Sugars: 25.89g; Protein: 8.09g

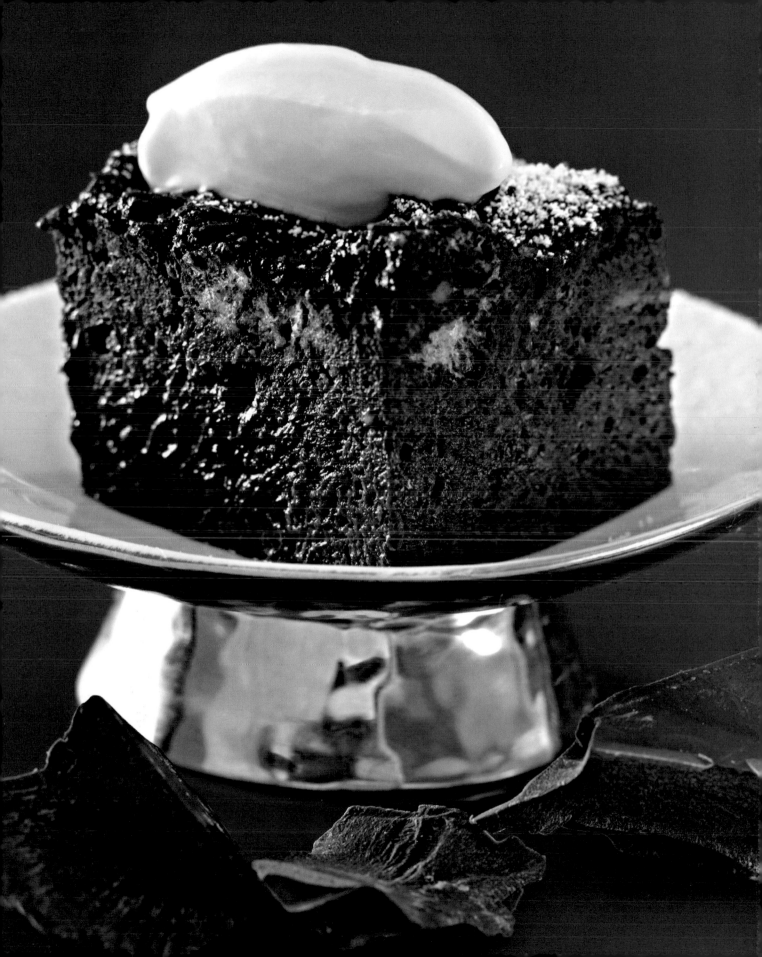

Cherry Cobbler with
Just a Little Shortcake Crust

SERVES 8

A thin topping of shortcake batter helps to produce a classic dessert far lower in fat than the original, but with great flavors and textures that don't compromise.

Shortcake Dough:

1 cup cake flour

2 tablespoons granulated sugar

1 teaspoon baking powder

¼ teaspoon kosher salt

3 tablespoons unsalted butter, chilled, cut into small chunks

5 tablespoons half-and-half

1 tablespoon unsalted butter, at room temperature

Filling:

2 pounds fresh cherries, pitted

¼ cup honey

¼ cup packed brown sugar

¼ teaspoon ground cinnamon

2 tablespoons cornstarch

1 tablespoon fresh lemon juice

1 tablespoon kirsch

To Assemble:

1 recipe Zesty Vanilla Nonfat Yogurt Sherbet (page 249) or 1 quart good-quality store-bought vanilla nonfat frozen yogurt

Confectioners' sugar, for dusting (optional)

Prepare the Shortcake Dough: In a food processor fitted with the stainless-steel blade, pulse the cake flour, granulated sugar, baking powder, and salt a few times to combine. Add the chilled butter and pulse the machine several times, until the butter is chopped up into small pieces the size of gravel. With the motor running, pour the half-and-half through the feed tube; stop processing the moment the dough barely begins to come together. Set the work bowl with the dough aside. Set aside the room temperature butter.

Preheat the oven to 375°F.

Prepare the Filling: In a medium saucepan, combine the cherries, honey, brown sugar, and cinnamon. Cook over low heat, stirring frequently, until the cherries begin to give up their juices and the mixture resembles a light compote, about 10 minutes. In a small bowl, stir together the cornstarch, lemon juice, and kirsch to form a fluid slurry. While stirring the cherries, drizzle in the slurry, and then continue cooking, stirring frequently, until the compote thickens.

Bake the Cobbler: Grease an 8-by-8-by-2-inch baking pan with the room temperature butter. Spoon the cherry filling into the buttered pan.

With a tablespoon, drop dollops of the shortcake dough evenly over the surface of the cherry mixture; use all the dough in the food processor bowl, carefully scraping off and including any dough sticking to the blade. Lightly spread the dough with the back of a spoon.

Bake until the shortcake is golden brown and the fruit is bubbly, 35 to 40 minutes. Remove from the oven and leave the cobbler to settle at room temperature for 10 minutes.

Assemble the dish: Use a large spoon to transfer portions of the cobbler to individual dessert plates or bowls. Add a scoop of Zesty Vanilla Nonfat Yogurt Sherbet or frozen yogurt on the side of each portion. If desired, spoon some confectioners' sugar into a fine-mesh sieve and tap the side over each portion to dust the cobbler. Serve immediately.

WOLFGANG'S HEALTHY TIPS

→ Look to this dessert for a good example of how a little bit of something good can go a long way. Rather than making a lighter version of a classic shortcake crust, I just halved the quantity and spread it thinner. So you still get a taste of delicious, rich crust in every bite of the cobbler.

→ Use this approach as the basis for making different cobblers with any fresh, juicy, in-season fruits you like, such as peaches, plums, nectarines, and all kinds of berries, simply substituting them for the cherries. Try mixing two or more fruit varieties, too.

Nutrition Facts Per Serving (including Zesty Vanilla Nonfat Yogurt Sherbet): Calories: 392; Calories from Fat: 60; Total Fat: 6.77g; Saturated Fat: 4.49g; Monounsaturated Fat: 1.91g; Polyunsaturated Fat: 0.38g; Cholesterol: 19mg; Sodium: 167mg; Total Carbohydrate: 73.83g; Dietary Fiber: 2.45g; Sugars: 54.75g; Protein: 7.43g

Teff Pie Dough

MAKES ENOUGH FOR 1 DOUBLE-CRUST 9-INCH PIE; 8 SERVINGS

Baker Christine Beard introduced me to this excellent dough featuring the ancient Ethiopian grain teff, which gives crusts made from the dough a deep brown color and rich, nutty flavor, along with a great combination of crispness and tenderness. Add the tantalizing hint of sweet flavor contributed by widely available Chinese five-spice powder, and you have a great crust for fresh fruit pies such as those made with the three fillings that follow.

1⅛ cups white spelt flour

¾ cup teff flour

1 tablespoon sugar

½ teaspoon Chinese five-spice powder

¾ teaspoon kosher salt

5 ounces (1¼ sticks) chilled unsalted butter, cut into ⅛-inch-thick slices

In a bowl, whisk together the spelt and teff flours, sugar, five-spice powder, and salt. Add the butter slices and toss lightly to coat them with the dry ingredients.

Turn out the mixture onto a clean, floured work surface. With a rolling pin, lightly roll the butter to flatten the slices into the flour mixture.

Using a dough scraper, gather up the mixture into a pile. Then, pound it with the rolling pin. Repeat the process three or four times, just until the mixture looks dry and flaky.

Use the scraper to scoop up and transfer the mixture back into the bowl. Add ⅓ cup water and stir with a sturdy spoon or a rubber spatula just until a loose dough forms. Turn out the dough onto the floured work surface and flatten and fold it over a few times by hand.

Form the dough into a flat disc. Wrap it in plastic wrap and refrigerate for at least 1 hour before rolling out.

WOLFGANG'S HEALTHY TIPS

→ Obviously, you still need a high enough proportion of butter to make this dough tender and flaky. But, once you've added a fruit filling such as those in the three recipes that follow, you'll achieve a surprisingly low-fat dessert.

→ Look for the spelt and teff flours in the baking section of well-stocked supermarkets and health food stores.

→ For pie à la mode, serve those made with this dough topped with a scoop of Zesty Vanilla Nonfat Yogurt Sherbet (page 249).

Nutrition Facts Per Serving: Calories: 243; Calories from Fat: 128; Total Fat: 14.33g; Monounsaturated Fat: 3.73g; Polyunsaturated Fat: 0.54g; Cholesterol: 38mg; Sodium: 30mg; Total Carbohydrate: 22.20g; Dietary Fiber: 3.75g; Sugars: 1.57g; Protein: 3.90g

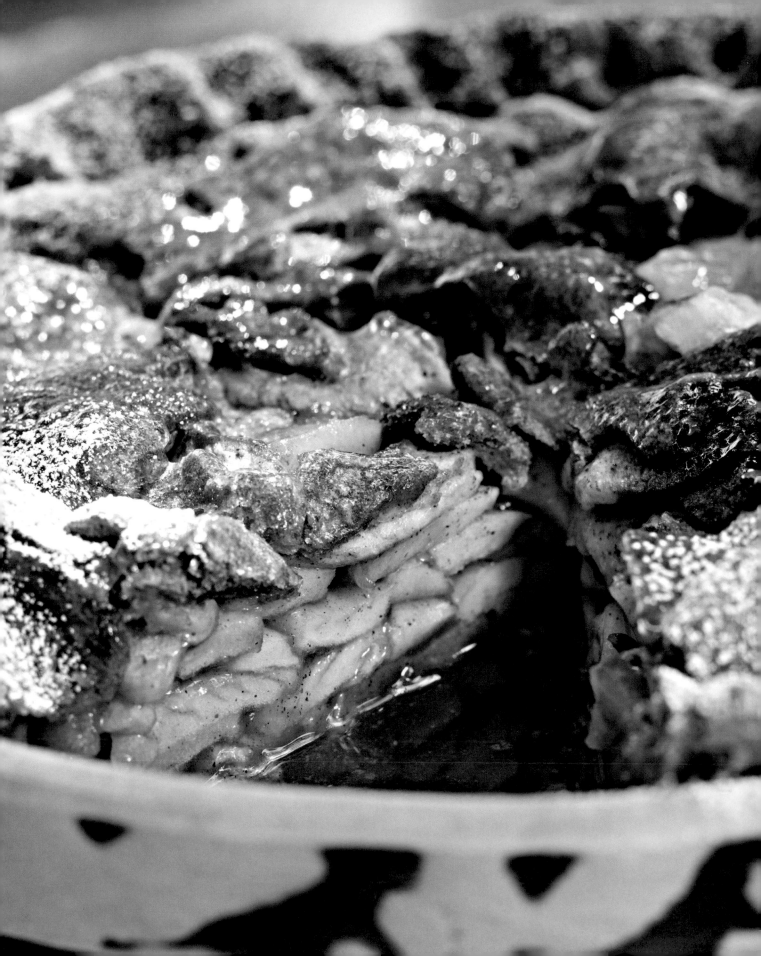

Apple Pie with Teff Pastry Crust

SERVES 8

A classic mix of sweet spices seasons this simple pie.

1 recipe Teff Pie Dough (page 259)

8 mixed medium baking apples, such as Granny Smith, Gala, and McIntosh

Zest of 1 lemon

Juice of 1 lemon

¾ cup sugar, plus more for sprinkling

1 tablespoon tapioca starch

½ teaspoon ground cinnamon

¼ teaspoon freshly grated nutmeg

¼ teaspoon kosher salt

⅛ teaspoon ground allspice

Confectioners' sugar, for dusting (optional)

Prepare the Teff Pie Dough as directed.

Divide the chilled dough in half. On a sheet of parchment paper, use a rolling pin to roll out one piece into a 12-inch circle. Loosely roll it up around the rolling pin, then unroll over a 9-inch pie plate. Gently press the dough into the plate. Roll out the remaining piece of dough, loosely roll it up around the rolling pin, and set aside.

Preheat the oven to 350°F.

Peel, halve, and core the apples. Cut into ¼-inch-thick slices. Put the slices in a bowl and toss with the lemon zest and juice.

In a separate bowl, stir together the sugar, tapioca, cinnamon, nutmeg, salt, and allspice. Sprinkle this mixture over the apples and toss thoroughly to coat.

Transfer the apples to the pie shell. Unroll the reserved rolled-out round of dough over the apples. With your fingers or the tines of a table fork, press down all around the rim to seal the top and bottom crusts together. With a small, sharp knife or kitchen scissors, trim the edge. Use the knife tip to cut a few slits in the top crust to vent steam during baking.

Lightly brush the top of the pie with a little cold water and then lightly sprinkle with sugar.

Transfer the pie to a baking sheet. Bake until the crust is nicely browned and the filling is bubbling, 40 to 50 minutes.

Set the pie on a wire rack and let cool to room temperature. If desired, spoon some confectioners' sugar into a fine-mesh sieve and tap the side over the rim all around the pie. Cut into eight wedges.

WOLFGANG'S HEALTHY TIPS

→ Feel free to add raisins, dried cranberries, or chopped nuts to the low-fat filling.

→ If you like, substitute some ripe but firm pears for some of the apples.

Nutrition Facts Per Serving (including Teff Pie Dough): Calories: 401; Calories from Fat: 130; Total Fat: 14.49g; Monounsaturated Fat: 3.75g; Polyunsaturated Fat: 0.62g; Cholesterol: 38mg; Sodium: 103mg; Total Carbohydrate: 64.10g; Dietary Fiber: 6.76g; Sugars: 36.07g; Protein: 4.53g

Blueberry Pie with Teff Pastry Crust

SERVES 8

Chinese five-spice powder, easily found in the seasonings aisle or Asian foods section of your market, contributes a very pleasant, slightly exotic flavor to the filling.

1 recipe Teff Pie Dough (page 259)

6 cups fresh blueberries, or frozen blueberries, thawed and thoroughly drained

¾ cup sugar, plus more for sprinkling

5 tablespoons tapioca starch

¼ teaspoon Chinese five-spice powder

Zest of 1 lemon

Pinch of kosher salt

1 tablespoon fresh lemon juice

Prepare the Teff Pie Dough as directed.

Divide the chilled dough in half. On a sheet of parchment paper, use a rolling pin to roll out one piece of dough into a 12-inch circle. Loosely roll it up around the rolling pin, then unroll over a 9-inch pie plate. Gently press the dough into the plate. Roll out the remaining piece of dough, loosely roll it up around the rolling pin, and set aside.

Preheat the oven to 350°F.

Put the blueberries in a bowl. In a separate bowl, stir together the sugar, tapioca, five-spice powder, lemon zest, and salt. Sprinkle this mixture over the blueberries along with the lemon juice. Toss thoroughly to coat.

Transfer the blueberry mixture to the pie shell. Unroll the reserved rolled-out round of dough over the blueberries. With your fingers or the tines of a table fork, press down all around the rim to seal the top and bottom crusts together. With a small, sharp knife or kitchen scissors, trim the edge. Use the knife tip to cut a few slits in the top crust to vent steam during baking.

Lightly brush the top of the pie with a little cold water and then lightly sprinkle with sugar.

Transfer the pie to a baking sheet. Bake until the crust is nicely browned and the filling is bubbling, 40 to 50 minutes.

Set the pie on a wire rack and let cool to room temperature before cutting into eight wedges.

WOLFGANG'S HEALTHY TIPS

→ Have fun varying the filling by substituting other berries from the farmers' market for some of the blueberries.

Nutrition Facts Per Serving (including Teff Pie Dough): Calories: 401; Calories from Fat: 131; Total Fat: 14.57g; Monounsaturated Fat: 3.78g; Polyunsaturated Fat: 0.70g; Cholesterol: 38mg; Sodium: 33mg; Total Carbohydrate: 62.90g; Dietary Fiber: 6.50g; Sugars: 31.42g; Protein: 4.74g

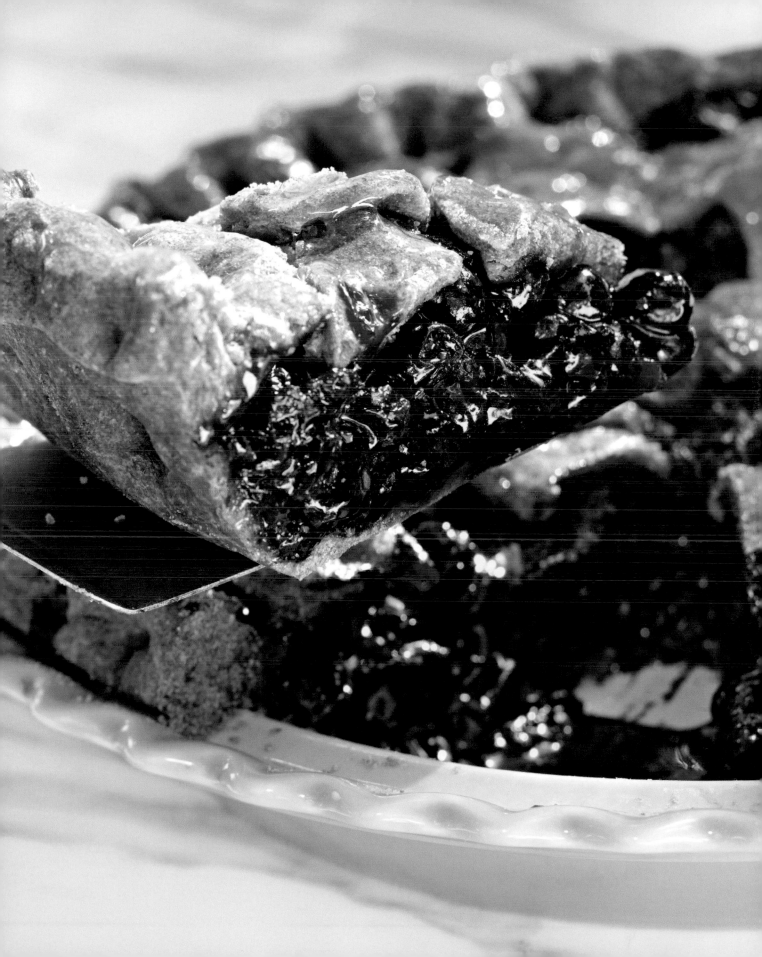

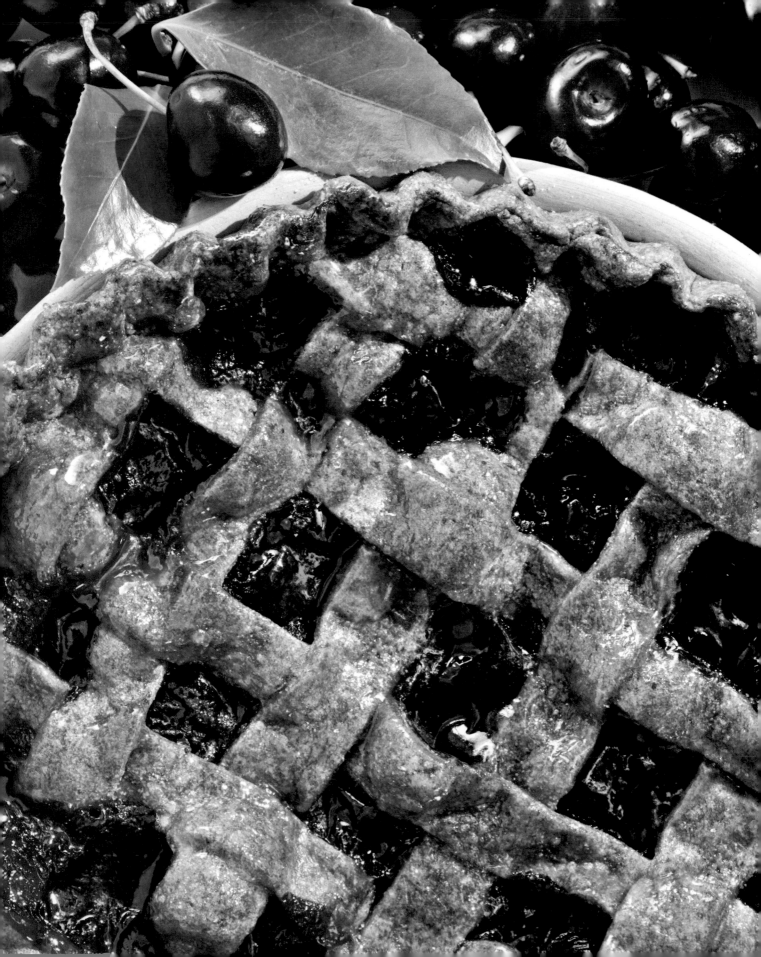

Cherry Pie with Teff Pastry Crust

SERVES 8

When fresh cherries are in season during late spring and early summer, nothing beats this easy pie. Touches of cinnamon and almond extract complement the fruit's flavor. If you like, cut the dough for the top crust into strips about ½ inch wide and weave them back and forth to make a lattice-top pie; or just make a regular top crust as directed in the instructions that follow.

1 recipe Teff Pie Dough (page 259)

6 cups pitted fresh sour "pie" cherries, or 3 (24 ounce) cans pitted Morello cherries, thoroughly drained

1½ cups sugar, plus more for sprinkling

⅓ cup tapioca starch

¼ teaspoon ground cinnamon

Pinch of kosher salt

¼ teaspoon almond extract

Prepare the Teff Pie Dough as directed.

Divide the chilled dough in half. On a sheet of parchment paper, use a rolling pin to roll out one piece of dough into a 12-inch circle. Loosely roll it up around the rolling pin, then unroll over a 9-inch pie plate. Gently press the dough into the plate. Roll out the remaining piece of dough, loosely roll it up around the rolling pin, and set aside.

Preheat the oven to 350°F.

Put the cherries in a bowl. In a separate bowl, stir together the sugar, tapioca, cinnamon, and salt. Sprinkle this mixture over the cherries along with the almond extract. Toss thoroughly to coat.

Transfer the cherry mixture to the pie shell. Unroll the reserved rolled-out round of dough over the cherries. With your fingers or the tines of a table fork, press down all around the rim to seal the top and bottom crusts together. With a small, sharp knife or kitchen scissors, trim the edge. Use the knife tip to cut a few slits in the top crust to vent steam during baking.

Lightly brush the top of the pie with a little cold water and then lightly sprinkle with sugar.

Transfer the pie to a baking sheet. Bake until the crust is nicely browned and the filling is bubbling, 40 to 50 minutes.

Set the pie on a wire rack and let cool to room temperature before cutting into eight wedges.

WOLFGANG'S HEALTHY TIPS

→ Low fat as the pie is, you can feel free to get a little extravagant if you like by sprinkling some semisweet chocolate chips among the cherries in the filling.

Nutrition Facts Per Serving (including Teff Pie Dough): Calories: 469; Calories from Fat: 131; Total Fat: 14.61g; Monounsaturated Fat: 3.83g; Polyunsaturated Fat: 0.64g; Cholesterol: 38mg; Sodium: 36mg; Total Carbohydrate: 79.91g; Dietary Fiber: 5.65g; Sugars: 48.87g; Protein: 5.07g

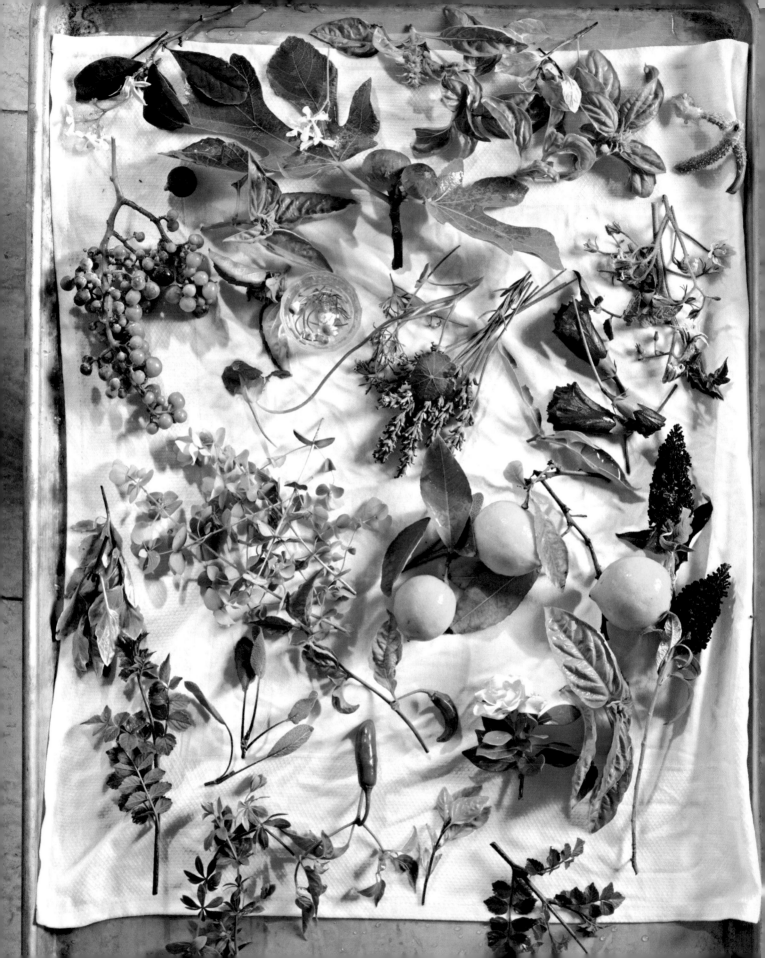

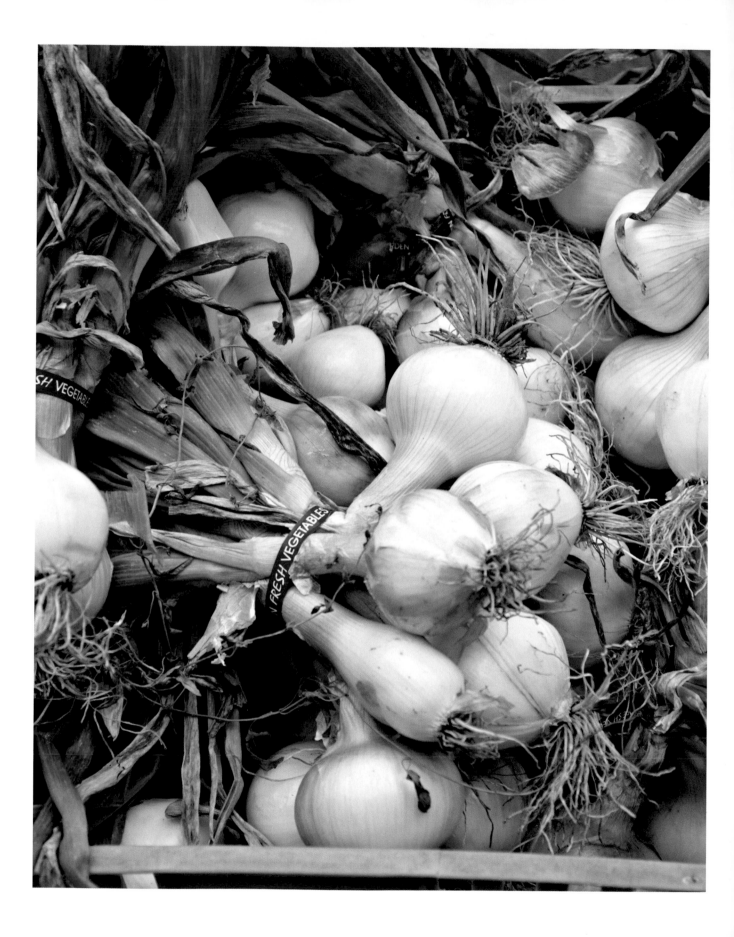

BASIC RECIPES AND TECHNIQUES

Any good cook depends on a handful of simple, go-to preparations that deliver reliable results again and again. That's what you'll find in this chapter—everything from the stocks that moisten and flavor so many savory dishes to versatile salad dressings and basic seasoning mixtures to standard ways of prepping common ingredients that maximize their flavor, texture, and appearance.

It's surprising to me how many people bypass such basics in their daily cooking. But once you try them and see what a simple yet dramatic difference they can make in enhancing the pleasure you get from the healthy meals you cook, I'm sure you'll become a convert.

Basic Recipes

MAKING STOCK

More and more serious chefs are preparing their stocks in pressure cookers, and it makes sense for home cooks to do so, too. In as little as a quarter of the time it would take to simmer a stock on the stovetop, you get rich, full-bodied, flavorful stock. And the pressure miraculously prevents the release of the albumen and other impurities that ordinarily require diligent skimming from the surface of simmering liquid to keep them from making the stock cloudy. The result is the easiest, most flavorful stock imaginable—reason alone, in my way of thinking, to buy yourself one of the convenient, automatic electric countertop pressure cookers available today.

The four easy recipes that follow should cover all your needs for stocks to moisten and flavor a wide range of soups, stews, braises, and other dishes. Make a batch or more in advance and keep it in the refrigerator or in small containers in the freezer. Of course, in a pinch, you can also use good-quality canned low-sodium, low-fat stocks or broths instead.

Pressure Cooker
Chicken Stock

MAKES ABOUT 2 QUARTS

Ask your butcher for the bones you'll need for this stock. Or save bones in a freezer bag whenever you bone chicken at home or have a leftover carcass or bones from a roast or other dish.

5 to 6 pounds chicken bones, including necks and feet, coarsely chopped

1 medium carrot, cut into large chunks

1 medium onion, quartered

1 small celery stalk, cut into large chunks

1 small leek, slit in half lengthwise and thoroughly cleaned, cut into large chunks

3 sprigs fresh flat-leaf parsley with stems

1 sprig fresh thyme

1 bay leaf

½ teaspoon whole white peppercorns

Put the chicken bones, carrot, onion, celery, leek, parsley, thyme, bay leaf, and peppercorns in the pressure cooker pot and add cold water to cover. Secure the lid.

Turn on the pressure cooker. When pressure has been reached, cook for 30 minutes. Turn off the pressure cooker and let the pressure release naturally.

Carefully strain the liquid through a fine-mesh strainer set over a clean bowl. Discard the solids. Leave the liquid to cool, then cover with plastic wrap and refrigerate for several hours.

With a large spoon, remove and discard the fat that has congealed on the surface. Store the stock in the refrigerator for up to 2 days; or seal in freezer containers and keep for up to 1 month.

Nutrition Facts Per 1 Cup: Calories: 20; Calories from Fat: 0; Total Fat: 0g; Saturated Fat: 0g; Monounsaturated Fat: 0g; Polyunsaturated Fat: 0g; Cholesterol: 0mg; Sodium: 130mg; Total Carbohydrate: 4g, Dietary Fiber: 0g, Sugars: 1g; Protein: 1g

Pressure Cooker
Beef Stock

MAKES ABOUT 2 QUARTS

Ask the butcher for the meaty bones you'll need and to cut them into chunks for you.

1 tablespoon extra-virgin olive oil

4 pounds meaty beef or veal bones, such as shanks, cut into 2-inch chunks

1 medium onion, coarsely chopped

1 medium carrot, coarsely chopped

1 celery stalk, coarsely chopped

1 leek, cleaned and coarsely chopped

1 large tomato, quartered, or ¼ cup tomato paste

1 cup dry red wine

½ teaspoon whole black peppercorns

1 bay leaf

1 sprig fresh thyme

Put the olive oil in the pressure cooker pot. Turn on the pressure cooker, uncovered. When the oil is hot, add half of the beef bones and sear until browned, turning occasionally, about 6 minutes. Transfer them to a bowl and repeat with the remaining bones; when browned, transfer them to the bowl as well. Add the onion, carrot, celery, and leek to the pressure cooker and sauté, stirring occasionally, until they begin to soften, about 5 minutes. Stir in the tomato or tomato paste and cook, stirring, 1 to 2 minutes more.

Add the red wine and stir and scrape with a wooden spoon to deglaze the pot. Return the beef bones to the pot and add the peppercorns, bay leaf, and thyme. Add enough cold water to cover all the ingredients. Secure the lid.

Turn on the pressure cooker. When pressure has been reached, cook for 1 hour. Turn off the pressure cooker and let the pressure release naturally.

Carefully strain the liquid through a fine-mesh strainer set over a clean bowl. Discard the solids. Leave the liquid to cool, then cover with plastic wrap and refrigerate for several hours.

With a large spoon, remove and discard any fat that has congealed on the surface. Store the stock in the refrigerator for up to 2 days; or seal in freezer containers and keep for up to 1 month.

Nutrition Facts Per 1 Cup: Calories: 20; Calories from Fat: 0; Total Fat: 0g; Saturated Fat: 0g; Monounsaturated Fat: 0g; Polyunsaturated Fat: 0g; Cholesterol: 0mg; Sodium: 140mg; Total Carbohydrate: 4g; Dietary Fiber: 0g; Sugars: 1g; Protein: 1g

Pressure Cooker
Fish Stock

MAKES ABOUT 1 QUART

Seafood shops, and the fish departments of well-stocked super-markets, will often keep the carcasses from fish they fillet, so the bones are available for customers who need them for stock making.

1 tablespoon extra-virgin olive oil

2 pounds fish bones, cut into pieces (use any saltwater fish except oily fish like salmon or mackerel)

1 medium carrot, cut into large chunks

1 shallot, cut into ¼-inch slices

½ medium onion, quartered

½ celery stalk, cut into large chunks

2 cups dry white wine

2 sprigs fresh flat-leaf parsley with stems

1 sprig fresh thyme

1 bay leaf

¼ teaspoon whole white peppercorns

Put the olive oil in the pressure cooker pot. Turn on the pressure cooker, uncovered. When the oil is hot, add the fish bones, carrot, shallot, onion, and celery. Sauté, stirring occasionally, for 10 minutes.

Add the white wine and stir and scrape with a wooden spoon to deglaze the pot. Add the parsley, thyme, bay leaf, and peppercorns. Add enough cold water to cover all the ingredients. Secure the lid.

Turn on the pressure cooker. When pressure has been reached, cook for 10 minutes. Turn off the pressure cooker and let the pressure release naturally.

Carefully strain the liquid through a fine-mesh strainer set over a clean bowl. Discard the solids. Leave the liquid to cool, then cover with plastic wrap and refrigerate for several hours.

With a large spoon, remove and discard any fat that has congealed on the surface. Store the stock in the refrigerator for up to 2 days; or seal in freezer containers and keep for 2 to 3 weeks.

Nutrition Facts Per 1 Cup: Calories: 17; Calories from Fat: 0; Total Fat: 0g; Saturated Fat: 0g; Monounsaturated Fat: 0g; Polyunsaturated Fat: 0g; Cholesterol: 0mg; Sodium: 20mg; Total Carbohydrate: 4g; Dietary Fiber: 0g; Sugars: 2g; Protein: 0.25g

Pressure Cooker Vegetable Stock

MAKES ABOUT 2 QUARTS

If you like, include the stems from ½ pound wild mushrooms to make an earthy-tasting mushroom stock.

1 pound yellow onions, coarsely chopped

¾ pound carrots, cut into large chunks

½ pound celery stalks, cut into large chunks

1 head garlic, cloves separated but left unpeeled, coarsely smashed

1 ounce fresh ginger, peeled and cut into ¼-inch slices

1½ teaspoons whole white peppercorns

1 bay leaf

Put the onions, carrots, celery, garlic, ginger, peppercorns, bay leaf, and 3 quarts cold water in the pressure cooker pot. Secure the lid.

Turn on the pressure cooker. When pressure has been reached, cook for 30 minutes. Turn off the pressure cooker and let the pressure release naturally.

Carefully strain the liquid through a fine-mesh strainer set over a clean bowl. Discard the solids. Leave the liquid to cool, then cover with plastic wrap and refrigerate.

Store the stock in the refrigerator for up to 2 days; or seal in freezer containers and keep for up to 1 month.

Nutrition Facts Per 1 Cup: Calories: 12; Calories from Fat: 0; Total Fat: 0g; Saturated Fat: 0g; Monounsaturated Fat: 0g; Polyunsaturated Fat: 0g; Cholesterol: 0mg; Sodium: 20mg; Total Carbohydrate: 3.07g; Dietary Fiber: 0g; Sugars: 2.04g; Protein: 0g

Dijon-Balsamic Vinaigrette

MAKES ABOUT ½ CUP; FOUR
SCANT 2-TABLESPOON SERVINGS

One of the most basic salad dressings you can make, this goes well with any combination of fresh seasonal vegetables, including my Chino Chopped Vegetable Salad (page 74).

½ tablespoon Dijon mustard

1½ tablespoons balsamic vinegar

1 tablespoon sherry vinegar

2 tablespoons extra-virgin olive oil

1 tablespoon safflower oil

Kosher salt

Freshly ground black pepper

In a bowl, whisk together the mustard, balsamic vinegar, and sherry vinegar. Whisking continuously, slowly drizzle in the oils to form a smooth emulsion. Season to taste with salt and pepper. Use immediately or cover and refrigerate for up to 1 week.

> **WOLFGANG'S HEALTHY TIPS**
> → All of the fat here comes from heart-healthy oils, and a little of this very flavorful dressing packs a big punch.

Nutrition Facts Per Serving: Calories: 96; Calories from Fat: 89; Total Fat: 9.89g; Saturated Fat: 1.22g; Monounsaturated Fat: 7.36g; Polyunsaturated Fat: 1.32g; Cholesterol: 0mg; Sodium: 22mg; Total Carbohydrate: 1.13g; Dietary Fiber: 0.06g; Sugars: 0.91g; Protein: 0.11g

Dijon-Sherry-Tarragon Vinaigrette

MAKES ABOUT ½ CUP; FOUR
SCANT 2-TABLESPOON SERVINGS

This simple salad dressing combines a lot of intriguing flavors—the woody tang of sherry vinegar, the smooth bite of Dijon mustard, the mellow sweetness of honey, the perfume of tarragon, and the fruitiness of olive oil. Try it on any salad, such as my Autumn Greens Salad (page 78).

2 tablespoons sherry vinegar

1 tablespoon Dijon mustard

1 tablespoon honey

1 teaspoon finely chopped fresh tarragon

Kosher salt

Freshly ground black pepper

2 tablespoons extra-virgin olive oil

In a small bowl, whisk together the sherry vinegar, mustard, honey, tarragon, and salt and pepper to taste. Whisking continuously, slowly pour in the olive oil to form a thick, smooth dressing. Taste and adjust the seasonings, if necessary, with more salt and pepper and even a little more mustard or vinegar. Use immediately or cover and refrigerate for up to 1 week.

> **WOLFGANG'S HEALTHY TIPS**
> → Remember that you don't need much dressing per serving, so the total fat and calories from fat it contributes to a salad will be relatively unimportant in the overall count of an entire meal or your day's eating.

Nutrition Facts Per Serving: Calories: 79; Calories from Fat: 60; Total Fat: 6.72g; Saturated Fat: 0.94g; Monounsaturated Fat: 5.02g; Polyunsaturated Fat: 0.75g; Cholesterol: 0.15mg; Sodium: 43mg; Total Carbohydrate: 4.62g; Dietary Fiber: 0.15g; Sugars: 4.34g; Protein: 0.22g

Lemon Vinaigrette

MAKES ABOUT ½ CUP; FOUR
SCANT 2-TABLESPOON SERVINGS

Use this basic, easy-to-make dressing to brighten any salad, including the Frisée and Apple Salad (page 82).

1 tablespoon grated lemon zest

2 tablespoons fresh lemon juice

2 teaspoons Dijon mustard

1 teaspoon sugar

3 tablespoons extra-virgin olive oil

Kosher salt

Freshly ground black pepper

In a small nonreactive bowl, combine the lemon zest, lemon juice, Dijon mustard, and sugar. Stir with a whisk until thoroughly blended. Whisking continuously, slowly drizzle in the olive oil to form a smooth emulsion. Season to taste with salt and pepper. Use immediately or cover and refrigerate for up to 1 week.

WOLFGANG'S HEALTHY TIPS

→ As in many salad dressings, most of the calories here come from fat, but that fat is heart-healthy olive oil. And a little of the tangy dressing goes a long way: Add it to most salads and the overall percentage of fat from calories will go way down.

Nutrition Facts Per Serving: Calories: 97; Calories from Fat: 89; Total Fat: 9.95g; Saturated Fat: 1.41g; Monounsaturated Fat: 7.45g; Polyunsaturated Fat: 1.09g; Cholesterol: 0mg; Sodium: 28mg; Total Carbohydrate: 1.95g; Dietary Fiber: 0.26g; Sugars: 1.32g; Protein: 0.16g

Orange Vinaigrette

MAKES ABOUT ½ CUP; FOUR
SCANT 2-TABLESPOON SERVINGS

The bright, tangy flavors in this
dressing really spark up combina-
tions like my Baby Beet Salad
(page 80).

½ cup fresh orange juice

1 tablespoon balsamic vinegar

¼ teaspoon minced fresh thyme leaves

½ tablespoon minced shallot

1½ tablespoons extra-virgin olive oil

Kosher salt

Freshly ground black pepper

In a small saucepan, bring the orange
juice to a boil over medium heat, then
reduce the heat to medium-low and
simmer briskly until the juice has
reduced to about 4 tablespoons. Pour
the juice into a heatproof nonreactive
bowl. Let cool to room temperature.

Whisk in the vinegar, thyme, and
shallot. Whisking continuously, slowly
drizzle in the olive oil to form a smooth
emulsion. Season to taste with salt and
pepper. Use immediately or cover and
refrigerate for up to 1 week.

WOLFGANG'S HEALTHY TIPS

→ Reducing the orange juice in the
dressing helps give the dressing a more
intense flavor and thicker consistency
with less oil.

→ Try experimenting with a mixture
of different citrus juices, though you
may have to add a touch of honey to
compensate for those of more sour
fruits like lemon or grapefruit.

Nutrition Facts Per Serving: Calories: 62;
Calories from Fat: 44; Total Fat: 4.96g;
Saturated Fat: 0.71g; Monounsaturated Fat:
3.71g; Polyunsaturated Fat: 0.55g; Cholesterol:
0mg; Sodium: 1mg; Total Carbohydrate: 4.13g;
Dietary Fiber: 0.07g; Sugars: 3.20g; Protein:
0.27g

Coconut-Lime Vinaigrette

MAKES ABOUT 1½ CUPS; TWELVE
2-TABLESPOON SERVINGS

Asian flavors bring excitement to this dressing, perfect for main-dish salads like my Thai Grilled Chicken Salad (page 89). In order to achieve the right balance and concentration of ingredients, the yield here is larger than my other dressing recipes.

4 tablespoons peanut oil
or vegetable oil

2 tablespoons coarsely
chopped garlic

1 tablespoon coarsely chopped
fresh ginger

2 (1-inch) pieces tender inner
leaves of fresh lemongrass

¼ teaspoon Thai green curry paste

¼ cup plum wine

2 tablespoons sake

½ cup canned coconut milk

3 tablespoons fresh lime juice

Kosher salt

Freshly ground black pepper

In a small saucepan, heat 2 tablespoons of the oil over medium-high heat. Add the garlic, ginger, and lemongrass and sauté, stirring continuously, until fragrant, about 2 minutes. Reduce the heat to medium, add the curry paste, and sauté until fragrant and slightly darkened in color, about 1 minute, taking care not to let it burn.

Add the plum wine and sake and stir and scrape with a wooden spoon to deglaze the pan. Stir in the coconut milk, raise the heat, and continue boiling until the liquid has reduced to a thick, creamy consistency.

Pour the reduced liquid through a fine-mesh strainer set over a bowl. With a rubber spatula, press down on the solids. Discard the solids. Let the liquid in the bowl cool to room temperature.

Transfer the cooled liquid to a blender. With the blender running on high speed, drizzle in the remaining oil to form a thick emulsion. Pulse in the lime juice and salt and pepper to taste.

This dressing can be made up to several hours in advance of serving—just refrigerate until ready to use. Remove the dressing from the refrigerator 30 minutes before serving and stir well before use. Use within 3 to 4 days.

> WOLFGANG'S HEALTHY TIPS
> → When you've made this dressing for another recipe, keep the rest on hand in the refrigerator to dress a quick salad made with shredded leftover roast or rotisserie chicken (with all skin removed), whatever salad leaves you have on hand, and small slices of any fruit you like.

Nutrition Facts Per Serving: Calories: 72; Calories from Fat: 55; Total Fat: 6.18g; Saturated Fat: 3.05g; Monounsaturated Fat: 2.17g; Polyunsaturated Fat: 1.47g; Cholesterol: 0mg; Sodium: 1mg; Total Carbohydrate: 1.99g; Dietary Fiber: 0.07g; Sugars: 0.31g; Protein: 0.33g

Low-Fat Green Goddess Dressing

MAKES ABOUT 2½ CUPS; TEN ¼-CUP SERVINGS

Named for its bright green color, and originally developed almost a century ago as a San Francisco chef's tribute to a popular play called *The Green Goddess*, this dressing traditionally gets its creamy richness from fat-rich mayonnaise and sour cream. Here, fat-free plain yogurt delivers similar results, plus extra tanginess.

1¼ cups nonfat plain Greek yogurt

½ cup packed baby spinach leaves

2 tablespoons packed chopped fresh flat leaf parsley leaves

2 tablespoons packed chopped fresh basil leaves

2 tablespoons packed chopped fresh chives

2 tablespoons packed chopped fresh chervil leaves

2 tablespoons fresh lemon juice

½ ripe Hass avocado, pitted

1 garlic clove, coarsely chopped

Kosher salt

Freshly ground white pepper

In a blender, combine the yogurt, spinach, parsley, basil, chives, chervil, and lemon juice. With a tablespoon, scoop the avocado flesh out of the skin into the blender. Add the garlic and a little salt and pepper to taste. Blend, pulsing the machine on and off and stopping as necessary to scrape down the bowl with a spatula, until a smooth dressing forms. Taste and pulse in more salt and pepper if necessary.

Transfer to a nonreactive container, cover, and refrigerate until ready to use. Serve within 3 to 4 days.

WOLFGANG'S HEALTHY TIPS

→ Use this as you would regular Green Goddess, to dress any small or large salad you like, however simple or elaborate.

→ The dressing has enough body to be served as a dip, too. Present it with vegetable crudités, with the dressing cupped inside a radicchio or iceberg lettuce leaf or a hollowed-out whole bell pepper. Or serve it with Steamed Whole Artichokes (page 37).

→ Once you've tried the original recipe, feel free to vary the herbs and their proportions. Use more chives, or even some scallion greens, for a more oniony dressing, for example. Add tarragon for its sweet perfume, or cilantro for a Latin flavor.

Nutrition Facts Per Serving: Calories: 30; Calories from Fat: 9; Total Fat: 1.01g; Saturated Fat: 0.18g; Monounsaturated Fat: 0.69g; Polyunsaturated Fat: 0.13g; Cholesterol: 0mg; Sodium: 25mg; Total Carbohydrate: 3.43g; Dietary Fiber: 0.58g; Sugars: 2.47g; Protein: 2.04g

Cilantro-Mint-Yogurt Dressing

MAKES ABOUT 2 CUPS; EIGHT 1/4-CUP SERVINGS

Virtually fat free, this dressing gets its rich body from nonfat yogurt and its lively flavor from a variety of Asian seasonings. Try it on meaty salads such as my Chinois Grilled London Broil Salad (page 95).

3 tablespoons rice wine vinegar

¼ cup coarsely chopped fresh mint leaves

¼ cup coarsely chopped fresh cilantro leaves

¼ cup coarsely chopped fresh flat-leaf parsley leaves

1 tablespoon honey

½ tablespoon minced fresh ginger

1 cup nonfat plain yogurt

Kosher salt

Freshly ground black pepper

In a blender or food processor, combine the vinegar, mint, cilantro, parsley, honey, and ginger. Blend or process until the herbs are finely chopped and a smooth paste has formed. Put the yogurt in a bowl and stir the herb-ginger mixture into the yogurt. Season to taste with salt and pepper. Use immediately or store in the refrigerator, covered, and use within 3 to 4 days.

WOLFGANG'S HEALTHY TIPS

→ This simple dressing offers excellent proof that our cravings for rich, fatty foods can be satisfied by other ingredients—in this case, nonfat yogurt—that have a similar intensity of flavor and luxurious texture, especially when lively seasonings add to the overall impact.

→ Feel free to spice up the dressing with some red pepper flakes or minced fresh chile, or season it with other herbs.

Nutrition Facts Per Serving: Calories: 28; Calories from Fat: 0; Total Fat: 0.08g; Saturated Fat: 0.04g; Monounsaturated Fat: 0.03g; Polyunsaturated Fat: 0.01g; Cholesterol: 0mg; Sodium: 26mg; Total Carbohydrate: 4.95g; Dietary Fiber: 0.23g; Sugars: 4.57g; Protein: 1.91g

Light Pesto

MAKES ABOUT ½ CUP; FOUR
2-TABLESPOON SERVINGS

Try this lighter version of the classic Mediterranean sauce as a condiment for such dishes as Grilled Cauliflower Steaks (page 191) or as a flavorful ingredient in recipes like Roasted Tomatoes Provençal (page 180).

½ cup loosely packed fresh basil leaves

2 medium garlic cloves

1 tablespoon extra-virgin olive oil

1 teaspoon grated lemon zest

Kosher salt

Freshly ground black pepper

Put all the basil, garlic, olive oil, lemon zest, and 1 tablespoon cold water in a mini food processor, mini blender, or in the blending cup of an immersion blender. Process until smooth. Pulse in salt and pepper to taste.

Nutrition Facts Per Serving: Calories: 34; Calories from Fat: 30; Total Fat: 3.35g; Saturated Fat: 0.47g; Monounsaturated Fat: 2.47g; Polyunsaturated Fat: 0.41g; Cholesterol: 0mg; Sodium: 0mg; Total Carbohydrate: 0.89g; Dietary Fiber: 0.28g; Sugars: 0.07g; Protein: 0.48g

Variation: Light Sun-Dried Tomato Pesto

To add sweet, rich tomato flavor to the pesto, substitute ¼ cup drained sun-dried tomato pieces for half of the basil.

Nutrition Facts Per Serving: Calories: 47; Calories from Fat: 37; Total Fat: 4.19g; Saturated Fat: 0.60g; Monounsaturated Fat: 3.06g; Polyunsaturated Fat: 0.52g; Cholesterol: 0mg; Sodium: 18mg; Total Carbohydrate: 2.34g; Dietary Fiber: 0.58g; Sugars: 0.05g; Protein: 0.64g

WOLFGANG'S HEALTHY TIPS

→ Traditional pesto sauce recipes containing lots of olive oil, pine nuts, and Parmesan get almost all of their calories from fat. This recipe, however, is pared down to the basic elements of pesto flavor: the basil (or basil plus sun-dried tomatoes) and garlic, with just a hint of olive oil.

Caramelized Onions

MAKES ABOUT ¾ CUP; FOUR
3-TABLESPOON SERVINGS

Sautéing onions gently until they become tender and light golden in color caramelizes their natural sugars, turning them mild and savory-sweet.

Nonstick cooking spray

½ tablespoon extra-virgin olive oil

1 large yellow, red, or white onion (about ¾ pound), cut into ¾-inch pieces

1 teaspoon balsamic vinegar

Kosher salt

Freshly ground black pepper

Heat a 10-inch nonstick skillet or sauté pan over medium heat. Spray with non-stick cooking spray and add the olive oil. Add the onion, drizzle with the vinegar and cook, stirring frequently, until lightly browned, about 15 minutes.

Season to taste with salt and pepper. Use the onions immediately, or transfer them to a nonreactive bowl or container, cool to room temperature, cover, and refrigerate. Use as needed, within 2 to 3 days.

> WOLFGANG'S HEALTHY TIPS
>
> → A few spoonfuls of this rich-tasting condiment add intense savory-sweet flavor to sandwiches such as my Turkey-Mushroom Burgers (page 160).
>
> → Try them on other dishes, too, such as any of the mashed potato recipes on pages 194–195.

Nutrition Facts Per Serving: Calories: 30; Calories from Fat: 15; Total Fat: 1.67g; Saturated Fat: 0.25g; Monounsaturated Fat: 1.24g; Polyunsaturated Fat: 0.18g; Cholesterol: 0mg; Sodium: 1mg; Total Carbohydrate: 3.73g; Dietary Fiber: 0.64g; Sugars: 1.79g; Protein: 0.42g

Onion (or Onion and Garlic) Soubise

MAKES ABOUT ¾ CUP

Soubise is a traditional French sauce in which the most distinctive flavor ingredient is caramelized onion. But it's usually based on a buttery, floury béchamel. Here, I've pared it down to the basics to get an intensely delicious puree you can use to flavor and add body to many savory dishes.

½ tablespoon extra-virgin olive oil

1 medium yellow onion, thinly sliced

2 garlic cloves, finely chopped (optional)

1 tablespoon dark brown sugar

Kosher salt

Freshly ground black pepper

2 tablespoons homemade Chicken Stock (page 271), Vegetable Stock (page 274), or good-quality canned low-sodium broth

In a medium nonstick skillet or saucepan, heat the olive oil over medium heat. Add the onion and the garlic (if using, for Onion and Garlic Soubise). Sprinkle in the sugar and add salt and pepper to taste. Cook, stirring frequently, until the onions have softened and turned a deep caramel brown, 10 to 15 minutes.

Transfer the onions to a blender or food processor and add the broth. Pulse until pureed. Transfer to a nonreactive container and refrigerate until ready to use.

WOLFGANG'S HEALTHY TIPS

→ There's little difference nutrition wise if you include garlic in the mixture. The two cloves add only about 1 calorie per tablespoon.

→ Use the vegetable broth for a vegan version.

→ If you want a more buttery effect for a particular recipe, and are not vegan, by all means use unsalted butter instead of the oil. It will actually drop the calories by about 1 per serving (because of butter's water content) and add 1mg of cholesterol.

Nutrition Facts Per 1 Tablespoon (for Onion Soubise): Calories: 14; Calories from Fat: 5; Total Fat: 0.56g; Saturated Fat: 0.08g; Monounsaturated Fat: 0.43g; Polyunsaturated Fat: 0.07g; Cholesterol: 0mg; Sodium: 6mg; Total Carbohydrate: 2.47g; Dietary Fiber: 0.22g; Sugars: 1.66g; Protein: 0.20g

Roasted Garlic

MAKES ABOUT ¼ CUP

Roasting whole heads of garlic caramelizes the natural sugars in the individual cloves, making them sweet, mellow, and soft as butter. A little of the garlic can add a big flavor punch to all kinds of dishes.

4 whole heads garlic

⅓ cup extra-virgin olive oil

Preheat the oven to 375°F.

Arrange the garlic heads in a small roasting pan and drizzle with the olive oil, turning them to coat them well.

Roast until the garlic is very tender when gently squeezed with a hand protected with an oven glove, 45 minutes to 1 hour. Set aside at room temperature until cool enough to handle.

When the garlic is cool, cut the heads crosswise in half with a serrated knife. Remove the softened garlic pulp, either by squeezing each half or by scooping out the garlic with a tiny teaspoon or the tip of a knife.

Transfer the garlic to a container, cover, and refrigerate. Use as needed within 3 or 4 days.

WOLFGANG'S HEALTHY TIPS

→ Much of the small amount of oil in this recipe is absorbed by the papery garlic skins and is left behind when you squeeze out the garlic cloves.

→ Use this as a flavoring in recipes. Or serve a whole roasted head of garlic per person, first cutting it in half with a serrated knife, to be squeezed from the skins and spread on warm, crusty whole-grain bread.

Nutrition Facts Per 1 Tablespoon: Calories: 96; Calories from Fat: 30; Total Fat: 3.44g; Saturated Fat: 0.51g; Monounsaturated Fat: 2.47g; Polyunsaturated Fat: 0.47g; Cholesterol: 0mg; Sodium: 7mg; Total Carbohydrate: 14.88g; Dietary Fiber: 0.94g; Sugars: 0.45g; Protein: 2.86g

Curry Powder

MAKES ABOUT 1⅓ CUPS

For wonderful aromatic flavor in Indian dishes like Curried Lentil Soup with Mint-Lemon Yogurt (page 67) or Northern Indian Chicken Curry (page 155), nothing beats the flavor of your own homemade spice blend.

¼ cup whole coriander seeds

2 tablespoons whole green cardamom seeds

2 tablespoons whole cumin seeds

2 tablespoons whole yellow mustard seeds

1 tablespoon plus 1 teaspoon whole fenugreek seeds

2 teaspoons whole cloves

1 teaspoon whole black peppercorns

1 cinnamon stick, broken into several pieces

¼ cup ground turmeric

2 tablespoons ground ginger

½ tablespoon ground cayenne

One by one, in a small, dry skillet over medium heat, toast each of the whole spices—the coriander, cardamom, cumin, mustard, fenugreek, cloves, peppercorns, and cinnamon stick—stirring with a wooden spoon just until they are fragrant and darken slightly in color, about 5 minutes each. (Note that the seeds, when ready, will make popping noises.) Transfer all the spices to a bowl to cool.

In a spice mill or grinder, working in batches as necessary, grind the spices to a fine powder. Pass the ground spices through a fine-mesh sieve set over a bowl and press with a rubber spatula. Discard any chaff in the sieve.

Add the ground turmeric, ginger, and cayenne. Stir well.

Store the spice blend in an airtight container at cool room temperature or in a resealable plastic freezer bag in the freezer.

WOLFGANG'S HEALTHY TIPS

→ Robust seasonings like curry powder have the power to make low-fat foods extra satisfying. To preserve the strength of the seasonings, be sure to store them airtight and at cool temperatures. Just as important, never prepare—or buy—more of a seasoning than you'll use within a few months, as its flavor diminishes over time.

→ "Curry powder" is a Western term that covers a wide variety of different Indian seasoning blends. Once you've tried this version, experiment with your own mixtures, changing the proportions to emphasize the flavors you prefer.

→ For centuries, the golden-colored turmeric in curry powder has been believed to hold health benefits in traditional Indian Ayurvedic medicine. Now, Western medical studies are finding that curcumin, a chemical compound in turmeric, may reduce inflammation and possibly help prevent arthritis, memory loss, and some cancers.

Nutrition Facts Per 1 Tablespoon: Calories: 19; Calories from Fat: 5; Total Fat: 0.63g; Saturated Fat: 0.11g; Monounsaturated Fat: 0.36g; Polyunsaturated Fat: 0.15g; Cholesterol: 0mg; Sodium: 2mg; Total Carbohydrate: 3.38g; Dietary Fiber: 1.48g; Sugars: 0.13g; Protein: 0.77g

Tandoori Seasonings

MAKES ABOUT 5 TABLESPOONS

Based on homemade Curry Powder (page 285) or a good-quality store-bought brand, this seasoning blend can provide the authentic flavor of traditional Indian-style clay oven–grilled food to a wide range of dishes such as my Tandoori-Style Chicken Kabobs (page 156).

3 tablespoons Curry Powder (page 285) or good-quality store-bought curry powder

1 teaspoon Kashmiri chile powder or hot paprika

1 teaspoon ground turmeric

1 teaspoon ground coriander

1 teaspoon ground cumin

1 teaspoon sweet paprika

½ teaspoon freshly grated nutmeg

½ teaspoon ground ginger

¼ teaspoon ground cardamom

Put all the ingredients in a bowl and stir together. Store in an airtight container.

Nutrition Facts Per 1 Teaspoon: Calories: 6; Calories from Fat: 2; Total Fat: 0.25g; Saturated Fat: 0.06g; Monounsaturated Fat: 0.12g; Polyunsaturated Fat: 0.07g; Cholesterol: 0mg; Sodium: 0mg; Total Carbohydrate: 1.22g; Dietary Fiber: 0.65g; Sugars: 0.10g; Protein: 0.27g

Whole Wheat Yeast Dough

MAKES ONE 10-INCH ROUND FOCACCIA,
TWO 9-INCH LOAVES, OR FOUR 8-INCH PIZZAS

Use this flavorful, fiber-rich dough to make the pizzas on pages 119–121 and the focaccias and breads on pages 207–210.

Sponge:

1 tablespoon active dry yeast

1½ cups lukewarm (80°F) water

1 tablespoon honey

1 cup all-purpose flour

1 cup whole wheat flour

Dough:

¾ cup all-purpose flour

¾ cup whole wheat flour

1½ tablespoons kosher salt

5 tablespoons extra-virgin olive oil

Prepare the Sponge: In the bowl of a stand mixer fitted with the whisk attachment, stir together the yeast, water, and honey until the yeast has dissolved. Stir in the all-purpose and whole wheat flours just until a soft, loose dough forms. Cover with a clean towel and set aside at warm room temperature for 20 minutes.

Prepare the Dough: Add the all-purpose and whole wheat flours, the salt, and the olive oil to the sponge. Fit the stand mixer with the dough hook and attach the bowl with the dough. Mix on the second-lowest speed for 1 minute. Stop and scrape down the sides of the bowl with a rubber spatula. Continue mixing on medium speed until the dough looks well developed and elastic, 8 to 10 minutes more.

Remove the bowl from the mixer, cover with a damp kitchen towel, and set aside to rest for 10 minutes before proceeding with the recipe in which you will use the dough.

For pizzas: Divide the dough into 4 equal balls. On a floured work surface, work each ball with clean hands by pulling down all around its sides and tucking under the bottom of the ball, repeating this 4 or 5 times to form an even, compact ball. Then, on a smooth, unfloured surface, roll the ball under your palm until its top feels firm and smooth, about 1 minute. Cover the balls with a damp towel and leave to rest for 15 to 20 minutes. (At this point, if you like, you can wrap the balls in plastic wrap and refrigerate for up to 2 days. Remove from the refrigerator and let the dough come to room temperature before continuing.)

Techniques

Blanching

Blanching refers to precooking vegetables briefly in boiling water and then draining and instantly plunging them into ice water to chill them down and stop the cooking process, a step that sets the vegetables' hues at their most vivid. Once blanched, a vegetable can be cooked further however you like, without diminishing how beautiful it looks. Since they've already been cooked to an al dente, tender-crisp stage, blanched vegetables can also be served as part of a crudités selection.

If a recipe calls for blanching more than one vegetable, blanch them one variety of vegetable at a time.

To blanch vegetables, bring a saucepan of water to a boil, adding some salt if you like. Fill a mixing bowl with ice cubes and water and set it nearby.

Cut up or otherwise prepare the vegetables as directed in the recipe. If you'll be blanching more than one vegetable, put the first batch in a wire-mesh strainer and lower the vegetables into the boiling water. As soon as they turn bright in color, after about 1 minute, remove them (leaving the water boiling) and immerse them in the ice water. Drain well and continue with the recipe as directed.

Repeat with any remaining vegetables.

Peeling and Seeding Tomatoes

Many recipes that involve cooking fresh tomatoes call for first removing their indigestible skins and watery seed sacs. The process is simple.

Select a saucepan large enough to hold the tomatoes comfortably. Fill it with water and bring to a boil over high heat. Fill a large bowl with ice cubes and water and set it nearby.

With a small, sharp knife, cut out the cores of the tomatoes and, on the opposite end of each one, score a shallow X in its skin. When the water is boiling, use a slotted spoon or wire skimmer to lower the tomatoes into the water. When their skins begin to wrinkle, after about 10 seconds, lift them out with a slotted spoon or skimmer and transfer them to the ice water to cool.

As soon as the tomatoes are cool enough to handle, use your fingertips and, if necessary, a knife, to peel them, starting at the X.

Cut each peeled tomato crosswise in half and, with your fingertip or the handle of a small spoon, scoop out and discard their seed sacs.

Continue preparing the tomatoes as directed in the recipe.

Roasting, Peeling, and Seeding Peppers

When roasted, all kinds of peppers—whether mild bell peppers or spicy chiles—develop a tender, juicy texture and a fuller, more complex flavor. The act of roasting also blisters the skins of peppers, making them easy to peel.

To roast peppers, preheat a broiler or grill. Place the peppers a few inches from the heat and cook, checking diligently, until the skin on the side facing the heat blisters and blackens, several minutes. Using tongs, turn the peppers, continuing the process until they are blistered and blackened all over.

Transfer the roasted peppers to a tray and cover with a damp kitchen towel; or put them in a food-grade paper bag and loosely close the bag. Set aside until cool enough to handle.

When cool, with your fingers, peel the skins from the peppers. (If working with hot chiles, you may want to wear kitchen gloves to avoid contact with their spicy oils; or, if using your bare hands, be sure to wash your hands thoroughly with warm, soapy water after you've finished, and avoid touching any sensitive areas.) Then, with your fingers or a knife and working over a bowl to catch the flavorful juices, split open the peppers. Pull out and discard the stems and the veins, and use a spoon to scrape out any remaining seeds.

Use the peppers as directed in the recipe. Or cover the bowl with plastic wrap and refrigerate for up to 2 days.

Segmenting Citrus Fruit

Citrus segments are individual wedges of peeled fruit minus the membranes that separate them, making for attractive, pleasurable-to-eat ingredients and garnishes for sweet and savory dishes alike.

To prepare segments, first use a small, sharp knife (a serrated one may help you) to cut off the peel of the fruit thickly enough to remove not only the white pith but also the outer membrane of the segments underneath, exposing the fruit itself.

Then, holding the peeled fruit over a bowl to catch the juices and the individual segments, carefully cut down along either side of a wedge-shaped segment between the fruit pulp and the membrane, freeing the segment from the membrane, letting the segment fall into the bowl below. Continue with each segment until all have been cut free from their membranes. Squeeze the membranes over the bowl to release any remaining juice.

Use the segments as directed in a particular recipe, reserving the juice for drinking or another use if not called for in the recipe.

Toasting Nuts

Nuts of any kind gain a richer flavor, crunchier texture, and more attractive golden color when you toast them.

To toast nuts, put them in a small, heavy, ungreased skillet just large enough to hold them in a single layer. Over low heat, cook the nuts, stirring almost continuously to prevent scorching. When the nuts are fragrant and a shade or two lighter than the shade you desire, remove them from the heat and transfer to a heatproof bowl; their residual heat will continue to cook and darken them slightly as they cool.

Total toasting time may range from 2 minutes to several minutes, depending on the size of the nuts.

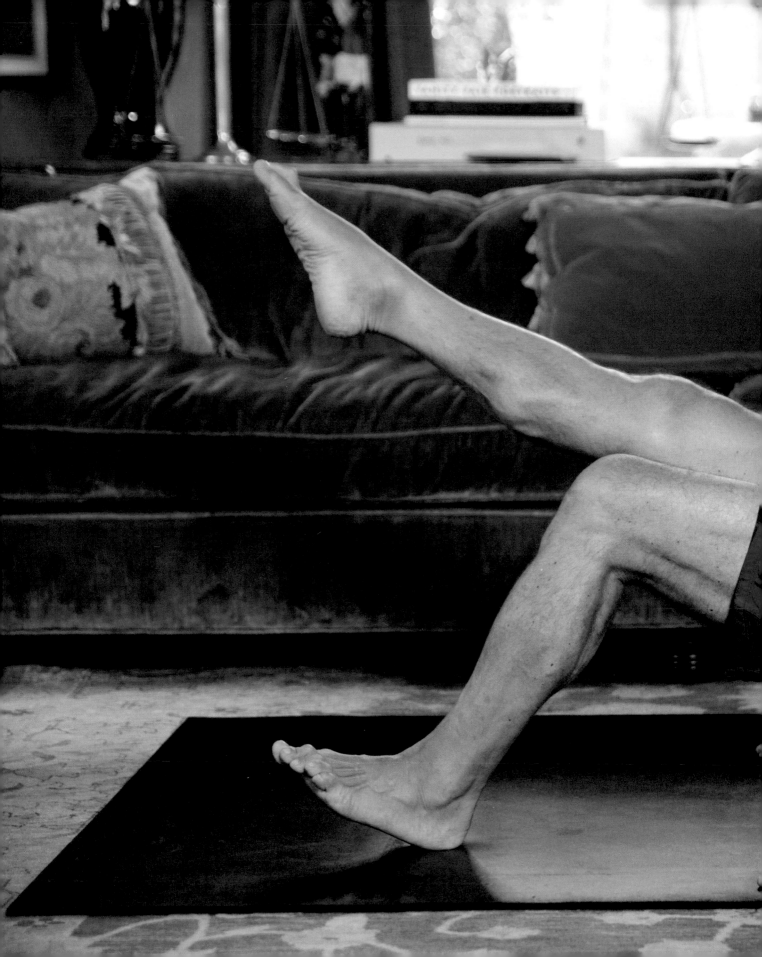

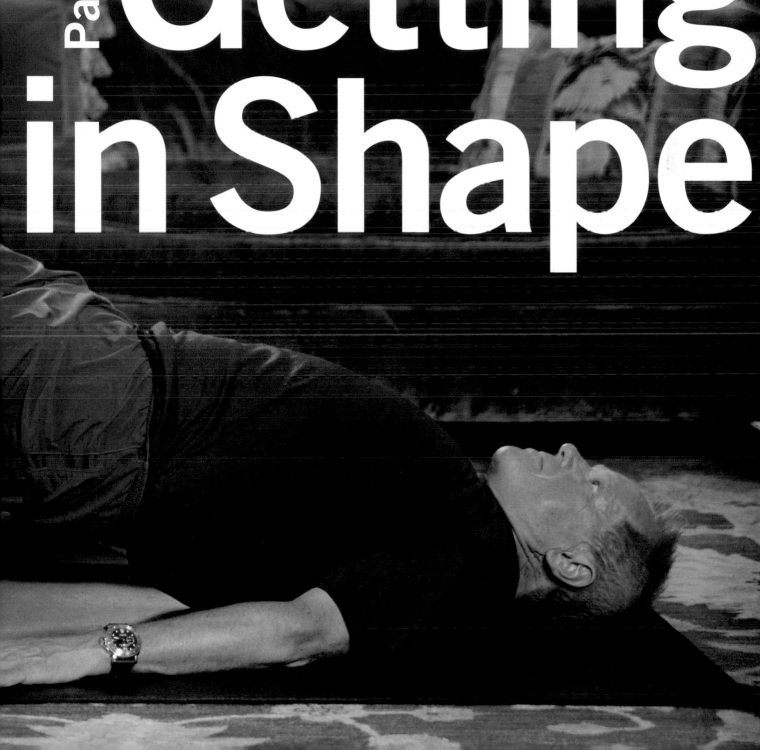

Part 3: Getting in Shape

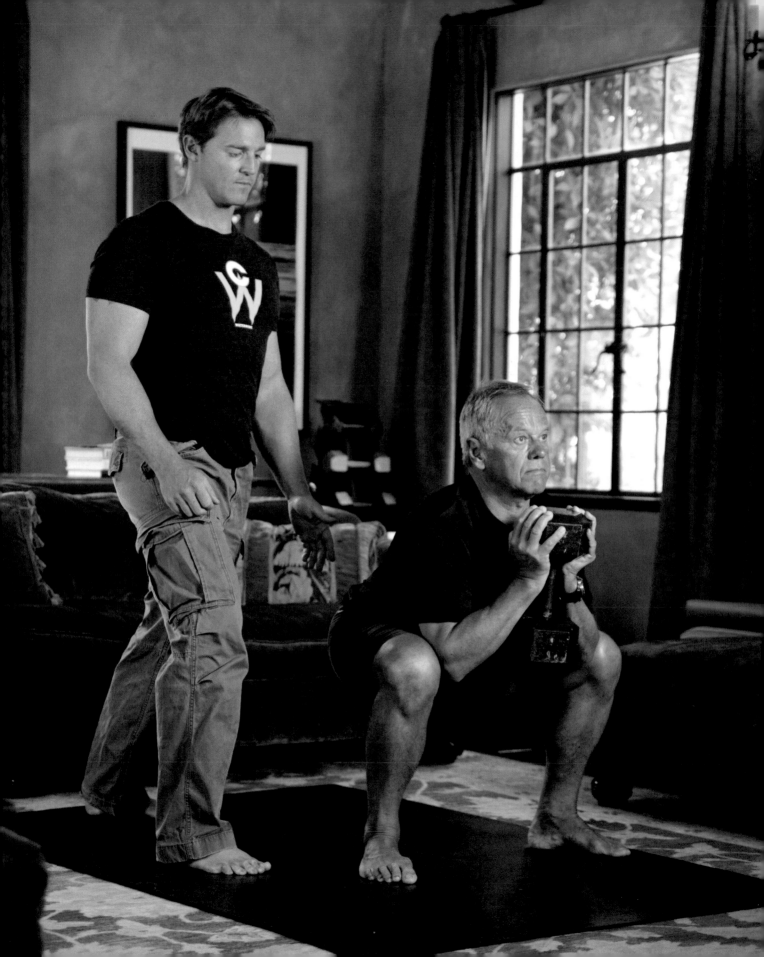

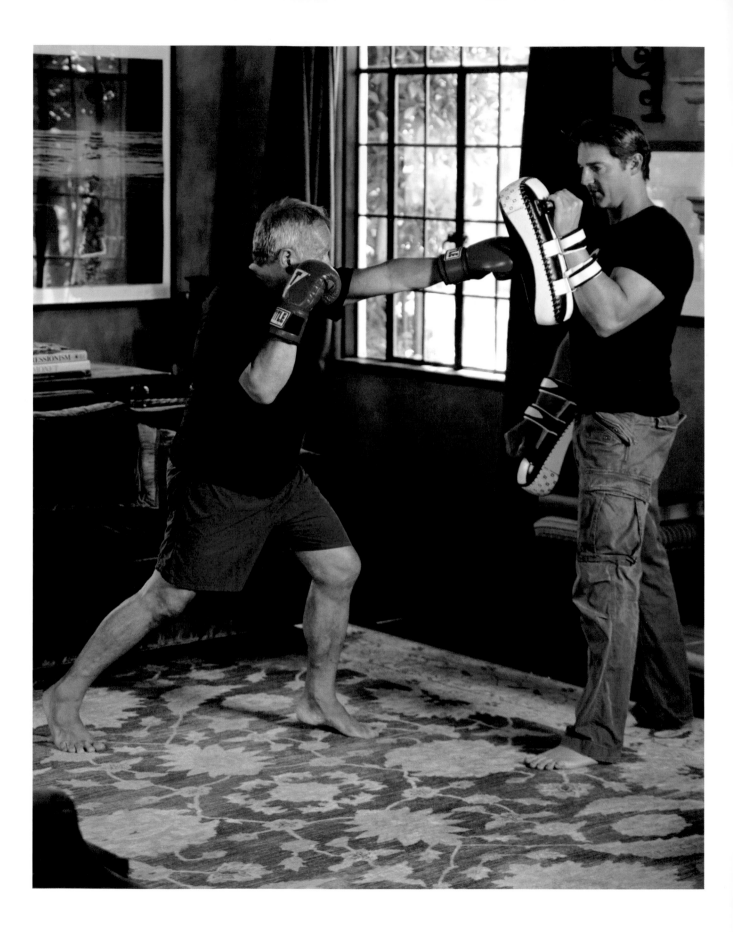

MY FITNESS PROGRAM

I started working with Chad, my trainer, when I was fifty-nine. I'd had a hip replacement after being in constant pain for several years, and I was still recovering from the surgery and wondering if I'd ever fully regain my flexibility or stamina. Unable to exercise as I might like, and working in a career in which I was constantly surrounded by food, my weight also concerned me. If I couldn't deal with these challenges, I was afraid I might have to give up skiing, my favorite sport.

Chad reassured me that we could address my concerns through a focused training program. He told me it wouldn't produce overnight results, and that I'd have to work hard. But he was confident that I could get into the best shape of my life. It sounded too good to be true.

It took only one workout for me to see it wasn't just talk.

Before working with Chad I had tried just about everything—gyms, workout machines, personal trainers. Most of the time I felt worse instead of better. But Chad's program was different. We started with a routine I could do, at an intensity level I could handle, instead of a routine Chad thought I should be able to do. That was a new experience for me.

We did our first workout in my living room. I had to start slow. I couldn't lift heavy dumbbells or do a lot of repetitions. I did only what I could. I gradually increased everything—repetitions, weight, the difficulty of the exercises Chad had me do. But by starting slow, I could see how quickly I made progress. Once my body got used to it, all of a sudden, better fitness felt possible. I kept on improving. After seven months I realized I could ski better at the age of sixty than I could at forty. Today the workouts I do with Chad are much more intense, but we still exercise in my living room, using hardly any equipment.

These workouts are different from any I'd seen or even heard about. But they aren't different just to be different. Chad has a reason for every single movement in his program, and he makes sure each one builds on the movement that comes before it while preparing your body for the next one. More than that, he can explain how it works in simple language. (He can also explain it in technical language—but believe me, you don't want to have that conversation!)

Now I'll turn this chapter and the next two over to Chad. He'll introduce you to his program and exercises and describe the minimal equipment you'll need. He'll explain how to adjust the program to fit your current level, how to make it more challenging as you increase your strength and develop better overall fitness, and finally how to take it on the road with a simple three-exercise workout you can do in a hotel room.

PROGRAM BASICS
BY CHAD WATERBURY

My passion is for human movement. I studied neurophysiology in graduate school, and no matter the age or circumstances of my client—whether it's a hardworking businessman like Wolfgang, a professional athlete, or anyone in between—my first goal is always to help them move better. To move better, you have to activate the right muscles in the right sequence. That's how I started with Wolfgang when we first trained together in 2009, using a program much like the one I'm about to show you. As you'll see, the workout has three distinct parts:

1. WARM-UP AND CORE ACTIVATION

You'll start each workout by rolling your bare feet over a golf ball. (If you don't have one, you can use a baseball. If that hurts your feet, you can start with a tennis ball.) The bottom of each foot has something like 150,000 nerve endings, and when you stimulate those, it helps wake up your entire nervous system. It also loosens the fascia, a section of strong connective tissue that's easily irritated. The older you are, and the more time you spend on your feet, the greater the risk that overly stiff fascia will lead to foot, knee, or hip pain. A third benefit: Rolling your feet over a ball sends a signal up through your calves, hamstrings, and back to improve flexibility. It sounds impossible, but you can test it yourself: Before you roll your feet over the ball, bend over from the hips and reach for the floor. (Don't push it; just bend as far as you can without discomfort.) After you roll, try it again. You'll see that unlocking the connective tissues in your feet gives those other muscles permission to move farther without risk of injury.

Now that we've turned up the volume on your nervous system, our next goal is to activate your core. These are the muscles of your abdomen, lower back, and hips—the ones that maintain your posture and protect your lower back. I include two core exercises here: the Side Plank and Hip Thrust. (All the exercises are fully described and illustrated in the next chapter.) Together they help keep your back and pelvis in a safe, stable position during the next part of the program.

> ## A BEGINNER'S GUIDE
> ## TO EXERCISE TERMINOLOGY
>
> **REP:** Short for "repetition," it means a single performance of an exercise. One Push-up is one rep.
>
> **SET:** A series of repetitions. If the chart says to do ten reps of an exercise, it means to do that exercise ten times, and then move on to the next one. If the exercise involves one arm or leg at a time, you'll do all the reps with each arm or leg without resting in between. When the chart specifies "alternating," that means you go right-left-right-left until you finish. If it doesn't, you do all the reps on one side, then switch to the other. In that case, you probably want to start with your weaker side and finish with the side that's stronger.
>
> **CIRCUIT:** A series of exercises you do consecutively, completing a set of each before you repeat the series.

2. STRENGTH

Our next goal is to help you get stronger. Most of us think of cardiovascular fitness as the key to a long, healthy life. That's true, but research shows that strength is also crucial. Not only do the strongest people live longer than people with less strength, they tend to have fewer disabilities as they get older. But a good strength-training program isn't just insurance against future problems. A stronger body will help you feel better *now*. As Wolfgang has told me many times, his increased strength improves his life in many ways. It's easier to work long hours on his feet. He has more stamina for his favorite sports, and even simple, everyday things like walking up stairs are now easier.

The total-body workout has an unusual structure. Instead of doing it the same old way—a few sets of this, a few sets of that, a few sets of something else—you'll do all six exercises sequentially, as a circuit, with a short amount of rest after each one. Then you'll repeat the circuit several times. Each time, you'll do one less repetition of each exercise. So if you start the first circuit with ten reps per exercise, you'll do nine per exercise for the second circuit, then eight, and so on.

A few reasons to do it this way:

→ A total-body workout is more demanding than a program that has you work individual muscles on different days (upper-body muscles one day, lower body the next, for example). You'll burn more calories each workout.

→ A total-body workout is more efficient. If you're pressed for time, it's better to work everything in a single workout three times a week than try to squeeze in four, five, or six workouts.

→ The circuit keeps your heart rate elevated. But because you alternate upper- and lower-body exercises, your muscles have time to recover between sets, which helps improve your performance.

→ You'll do the most work when your body is fresh. As you get fatigued, you'll do fewer repetitions per set of each exercise.

You'll start with just your body weight on two or three of the exercises. For the others, you'll need a set of adjustable dumbbells, or a range of fixed-weight dumbbells (see the next page). The goal is to get stronger from workout to workout and week to week, and you want to make sure your equipment allows you to do that.

The system gives you multiple ways to improve (which are explained in greater detail in Chapter 13):

→ You can do more repetitions on the first set—eleven instead of ten—and then work your way down.

→ You can do the same repetitions, but with heavier weights or more advanced versions of the Push-up. When you can't increase the difficulty of the exercise, you can still make it more challenging by adding a pause in the bottom position.

→ You can decrease the amount of rest between sets.

3. RECOVERY

While it's not a good idea to stretch at the beginning of a workout, it's a great idea to work on your flexibility at the end. Your body will be warm, and you'll probably feel better if you release some of the tension from your muscles by stretching them.

Rather than show you a bunch of stretches for individual muscles, some of which you probably know already, in the next chapter we'll show you a single flexibility exercise that improves the mobility of everything from your upper back to your thighs.

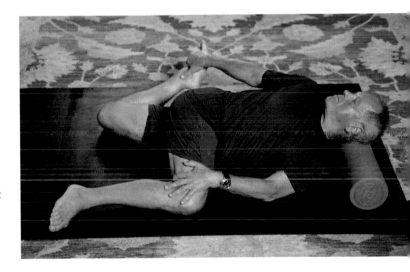

EQUIPMENT

The workouts are set up to make them easy to perform at home or in a gym. If you work out at home, you won't need traditional weightlifting equipment like a barbell and bench. But you will need access to a range of dumbbells, including weights that are heavier than you can use now, to accommodate your increasing strength.

DUMBBELLS

If you belong to a health club, this won't be a problem. Even bare-bones gyms typically have dumbbells that go from 5 to 50 pounds. Very few readers will need more than that, especially at the beginning. But if you work out at home, you'll need to get a range that works for you.

The easiest solution is an adjustable dumbbell set, which takes up the space of a single large pair. There are several different styles. Expect to pay at least $100 for two adjustable dumbbells that go from 5 to 25 pounds, and at least $200 for a set that goes up to 50 pounds per dumbbell. (If you shop online, search for a seller that offers free shipping.)

Alternatively, you may want to get individual pairs of dumbbells. The challenge is to accumulate enough of them to cover all your needs. For example, most readers will need at least twice as much weight for the Dumbbell Row, which uses the big muscles of your upper back along with the biceps, than they will for the Shoulder Press, which uses relatively small muscles.

GOLF BALL

If you don't have one sitting around your home, buy the cheapest you can find. Name brands offer no added benefit; your foot doesn't know the difference. You can also use a baseball to work out the tension in your feet—or if you prefer something softer, a tennis ball.

MAT OR PADDED SURFACE

You'll want to cushion your elbows and forearms when you do the Side Plank. You may also want to use it to protect your knees for one of the Push-up variations.

BOX, BENCH, STOOL, OR CHAIR (OPTIONAL)

Choose one that will support your weight. This comes in handy for Push-ups. Stronger readers can set their toes on the box to make the exercise more difficult, while those with less upper-body strength can rest their hands on it to make them easier.

KETTLEBELLS (OPTIONAL)

A kettlebell is an iron ball with a handle and a flat bottom. It's fun to use for the Swing in the strength circuit. You can pick them up anywhere these days, either online or in any sporting goods store. Even the big discount chains carry them. As with dumbbells, you don't want to limit yourself to just one size because you'll quickly outgrow it. Women probably want at least a 15-pound kettlebell to start, while men will want one that's at least 30 pounds.

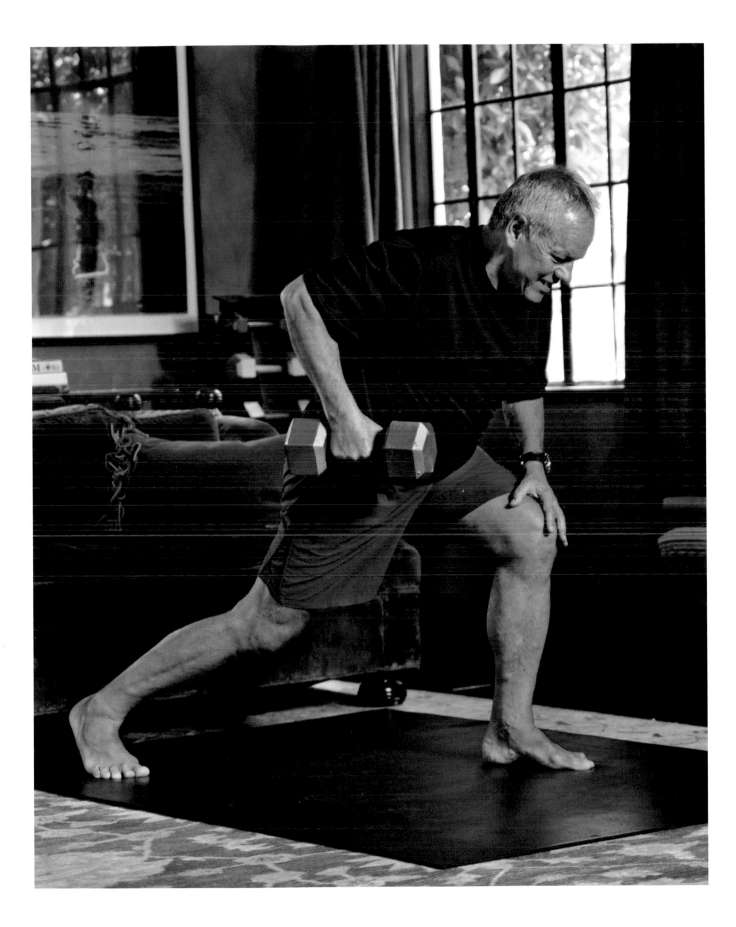

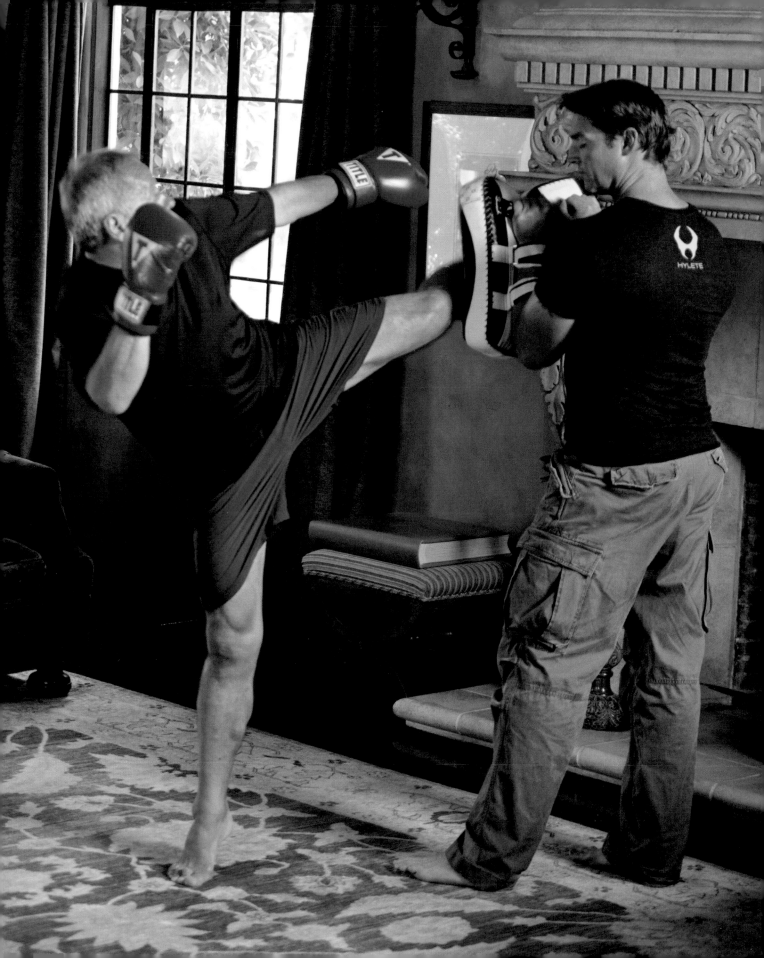

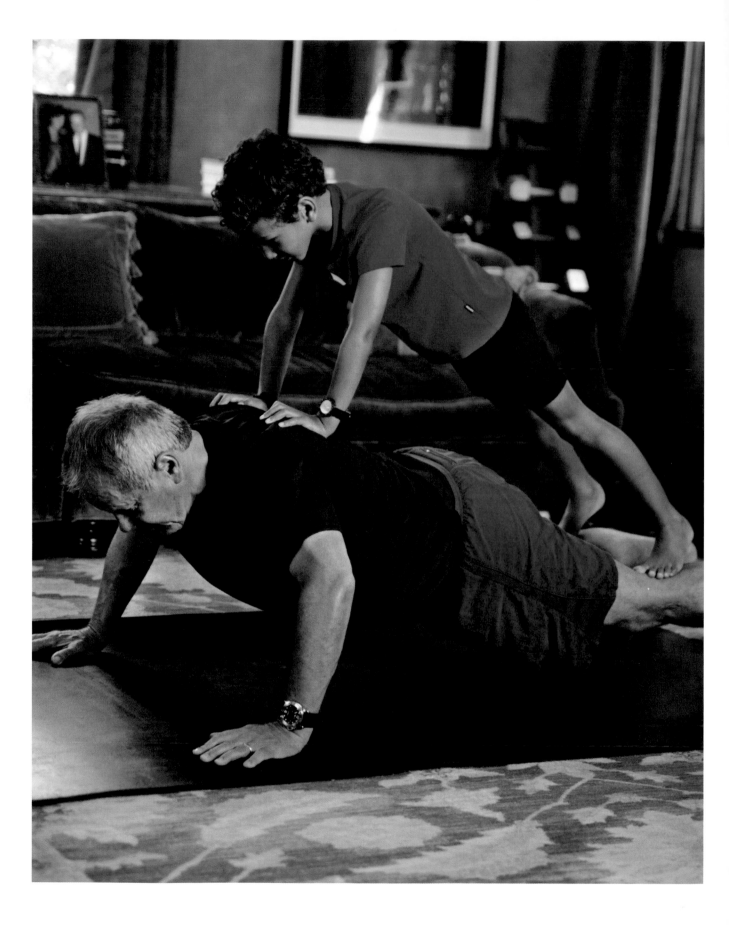

THE EXERCISES

Just as Wolfgang has done, you'll get the best results with my total-body program when you do the workout three times a week—Monday, Wednesday, and Friday, for example, or Tuesday, Thursday, and Saturday—with at least one full day in between to allow your muscles time to recover and adapt to the program by getting bigger and stronger. If that's too much, or if your schedule includes another type of exercise you prefer to do more frequently, you can use the total-body program twice a week.

On the days in between, you can do any type of exercise you like, as long as it doesn't work the same muscles in the same way. So you want to avoid heavy lifting, but everything else is open to you: walking or running, yoga or Pilates, spinning or martial arts classes, tennis or golf or any other sport.

We'll start this chapter with the basic workout and exercises, and then look at some of the many ways you can modify the system as you get stronger and need new challenges. Finally, we offer a simple workout you can do anytime, anywhere, without any equipment at all.

WARM-UP AND CORE ACTIVATION

Exercise	How to do it	Rest
Golf Ball Foot Roll	Roll each foot 45 to 60 seconds	No rest
Side Plank*	Hold 20 to 60 seconds per side	10 seconds
Single-Leg Glute Bridge*	5 reps per side	10 seconds

* If you have experience with the exercises, you can do a second set of the Side Planks and Glute Bridges.

Golf Ball Foot Roll

Stand with bare feet, or at most wearing socks. Set the golf ball on the floor. Roll one foot over the ball, focusing on any part of your foot that feels especially sensitive. You can lessen the pressure by sitting down, or by resting your heel on the floor while working the ball around. If that's still too intense, you can also use a tennis ball instead of a golf ball. Shoot for 45 seconds per foot, less if there's no discomfort at all, more if you have problem areas that require extra time.

Side Plank

1. Lie on your left side with your weight resting on your left elbow (you may want to put a pad or towel beneath the elbow) and the outside edge of your left foot.

2. Set your right foot on top of your left foot. Rest your right hand on your right hip.

3. Now lift your hips and set your body in a straight line from your nose to your navel. Make sure your hips are pushed forward and your right shoulder is directly over your left. You should feel your oblique muscles on the left side of your abdomen working to hold your body straight.

4. Hold that position for 20 seconds, then switch sides and repeat. In subsequent workouts try to increase the time you can hold this position, up to 60 seconds per side.

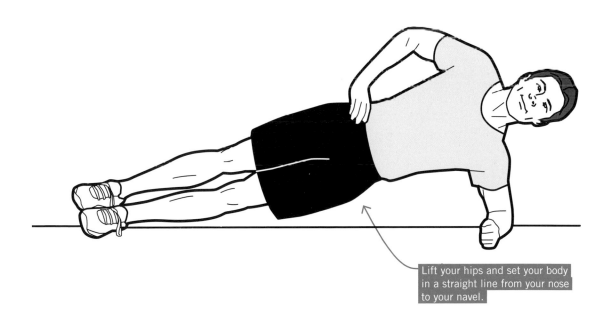

Lift your hips and set your body in a straight line from your nose to your navel.

Single-Leg Glute Bridge

1. Lie on your back with your knees bent, arms at your sides, and heels on the floor.

2. Lift your right foot off the floor and straighten your right leg so it's aligned with your left. This is your starting position.

3. Lift your hips off the floor until your body forms a straight line from your left knee to your shoulders, with your right leg staying aligned with your left. You should feel an intense contraction in your left glute. Hold that position for one second (count "one one thousand").

4. Lower your hips until they're close to the floor, but not touching it, and then raise your hips again for the next Glute Bridge. Do 5 reps, then switch legs and repeat.

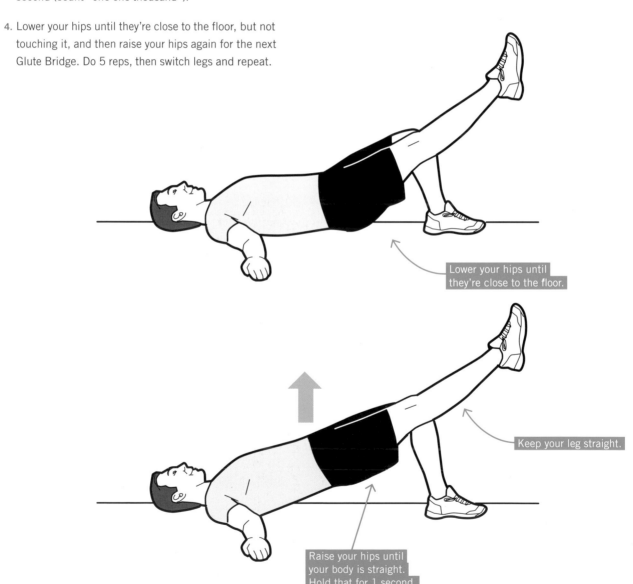

Lower your hips until they're close to the floor.

Keep your leg straight.

Raise your hips until your body is straight. Hold that for 1 second.

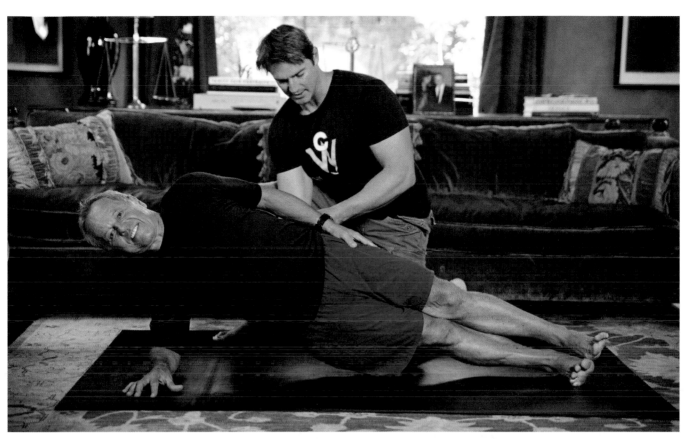

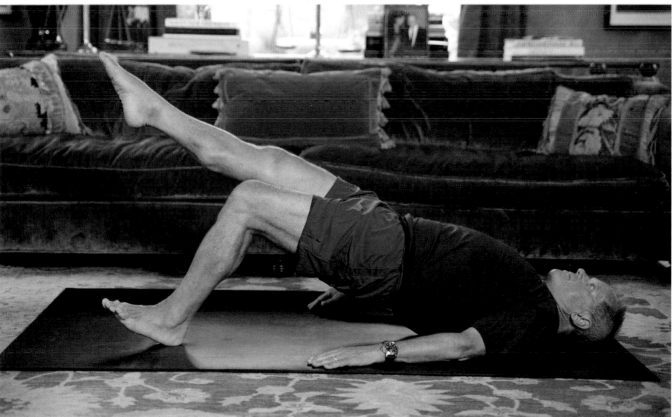

STRENGTH

Exercise	How to do it	Rest
Swing	10 reps	30 seconds
Push-up	10 reps	30 seconds
Dumbbell One-Arm Row*	10 reps each side	30 seconds
Dumbbell Alternating Shoulder Press and Twist	10 reps	30 seconds
Dumbbell Offset Reverse Lunge*	10 reps	30 seconds
Lying Leg Raise	10 reps	30 seconds

*no rest between sides

After doing each exercise as described, repeat the circuit, this time doing 9 reps of each. Do the next circuit with 8 reps, then 7, continuing until you do 5 reps of each.

Swing

1. Grab a kettlebell, if you have one, or a dumbbell if you don't, and hold it with both hands. If you're using a kettlebell, grip the handle with your thumbs next to each other. If you're using a dumbbell, interlock your fingers around the handle, just below one end of the weight. Stand with your feet wide apart and toes pointed out slightly. Let your arms hang straight down.

2. Push your hips back as you swing the weight behind you. Let your knees bend naturally as you lower your torso until it's at about a 45-degree angle to the floor.

3. Reverse the movement, thrusting your hips forward and squeezing your glutes hard when your body is straight. Your momentum will allow the weight to swing out in front of you. Don't worry about the height of your swings. If it rises to the height of your navel, that's good enough. You don't want to use your upper-body muscles to pull the weight to a predetermined height.

4. As the weight swings back down, push your hips back for the next repetition.

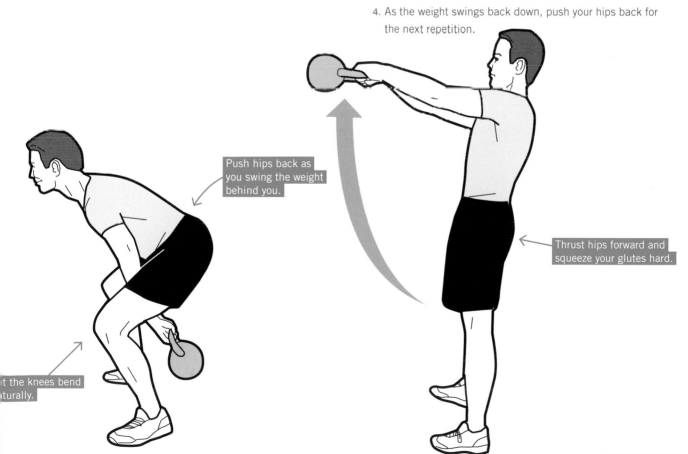

Push hips back as you swing the weight behind you.

Thrust hips forward and squeeze your glutes hard.

t the knees bend turally.

Push-Up

1. Get into the classic Push-up position, with your weight on your hands and toes, arms straight, and hands just outside your shoulders. You want your feet about hip-width apart, but if you struggle with the exercise, it's okay to set them wider. That will make it a bit easier to stabilize your body.

2. Set your body in a straight line from ankles to ears. It's crucial that your lower back remain in its natural arch. You don't want to let your belly sag, which will exaggerate the arch, or lift your hips so high that you flatten the arch.

3. Bend your elbows as you lower your entire body toward the floor, keeping the exact same alignment. Stop when your upper arms are parallel to your torso or your chest touches the floor. For most, your nose will be about 4 inches above the floor in the bottom position. Keep your chin tucked—that is, give yourself a double chin—throughout the movement.

4. Push back up to the starting position. The exercise works your chest, shoulder, and triceps muscles, but for the first few repetitions you'll feel it most in whatever muscles are weakest. For many that will be the triceps, but if you aren't used to doing core exercises, you may feel it first in the stabilizing muscles of your abdomen.

Performance Tips

→ If the classic Push-up is too challenging, you can elevate your hands on a step, bench, or anything else that won't move and is solid enough to support your weight. The higher the platform, the easier the exercise will be.

→ If it's too easy, raise your feet on a bench or step.

PUSH-UP VARIATIONS

There are easily enough Push-up variations to fill a book, many of which Wolfgang does in his workouts with me. More advanced exercisers who work out three days a week can do a different variation in each workout—the classic version along with these two:

Push-up with Hands Together

1. Set up in the classic Push-up position, but with your hands in the "triangle" position—thumbs and index fingers touching.

2. Do the exercise as described to the left, keeping your body aligned from your ankles through your neck. You should feel it much more in your triceps with your hands this close together. If you can't do all the repetitions, it's okay to move your hands a few inches apart. You should still shift some of the work from your chest and shoulders to your triceps.

Inverted Shoulder Press from Floor

1. Set up in the Push-up position, but with your hips elevated so your torso and legs form a 90-degree angle.

2. Lower the top of your head to the floor.

3. Push back up to the starting position, and repeat. You should feel this more in your shoulders than your chest, along with your triceps.

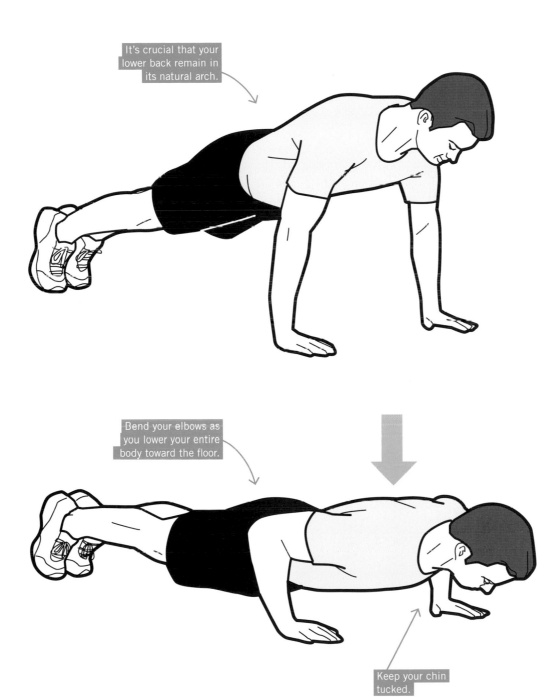

It's crucial that your lower back remain in its natural arch.

Bend your elbows as you lower your entire body toward the floor.

Keep your chin tucked.

Dumbbell One-Arm Row

1. Grab a dumbbell with your right hand, and take a long step forward with your left leg. (For suggested starting weights, see the sidebar on page 321.)

2. Bend forward at the hips so your body forms a straight line (more or less) from your shoulders through your torso, hips, and right leg. Your left knee should be bent about 120 degrees.

3. Rest your left hand on your left leg, just above the knee, and let the weight hang straight down from your right shoulder. This is your starting position.

4. Pull the weight straight up to the side of your torso. You should feel the contraction on the right side of your middle and upper back. By your final repetitions in each set you'll probably feel it in your biceps as well.

5. Lower the weight to the starting position. Do all your reps, then without resting, switch sides and repeat.

Performance Tips

→ If you're right-handed, you probably should start with your left arm. It's not a hard-and-fast rule, but if you're new to strength training, your dominant arm and leg are probably quite a bit stronger than your nondominant limbs. So you want to start each single-limb exercise with your weaker side until both sides are equally strong.

> ### ONE-ARM ROW VARIATIONS
>
> **1.** If you do this exercise with your palm facing forward, instead of turned in toward your torso, you'll feel it more in your biceps. You can use this variation in one workout a week.
>
> **2.** If you do the exercise with the palm turned back (that is, with your knuckles facing forward), you'll see that you do the exercise with your upper arm farther from your torso in the top position. This will shift some of the work to your upper-back muscles, including the trapezius (the muscle that controls your shoulder blades) and the rear part of your deltoid (the muscle that covers your shoulder joints).

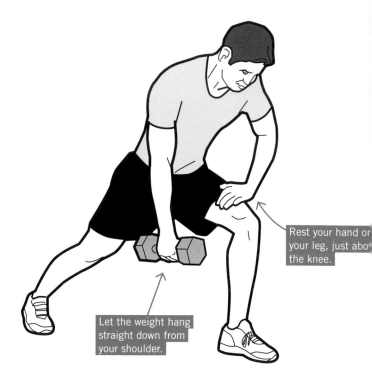

Rest your hand on your leg, just above the knee.

Let the weight hang straight down from your shoulder.

Pull the weight straight up to the side of your torso.

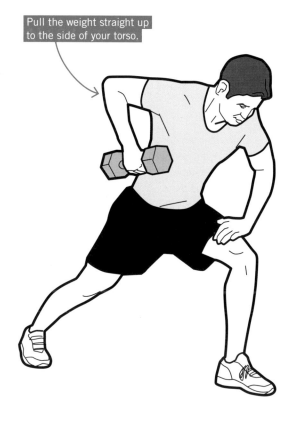

Dumbbell Alternating Shoulder Press and Twist

1. Grab a pair of dumbbells and stand holding them at your shoulders, with your feet shoulder-width apart and toes pointed straight ahead, and your palms facing each other.

2. Press the weight in your left hand straight up, while rotating your hips and shoulders to your right. Pivot on your left foot as you do this, but keep your right foot in place.

3. Turn back to the starting position as you lower the weight, and then immediately press the weight in your right hand straight up, while rotating your hips and shoulders to your left. Pivot on your right foot as you do this, but keep your left foot in place.

4. Alternate sides until you do all the repetitions with each arm.

SHOULDER PRESS VARIATIONS

As with the Push-ups, the most experienced lifters can modify the exercise so you do a different variation in each of your three weekly workouts.

One-Arm Shoulder Press

Start with a dumbbell in your left hand (or your right if you're left-handed), do all your repetitions, then repeat with your other side. By having the weight offset—that is, all on one side of your body, rather than balanced—you force your core muscles to work harder to keep you upright.

Dumbbell Shoulder Press

This is the most basic version of the exercise. You simply stand holding two dumbbells at your shoulders, and press them overhead simultaneously. Most of us can use slightly more weight, which helps speed up strength and muscle development.

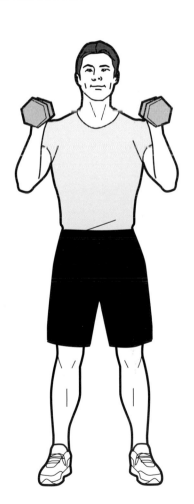

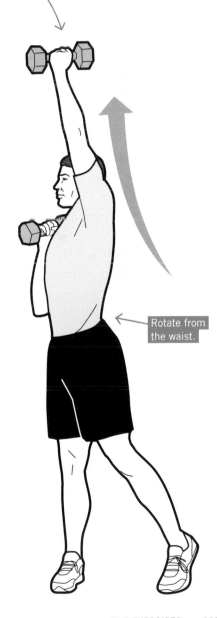

Press the weight in your hand straight up.

Rotate from the waist.

Dumbbell Offset Reverse Lunge

1. Stand holding a dumbbell in your left hand at shoulder height, with your feet about hip-width apart. It's the same setup as the One-Arm Shoulder Press described previously, only with your feet closer together.

2. Take a long step straight back with your left leg, lowering your body until your right knee (the one in front) is bent about 90 degrees and your left knee nearly touches the floor. Keep the weight in the same place at your shoulder.

3. Step back to the starting position, do all your repetitions, and then switch the weight to your right hand without stopping to rest. Do the same number of reps stepping back with your right leg.

REVERSE LUNGE VARIATIONS

1. If you're new to strength training, or simply unfamiliar with the Reverse Lunge, you can start with no weights. Hold your hands behind your head in what's called the prisoner grip. When you can do all the repetitions in the workout using just your body weight, shift to the Dumbbell Offset Reverse Lunge.

2. More advanced readers, on the other hand, can incorporate any number of lunge variations. You can hold any type of weight (dumbbell, kettlebell, or even a sandbag if you want to try something truly unconventional) in the offset position. Or you can hold that weight overhead, instead of at shoulder level, to change your center of gravity and force your core and shoulder muscles to adjust to the new challenge to your balance.

3. Another advanced option is to stand on a low step, perhaps 4 to 6 inches high, and step down to the floor as you do the Reverse Lunge. That extends the range of motion for your lower-body muscles, leading to improved mobility along with muscle development.

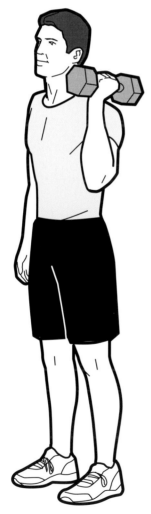

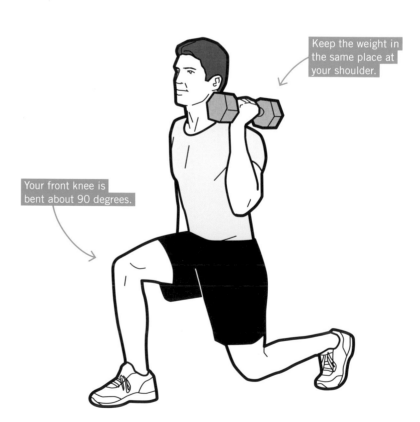

Your front knee is bent about 90 degrees.

Keep the weight in the same place at your shoulder.

Lying Leg Raise

1. Lie on your back with your legs straight up from your hips, with your feet together and arms at your sides. They should be at an approximately 90-degree angle to your torso.

2. Lower your legs, keeping them together, as far as you can. As soon as you feel your lower back start to rise off the floor, stop the movement.

3. Raise your legs again, and repeat to finish the set.

Performance Tips

→ As you get better, you should be able to bring your legs closer to the ground while keeping your lower back pressed against the floor.

→ If you can lower your legs all the way to the floor, stop just before they touch and lift them back to the starting position.

→ When you can complete all the reps on every set with the full range of motion, pause for 2 seconds in the bottom position. (Count "one one thousand, two one thousand" to make sure you don't cheat yourself.)

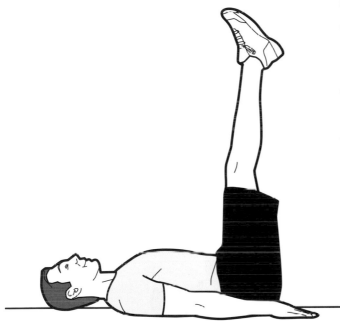

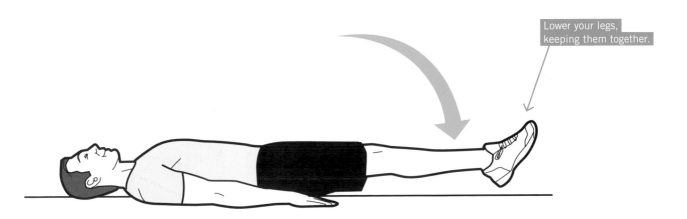

Lower your legs, keeping them together.

RECOVERY

Brettzel

Unlike the other two parts of the workout, here you'll do just one exercise: the Brettzel, which is named after strength coach Brett Jones. (The exercise was popularized by Gray Cook, a physical therapist and a friend of Jones.) Most of the stretches you've seen or used attempt to isolate one or two muscle groups. The Brettzel increases flexibility in your upper thighs, hips, and back. It's perfect for the end of the workout, when your body is warm and your joints will achieve a better range of motion than they would in a pre-workout stretch.

1. Lie on your right side with your head resting on a rolled-up towel or a small cushion. The goal is to elevate your head an inch or two above the floor and ensure that your neck is aligned with your spine.

2. Bend your right knee and grab your right ankle with your left hand. (If you can't reach it, you can loop a towel around the right ankle and hold on to the ends with your left hand.) Once you have a solid grip, pull your right heel toward your glutes.

3. Now lift your left thigh as close to your chest as you can (the angle of your thigh and torso has to be less than 90 degrees to avoid stress on your lower back), and hold it in place with your right hand, just above your left knee. Your left knee and the inside edge of your left foot should rest on the floor.

4. All that sets you up for the actual exercise, which has two parts. First, take a deep breath and try to straighten your right leg while you keep it in place with your left hand. Keep trying for 3 to 4 seconds.

5. Here comes the second and most important part: Exhale and turn your upper body to the left as far as you can, while keeping the inside of your left knee in contact with the floor.

6. Repeat this sequence—inhale; try to straighten your right leg; exhale; rotate—3 to 4 times. It should take you about a minute to complete 4 repetitions.

7. Switch sides and repeat.

OTHER RECOVERY TIPS

1. Another good way to take tension out of your muscles is to use a foam roller, a six-inch-wide cylinder that's usually 18 to 36 inches long. (You can buy a basic one online or in a sporting-goods store for $10 to $20.) You use it to work out the kinks that accumulate in muscles and connective tissues, keeping them supple and helping them function smoothly. Let's say you want to work on your hamstrings. You simply place the foam roller on the floor, place the back of both legs on it (with the roller positioned perpendicular to your legs), and push yourself over the roller, from one end of the muscle (just above the back of your knees) to the other (the gluteal crease at the top of your legs). Continue for 10 to 20 seconds. Your body weight provides all the pressure you need. It's easiest to use on your calves, hamstrings, quadriceps, and glutes.

2. A good strength workout speeds up your body's normal process of breaking down muscle protein and adding new protein to take its place. Your goal is to make sure you end up with a net gain in protein, which will give you stronger, more resilient, and better-looking muscles. So increasing the amount of protein in your diet, especially in the meal following your workout, will help you achieve that net gain. Wolfgang, for example, often likes to eat an egg-white omelet for breakfast after he works out with me.

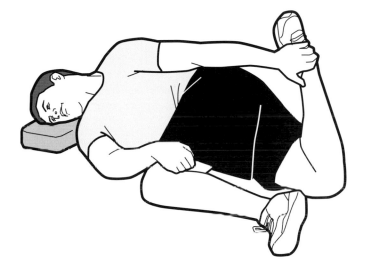

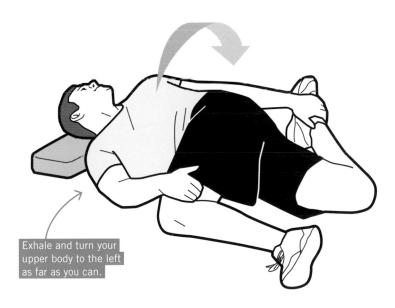

Exhale and turn your upper body to the left as far as you can.

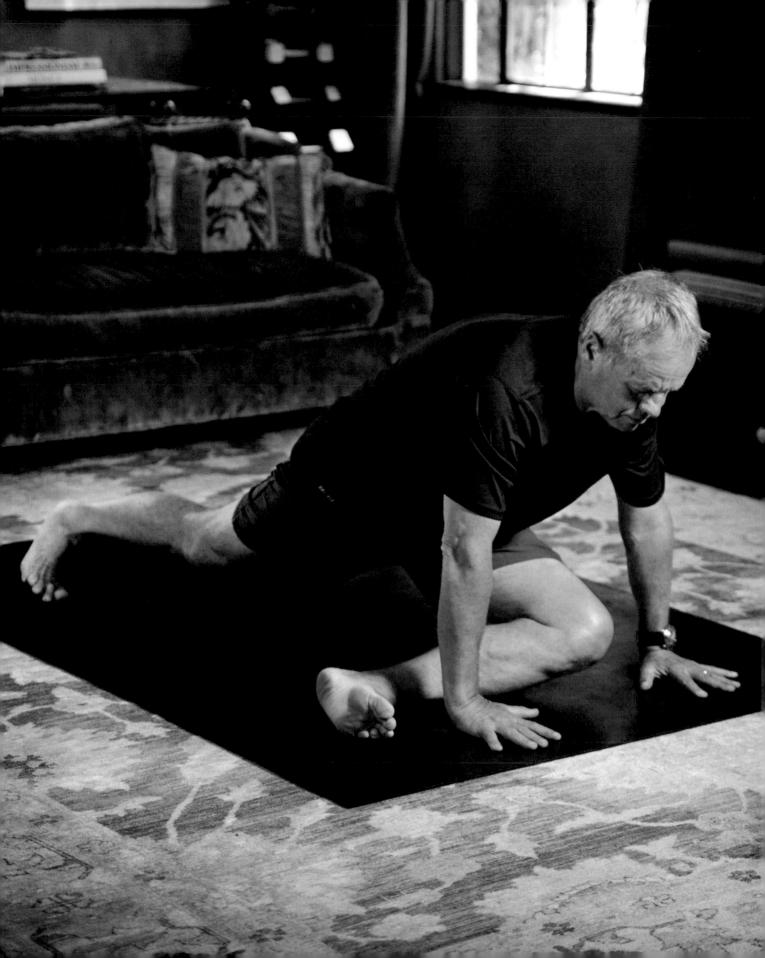

PROGRESS AND VARIETY

For most readers, the initial workouts will be challenging enough. It's safe to assume few will go through the program on Day One and find it easy. Even readers in top shape will probably need at least two weeks—six workouts—to fully adapt to the program as written.

You'll need to make small adjustments to the load as you go along. You may pick a weight that's too heavy or light for your first couple of workouts. Or you may gain strength in one or two exercises faster than the others. (See sidebar for more specific tips.) Eventually, even if it's for just one or two workouts, you'll reach a point at which each exercise is about equally challenging. When you get there, your first goal is to complete all the repetitions of every exercise. Then you can increase the challenge three different ways:

1. INCREASE THE NUMBER OF SETS
Instead of starting with 10 reps of each exercise, start with 11, and work your way down to 5. Then increase to 12 for your first set, and again work your way down to 5. By that point you're doing 68 reps of each exercise, and on single-limb exercises like rows and lunges you're doing 68 with each arm or leg. Your next challenge is to...

2. INCREASE THE RESISTANCE
Go up by at least 5 pounds on each exercise, and then reduce the reps to the original configuration—10 on the first set, 9 on the second, going down to a final set of 5. With Leg Raises and Push-ups, add a 2-second pause in the bottom position. When that starts to feel less challenging, you can either increase the weights again, or you can...

3. DECREASE THE REST BETWEEN EXERCISES
Take 20 seconds to catch your breath, instead of 30 seconds. Once again, start with 10 reps on the first set, working your way down to 5. Then increase to 11 on the first set, and finally 12.

By using all three of these methods, and by occasionally mixing in new exercises to keep things fresh, you can continue this program as long as you want.

SOME OPTIONS TO KEEP IT INTERESTING

"HOW MUCH WEIGHT SHOULD I USE?"

Human strength is almost as varied and unpredictable as human personality. All we can really say for certain is that you'll need a range of weights because you're going to be stronger in some exercises. For example, just about anybody, beginner or experienced, will be able to use at least twice as much weight for Rows as for Shoulder Presses. And yet, if you exercise in a commercial gym, you'll sometimes see healthy adults use the same weights for everything, no matter how big or strong the targeted muscles may be.

Some good starting weights:

SWING: The power for the Swing comes from your glutes and hamstrings. These are your body's strongest muscles, the ones you use for jumping, sprinting, and climbing. In the Equipment section we suggested that women start with at least a 15-pound kettlebell (you'd use about the same weight with a dumbbell), while men would use at least 30 pounds. You'll quickly outgrow those weights as you get used to the exercise, but the lighter kettlebell isn't destined to gather dust. Eventually, you'll be able to use it for One-Handed Swings, which you can substitute for the Swing in the program, which uses both hands. (Just make sure you do all the reps with each side.) You can also use a kettlebell for the Offset Reverse Lunge.

SHOULDER PRESS: A few years ago, one of my personal training colleagues did a strength-training workshop for a group of twelve-year-old Girl Scouts working on a fitness badge. He brought along a pair of 10-pound dumbbells to demonstrate exercises. As soon as he put them down, the girls rushed over and tried to lift them. Every single girl, big or tiny, managed to press the two weights overhead at least a couple of times. It's instructive because so many adults use lighter weights in their own workouts, even though they're clearly strong enough to use more.

For the higher reps in this program, most men and many women should be able to start with at least 10 pounds, unless you're recovering from an illness or working around an injury. For women, 5 pounds is probably the minimum.

ROW: This exercise is powered by your biggest, strongest upper-body muscles. For women, 15 to 20 pounds is a reasonable starting weight. For men, 30 to 40 should work. Your strength should improve rapidly.

You don't have to do the strength workout as a six-exercise circuit. You can break it up into two circuits of three exercises:

> **Circuit 1:** Swing, Push-up, Row
>
> **Circuit 2:** Shoulder Press, Lunge, Leg Raise

Or you can do it as three exercise pairs:

> 1. Swing + Push-up
> 2. Row + Shoulder Press
> 3. Lunge + Leg Raise

Breaking it up this way allows you to put more focus on the exercises. Most of us can probably use more weight on the exercises when we do it this way, especially on the first circuit or pair of exercises. It's also better when you're working out in a commercial health club where space is limited, or in a hotel gym with minimal equipment.

THE HOTEL-ROOM WORKOUT

Finally, here's a quick three-exercise circuit you can do anywhere, with no equipment and less space than you'd need to unroll a sleeping bag.

Exercise	How to do it	Rest
Jumping Jack	20 reps	15 seconds
Reverse Lunge, Alternating, with Overhead Reach and Side Bend	10 reps per side	15 seconds
Push-up with Mountain Climber	10 reps	15 seconds

After doing each exercise as described, repeat the circuit, this time doing 9 reps of Lunges and Mountain Climbers, then 8, then 7, continuing until you do 5 reps of each. You'll still do 20 Jumping Jacks each time.

Jumping Jack

1. Stand with your feet together and hands at your sides.

2. Jump straight out to the sides with both feet as you bring your hands together over your head.

3. Jump back and repeat. Just like gym class!

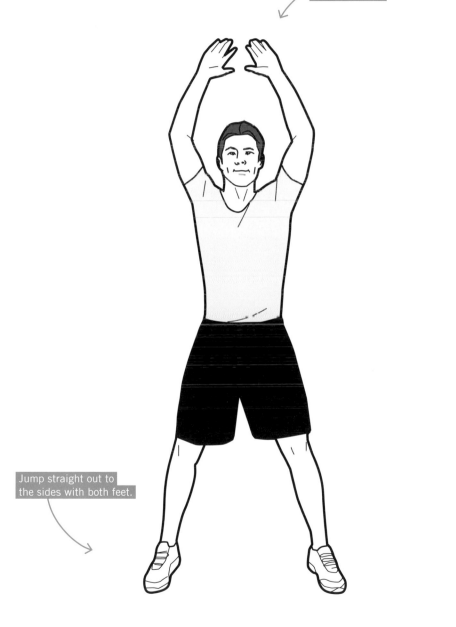

Your hands come together over your head.

Jump straight out to the sides with both feet.

Reverse Lunge, Alternating, with Overhead Reach and Side Bend

1. Stand with your feet hip-width apart and your arms at your sides.

2. Take a long step back with your left leg. At the same time, reach over the top of your head with your left hand as you bend your torso to the right. You should feel a good stretch all along your left side.

3. Step back to the starting position and repeat with your right leg stepping back and a bend and reach to your left.

4. Alternate until you finish all the repetitions with each side.

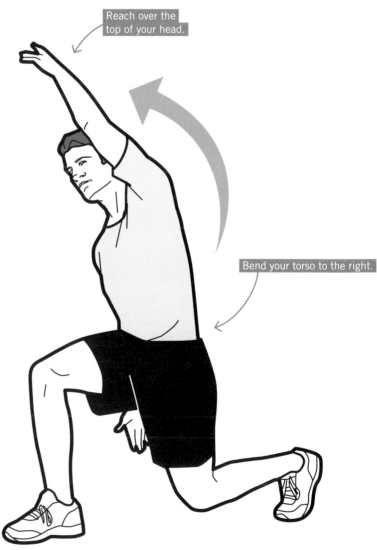

Reach over the top of your head.

Bend your torso to the right.

Push-up with Mountain Climber

1. Set up in the Push-up position described earlier: hands directly beneath your shoulders, toes on the floor, body straight from neck to ankles.

2. Do a Push-up.

3. When you return to the starting position, lift your right knee up toward your chest while keeping your body straight.

4. Lower your right leg, and raise your left knee toward your chest.

5. Lower your left leg so you're back in the original Push-up position. That's one repetition: a Push-up plus a Mountain Climber with each leg. Repeat until you finish all the reps.

> **MODIFIED VERSION (FOR THOSE WHO CAN'T DO CLASSIC PUSH-UPS)**
>
> You can modify the Push-up by raising your hands onto anything solid that will hold your weight. Most hotel rooms, for example, will have a desk that's braced against a wall. Lean forward with your hands on the edge of the desk and your body straight from neck to ankles. Lower your chest toward the desk, then push back to the starting position. Then do the Mountain Climber as described with each leg, and continue until you finish all your repetitions.

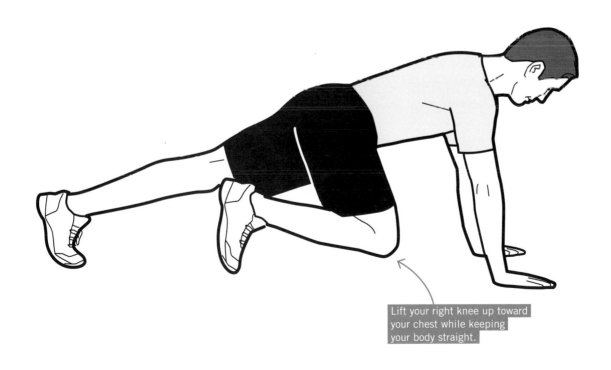

Lift your right knee up toward your chest while keeping your body straight.

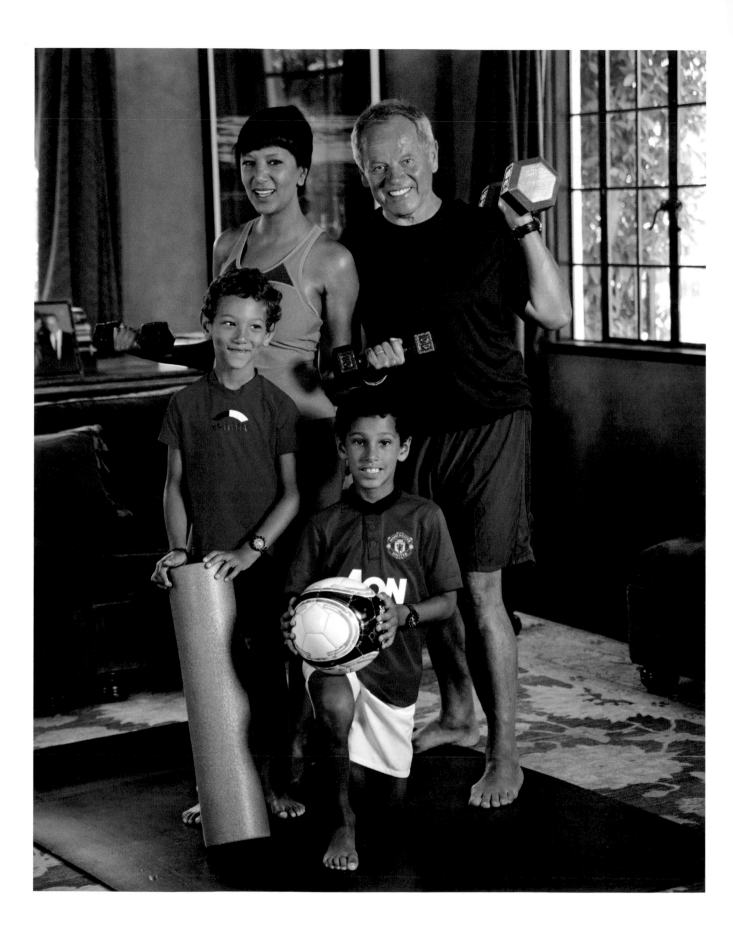

ACKNOWLEDGMENTS

Just like a great restaurant meal, this book resulted from a team effort. So, I would like to acknowledge all the many people who worked on it with me.

First, I give sincere thanks to Chad Waterbury. He revolutionized the way I think about exercise, in the process, helping me to feel more energetic and fit than I have in my life. Chad also inspired me to think more than ever before about the importance of healthy cooking and eating. This book is the result.

Norman Kolpas worked with me from start to finish on developing, writing, and editing the book's recipes and its narrative text. Without Norman, this book project would have started but never finished. Thank you, Norman, for keeping us on schedule, even though I changed the schedule all the time. You are the man. You made it happen.

Thanks to Matt Bencivenga, my partner and head chef at Wolfgang Puck Catering, an outstanding cook and good man who always goes above and beyond what I ask of him. And thanks to Matt's dedicated team—including Justin Campbell, Christine Beard, Jen Fox Robles, Hipolito Arias, Karl Matz, George Quintana, Adam Del Bado, Jason Lemonnier, and Frank Bonventre—who not only cooked all the recipes for testing but also worked with Matt and me to prep all the food for photography. Also instrumental in preparing the food and providing logistical support for photography was the entire team at Hotel Bel-Air: Executive Chef Sonny Sweetman, Chef Raymond Weber, Food and Beverage Director Stephane Lacroix, Restaurant General Manager Adam Crocini, and Hotel General Manager Denise Flanders. I also want to thank the team at Spago Beverly Hills, including Partner and Executive Chef Lee Hefter, General Manager Tracey Spillane, Chef de Cuisine Tetsu Yahagi, Pastry Chef Della Gossett, Executive Sous Chef Justin Katsuno, Chef Karo Patpatyan, and Sous Chef Ryan Riedy.

I send special thanks to the entire Chino family—including Tom, Koo, Kay, Fred, and Frank—at Chino Family Farm in Rancho Santa Fe, California. You've provided your outstanding produce to Spago and my other L.A.-area restaurants since the early 1980s, and you welcomed us warmly to your farm, as you always do, to take some of the photos for this book. The Chinos feel like my family, too.

Photographer Carin Krasner was an ideal collaborator on the visuals for this book. Thank you, Carin, and your hardworking assistants: Digital Technician Juvenia Tso-Wheeler; Photography/Lighting Assistant Derek Johnston; and Lighting Assistant Sam Haligman. Prop Stylist Kim Wong also helped find many of the beautiful tabletop items that appear in the photos.

Many more people also played important roles in turning an idea into a book. My agent, David Black, helped the book find an excellent home with Grand Central Life & Style and its Vice President and Editorial Director, Karen Murgolo. My thanks to both Karen and David and to their capable teams. Writer Lou Schuler worked with Chad Waterbury to make the fitness information and exercise instructions so intelligent and clear; and Jason Lee created illustrations that help make the exercises even easier to follow.

Special thanks go to my executive assistant, Maggie Boone. For many years now, Maggie has kept my demanding work life superbly organized, and she does it always with good humor, grace, and kindness. Her logistical skills were instrumental in helping this book come to life.

INDEX

ABOUT THE AUTHORS

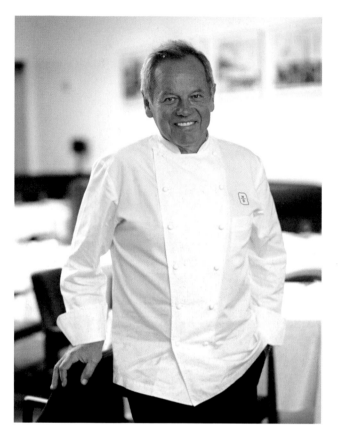

WOLFGANG PUCK has been a leading innovator in modern American cooking since the mid-1970s, when he first rose to prominence as chef of Ma Maison in Los Angeles before opening his flagship restaurant Spago in 1982. He has been at the forefront of defining the way people dine out, shop, and cook at home today, including championing the farm-to-table and farmers' market movements, supporting sustainably raised and organic ingredients, and leading the shift from formal course-by-course dining to more casual sharable plates. And now Puck is dedicating himself to spreading an ever-wider awareness of how important it is to cook, eat, and live more healthfully.

In addition to his dozens of fine-dining, casual, and quick-service restaurants worldwide, Puck spearheads a catering company with venues in fifteen cities across the country, most widely known for the gala Governors Ball following each year's Oscars ceremony in Hollywood. He is widely seen through his frequent cooking demonstrations on ABC's *Good Morning America* and other news and talk shows; cameo performances as himself in TV series and movies; and regular appearances on the Home Shopping Network in the U.S. and The Shopping Channel in Canada, demonstrating his professional-quality cookware, tools, and appliances designed for home cooks. Puck has also developed his own lines of gourmet soups, pasta sauces, bottled iced coffee drinks, estate-grown coffees, and fine wines.

The author of six previously published cookbooks, Puck also writes a syndicated newspaper column, "Wolfgang Puck's Kitchen," which reaches more than 5.3 million home cooks every week across the U.S. and Canada.

CHAD WATERBURY is a high-performance strength coach and personal trainer based in Santa Monica, California. His clients include MMA champion Ronda Rousey and other athletes. He has a master's degree in physiology from the University of Arizona and is the author of *Huge in a Hurry*.